Physical Therapy Professional Foundations

KEYS TO SUCCESS IN SCHOOL AND CAREER

Physical Therapy Professional Foundations

KEYS TO SUCCESS IN SCHOOL AND CAREER

Kathleen A. Curtis, PhD, PT
California State University, Fresno

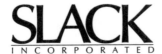

An innovative information, education and management company
6900 Grove Road • Thorofare, NJ 08086

The procedures and practices described in this book should be implemented in a manner consistent with the professional standards set for the circumstances that apply in each specific situation. Every effort has been made to confirm the accuracy of the information presented and to correctly relate generally accepted practices. The author, editor, and publisher cannot accept responsibility for errors or exclusions or for the outcome of the application of the material presented herein. There is no expressed or implied warranty of this book or information imparted by it.

The work SLACK publishes is peer reviewed. Prior to publication, recognized leaders in the field, educators, and clinicians provide important feedback on the concepts and content that we publish. We welcome feedback on this work.

Curtis, Kathleen A.
    Physical therapy professional foundations: keys to success in school and career /
Kathleen A. Curtis.
        p. cm.
    Includes bibliographical references and index.
    ISBN 1-55642-411-6 (alk. paper)
    1. Physical therapy--Practice. 2. Physical therapy--Vocational guidance. 3. Medical
care--United States. I. Title.

RM705 .C87 2001
615.8'2'068--dc21

                                                                2001040023

Printed in the United States of America

Published by: SLACK Incorporated
                 6900 Grove Road
                 Thorofare, NJ 08086 USA
                 Telephone: 856-848-1000
                 Fax: 856-853-5991
                 www.slackbooks.com

Contact SLACK Incorporated for more information about other books in this field or about the availability of our books from distributors outside the United States.

Last digit is print number: 10   9   8   7   6   5   4   3   2

Dedication

To Linda Crane, Huber Yesid Garcia, and El Dulce Kona,
my dear friends who all lived with sweetness, joy, and love.

Contents

Acknowledgments

I have traveled an interesting path while first thinking about and finally writing this book. Sandra Graham and Bernard Weiner at University of California, Los Angeles initially helped me see that choosing a strategy is the one choice that we have within our control. My doctoral work helped me to establish the power of choice in the real world of problems and challenges I had experienced early in my career. Thank you both for helping me find ways to apply attribution theory in my work with practicing health professionals. My ongoing research continues to support the power of conscious choice, reflection, intention, and strategy in fundamentally changing the nature of our professional lives and career experiences.

Amy Drummond and John Bond at SLACK Incorporated first helped this book come alive through their encouragement and support for these ideas. Kianna Modir-Fatemi spent many hours in the library helping me research and find the resources I needed. ChrisTina Buettell has been exceptionally helpful in her feedback, suggestions, and contributions to this text. Her own journey as a student through the professional education process while I was developing the content for this book illuminated my path in so many ways. James Moore and Colleen Elkin, two shining examples of the future of physical therapy, ensured my accuracy about the American Physical Therapy Association (APTA) Student Assembly.

Laurie Haston, Linda Crane, Carol Davis, Bob Gailey, and my many colleagues at the University of Miami were so much a part of the evolution of my ideas and approaches as an educator. Darlene Stewart, professor emeritus at California State University, Fresno, created a curriculum that provided a time to teach all that I felt was critical to the future of our field and then invited me to come to teach it. Ethylynda Harding, director of the Center for the Enhancement of Teaching and Learning; Benjamin Cuellar, Dean of the College of Health and Human Services; Vivian Vidoli, dean of the Division of Graduate Studies; and J. Michael Ortiz, provost and vice-president of Academic Affairs at California State University have created an institution that supports innovation and choice during professional education in physical therapy.

On a personal note, I must acknowledge Kona (my enthusiastic chocolate Lab) for the hours he lay close by while I sat at the computer, and Behzad Setoodeh for his constant encouragement. And finally, Maria Nora Peña provided her patience and efficiency in helping me revise and edit the final manuscript during a very busy academic year.

My gratitude to all.

About the Author

Dr. Kathleen Curtis is professor and chairperson of the Physical Therapy Department at California State University, Fresno. Dr. Curtis received her bachelor of science degree in physical therapy at Northeastern University, Boston, Mass. She received her master's degree in health science from San Jose State University and received her PhD in education at University of California, Los Angeles. She taught courses in physical therapy professional issues, communication, career development, research methods, and psychosocial considerations in health care.

Her background includes a wide variety of experiences in clinical practice, staff development and supervision, clinical research, and clinical and academic teaching in physical therapy. Her research on interprofessional role conflict, helping behavior, early career development, and role satisfaction has received wide exposure across the health care fields. She co-authored and serves on the Advisory Board of California State University, Fresno's Certificate of Advanced Study in Interprofessional Collaboration. She cofounded and currently directs the interdisciplinary Disability Studies Institute at California State University, Fresno. She also coordinates an annual Graduate Student Success Seminar for incoming graduate students, a program designed to ensure that they have the skills to succeed in physical therapy professional education.

She is a well-known speaker and author. She has published extensively in the rehabilitation literature and serves as a manuscript reviewer for several journals. She is a recipient of the California Physical Therapist Faculty Research Award and her book, *The Physical Therapist's Guide to Health Care,* has been used as a text in a majority of college and university physical therapy education programs.

Contributing Author

ChrisTina Buettell, MPT

ChrisTina Buettell is staff physical therapist at Town Center Village, a retirement community and outpatient clinic, and Generations Home Care, an independent home care agency, both located in Portland, Ore. She also teaches yoga and dance, cofacilitates wellness programs at a retreat center, volunteers as a hippotherapy assistant with Shriners' Hospital, and advises high school cross-country runners.

Preface

Physical Therapy Professional Foundations is a comprehensive guide for physical therapy students as they enter and progress through the educational program and prepare for licensure and transition to clinical practice.

As health care professionals, we are faced with a multitude of choices every day of our professional lives. Many of those choices fundamentally change the nature of our experience from moment to moment. It is much more than the simple perspective of "Is the glass half empty or half full?" We have choices in how to allocate precious resources such as time and energy, whether to choose effective or ineffective strategies, and if, when, and how to take advantage of the opportunities that are available to us. We can choose to nurture the relationships that support us and to learn to say "No" to the challenges that drain our resources. Students face numerous choices, challenges, opportunities, and obstacles during the professional education process. This book offers an array of strategies for success in physical therapy professional education and clinical practice.

The first few chapters provide both an introduction to the physical therapy profession and a context by describing the current health care environment and the changing roles of physical therapists. The text then includes a comprehensive path through professional education in physical therapy, including financial considerations, professional behavior, performance expectations, requirements, and challenges students face in the graduate education process. Following this are strategy-based approaches for success that address common issues in learning and skill acquisition, performance anxiety, personal management decisions, ethical challenges, and legal considerations for students in physical therapy professional education. Another component includes special coverage of issues of concern to re-entry students, students with disabilities, and students whose first language is not English.

An entire section is devoted to cutting-edge professional issues, including an introduction to evidence-based practice and critical thinking, essentials of information competence, interprofessional collaboration, cultural competence, active participation in professional conferences, and student roles in the American Physical Therapy Association. The final few chapters address the transition from student life to professional practice, including preparing for the licensure examination, entering the job market, and common challenges for new graduate physical therapists, including planning for career development.

This book was written to help preprofessional students make healthy choices about entering the field of physical therapy, to assist physical therapy students to establish sound habits and realistic expectations, and to facilitate success for new graduates in the transition from the academic setting to clinical practice. Clinical and academic faculty may also find these ideas useful in advising students at various stages in the professional education process. The "Putting It Into Practice" exercise at the end of each chapter encourages students to use the resources and tools available to them to make well-informed choices that will facilitate their success.

I welcome your feedback and ideas on how we can make this journey more successful and more fulfilling. The future of the profession of physical therapy rests in the hands of the students and new graduates who choose to practice in our current and ever-changing health care environment. I wish you all the best and hope that in some small way this book has made the journey better.

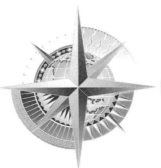

Part One

The Physical Therapy Profession in the Changing World

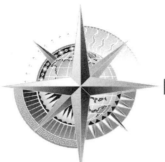

Chapter 1

The Profession of Physical Therapy

Angela G. nervously awaited her interview for admission to the physical therapy program. She had visualized this day for years, since she first volunteered at the local hospital after school in high school. Now the day had finally come. During her interview, a faculty member asked her, "How would you describe the profession of physical therapy?" She answered, "It's a flexible profession with lots of opportunities for career growth and a variety of practice sites for part-time or full-time employment."

Jennifer B. also awaited her interview following Angela. When asked the same question, she answered, "I've always wanted to help people; I'm a 'people-person' and this is a great profession that really makes a difference in people's lives."

Which answer do you prefer? How do you think they scored in the interviewer's assessment? Are these interviewees talking about *jobs* or the *profession of physical therapy*? How would you answer the same question?

Let's first look at what defines a profession and how physical therapy fits into these criteria.

What Is a Profession?

1. A profession is a special kind of occupation, distinct from other occupations in that it has *auton-omy*, the right to control its own work, its members, and the rules that govern it.

2. A profession has *prolonged and specialized training in an abstract body of knowledge* unique to that profession.

3. Persons in a profession are *oriented toward service*.

4. Those who are members of the profession *work in accordance with specific guidelines, laws, or regulations which govern the practice* of that profession.[1,2]

Many characteristics of a profession relate to autonomy in exercising professional judgment and are outlined in Table 1-1.

Professions typically have standards for professional education and requirements for accreditation of programs that provide education for individuals entering the profession. Many professions require extended periods of training beyond an academic degree, such as periods of internship or residency.

Professionalism in Physical Therapy

Pellegrino defined professionals as "those whose functions bring them into direct personal contact with the vulnerable patient and call for direct participation in the healing relationship."[3] Physical therapists clearly fit within this definition.

Professionalism is characterized by formal educa-

Table 1-1
SOME CHARACTERISTICS OF A PROFESSION[2]

1. The profession possesses a specialized and unique body of abstract knowledge.
2. The profession provides a service to society.
3. The profession determines its own standards of education and training.
4. Professional practice is governed by a code of ethics that is determined by the profession.
5. Professional practice is often legally recognized by some form of licensure.
6. Members of the profession serve on licensing and admission boards.
7. Most legislation concerning the profession is shaped by that profession.

tion, expertise, autonomy, commitment, and responsibility.[4] These values are clearly characteristic of the nature of the work that physical therapists perform. Let's look further at how the profession of physical therapy has defined itself.

What is Physical Therapy?

Physical therapy is the care and services that are provided under the direction and supervision of a physical therapist. Over 90,000 physical therapists practice in the United States today, treating an estimated one million people every day.[5] The physical therapy profession was founded in the belief that improved physical function makes our lives better.

How Does the Profession Define the Practice of Physical Therapy?

The opening sentence of the *Guide to Physical Therapist Practice* characterizes the physical therapy profession using the following definition:

"Physical therapy is a dynamic profession with an established theoretical base and widespread clinical applications in the preservation, development, and restoration of optimal physical function."[5]

Physical therapists carry out varied roles in many different types of health care, educational and occupational settings including hospitals and rehabilitation centers, outpatient clinics, patient's homes, schools, and professional, corporate, athletic, industrial, and community organizations.

The Model Definition of Physical Therapy for State Practice Acts (Appendix A) refers to four distinct areas of physical therapy, including:

1. Examining individuals with impairment, functional limitation, and disability to determine a diagnosis, prognosis, and plan of intervention.
2. Alleviating impairment, functional limitations, and disabilities by designing, implementing, and modifying therapeutic interventions.

3. Reducing the risk of injury, impairment, functional limitation, and disability.
4. Engaging in administration, consultation, education, and research.[5]

The functions in #4, unless provided *by a physical therapist or under the direction and supervision of a physical therapist*, are not physical therapy and should not be represented or reimbursed as such.

Only physical therapists can provide physical therapy and use the initials "PT" after their names to designate their licensure as physical therapists. The initials "LPT" and "RPT" were used in the past (and still may be used by some therapists). Services that are provided by support personnel such as physical therapist assistants or physical therapy aides may be designated by the term *physical therapy* only if they are provided under the direction and supervision of a physical therapist.

Who Works in Physical Therapy?

Physical Therapists

Physical therapists, or PTs, are graduates of physical therapist professional education programs at the college or university level and are required to be licensed in the state in which they practice. Professional education for physical therapists must be at the post-baccalaureate level, effective in 2002.

Physical therapists evaluate and establish a plan of care for people with health problems resulting from injury or disease. They evaluate joint motion, muscle strength and endurance, cardiopulmonary function, and performance of activities of daily living, among other responsibilities. They provide intervention that may include therapeutic exercise, cardiovascular endurance training, and training in activities of daily living.

They are involved in collaboration with other professionals, consultation in many capacities, education, research, and administration. Physical therapists are responsible for the supervision of physical therapy support personnel, including physical therapist assistants and physical therapy aides.

Physical Therapist Assistants

Physical therapist assistants, or PTAs, are graduates of physical therapist assistant associate degree programs. Many, but not all, states require licensure for PTAs. Physical therapist assistants provide physical therapy services only under the supervision of physical therapists.

PTAs assist physical therapists in implementing treatment programs such as therapeutic exercise and activities of daily living. PTAs carry out various portions of the plan of care and maintain open communication with the physical therapist.

In addition to direct patient care, the PTA often performs functions such as patient transport, maintenance of equipment, and other clinic needs. Specific conditions for supervision of the PTA are outlined in each state's physical therapy practice act.

Physical Therapy Aides

Physical therapy aides are *nonlicensed personnel* who are usually trained on-the-job under the direction of a physical therapist. The physical therapy aide performs routine tasks either delegated by the physical therapist or, if permitted by state law, by the physical therapist assistant. The aide is permitted to perform specific patient-related duties only with continuous onsite supervision by the physical therapist or, if permitted by state law, the physical therapist assistant. The physical therapist or physical therapist assistant must be in the immediate area to provide continuous onsite supervision.

Other Personnel

Other personnel, such as massage therapists, exercise physiologists, or athletic trainers, sometimes work with physical therapists in providing care. Depending on state law, these personnel may be licensed or may hold certifications from professional organizations. These personnel should be employed under their appropriate title.

Their roles in patient or client care should be defined by the scope of their education and relevant laws and regulations. The specific physical therapy-related services that are provided by these types of personnel are determined by the physical therapist and must be in compliance with state and federal laws and regulations.

Becoming a Professional

Professionals go through a distinct period of *role socialization* during which they acquire the specialized knowledge, values, attitudes, and skills of the profession. In addition to knowledge, skills, and attitudes, the developing professional also develops a distinct language. Let's look at the following note, found in a patient's medical record.

> *Barry H., a new graduate physical therapist, documented patient progress in the patient's medical record by writing: "Pt. amb 40' PWB ⓛ c̄ FWW and VC"*
>
> *The patient's physician is overheard at the nurses' station after reading the chart muttering, "I can never tell whether that's good or bad."*

Some sociologists have described professions as social constructs with their own languages, belief systems, and symbolic lives. The above example shows a message in a language intelligible only to members of the professional culture.

> *What does this mean? Pt. amb 40' PWB ⓛ c̄ FWW and VC*
>
> *Translation: Patient ambulated 40 feet partial weight-bearing on the left leg with front-wheeled walker and verbal cueing.*

The role socialization period for health professionals extends for a period of as long as 2 years following graduation and entry into the professional field. Research on role socialization in physical therapy shows that clinical role models are likely to be the most powerful determinants of professional values for new graduate physical therapists.[6,7]

Becoming a Physical Therapist

Physical therapists must complete a post-baccalaureate (masters or doctorate) degree in physical therapy from an accredited education program. At present, there are over 200 colleges and universities nationwide that offer professional education programs in physical therapy. Most of these programs

Table 1-2

EARLY EVENTS IN THE EVOLUTION OF THE PHYSICAL THERAPY PROFESSION[10-12]

1914, 1916	Widespread polio epidemics occurred. Physical modalities, massage, and corrective exercise were applied by nonphysician personnel trained in physical education.
1915	Mary McMillan was recognized as the first physical therapist in the United States. She received her training in England and returned to the United States in 1915.
1917-1918 (World War I)	Reconstruction aides were employed in Army hospitals. They were women, most from backgrounds in physical education, who participated in 3-month courses during the war to train them in military massage and muscle re-education. They worked in Army and veteran's hospitals during the war.
1918	First physical therapy course was organized at Walter Reed Hospital to train reconstruction aides. Courses were soon established in 14 institutions, the largest of which was Reed College in Eugene, Ore. Standards were administered by the Surgeon General's Office.
1921	The American Women's Physical Therapeutic Association was founded by Mary McMillan. *PT Review*, a professional journal, began in March 1921.
1922	Name change from American Women's Physical Therapeutic Association to American Physiotherapy Association (APA).
1928	In the 1920s, a Council on Physical Therapy was established in the American Medical Association (AMA). By 1928, they had established a standard for schools: a course length of 9 months and 1200 hours of theory and practice. Entry requirement was graduation from a school of physical education or nursing. From 1936 to 1977, the standards for training and education of physical therapists remained under the purview of the AMA and House of Delegates of the AMA.

continued

encompass six or more semesters of academic coursework including or followed by a period of extended clinical internship.[8]

After graduation, candidates must successfully pass an examination administered by each state. There are additional requirements for physical therapy practice that vary from state to state by individual state physical therapy practice acts or state regulations that govern the practice of physical therapy.

Becoming a Physical Therapist Assistant

Physical therapist assistants complete a 2-year college education program and receive an associate's degree upon graduation. Physical therapist assistant programs are usually offered at community colleges. The academic program usually includes 1 year of general education and 1 year of coursework, including physical therapy procedures and clinical experience. At present there are 266 accredited physical therapist assistant education programs in the United States.[9]

More than half of all states have practice acts that require physical therapist assistants to meet specific educational and examination criteria. In these states, physical therapist assistants must be licensed, registered, or certified. Regardless of state licensure, physical therapist assistants may only work under the supervision of physical therapists.

The Evolution of the Physical Therapy Profession

The physical therapy profession had its origins in the post-World War II era rehabilitation needs of returning veterans. In over 75 years, the profession has grown, developed, expanded, and increased its autonomy.

Detailed histories are available both in written and oral forms from the American Physical Therapy Association (APTA). The APTA will loan copies of videotapes, audiotapes, and transcripts of oral histories by leaders in the profession. See the following site for more information: http://www.apta.org/Research/factsheet_tips/sourcesofinformation/OralHistories

Table 1-2 indicates some of the key events and per-

Table 1-2, continued

1934	The American Registry of Physical Therapy Technicians was established by the American Congress of Physical Therapy (an organization of physicians specializing in use of physical therapy). It involved a written examination. Passing the examination allowed one to use the title Registered Physical Therapist (RPT), not to be confused with legal licensure allowing one to call oneself RPT. It was not until the 1950s that widespread legislation was enacted on a state-by-state basis.
1935	Standards for ethics and discipline were adopted, which addressed the expected behavior in therapeutic intervention and the exclusive responsibilities of the physician for diagnosis, prognosis, and prescription. The physician was considered critical in establishing the legitimacy of the work in physical therapy.
1944	The medical specialty of physical medicine was developed; physicians dropped the name physical therapist (changed to physiatrist), which allowed physical therapist technicians to drop the technician title and use physical therapist as their name.
1940-1945	Rehabilitation concepts introduced in WWII fostered the growth of the physical medicine specialty. In many institutions, physical therapy services were only available via referral to the physiatrist.
1947	Name change to American Physical Therapy Association (APTA). By 1946, the organization had more than 3000 members.
1960s	Amendments to the Social Security Act necessitated an increase in manpower. The physical therapist assistant was developed to help meet needs of health care personnel. Curriculum changes were instituted to reflect the evolution of the practice of physical therapy. Practitioners needed to not only be skilled in use of PT procedures but also understand the rationale for application. Standards increased breadth and depth of coursework as the foundation of the profession.
1970s	The APTA House of Delegates adopted a new document that departed from the course titles, clock hours, and semester hours included in earlier versions. Standards for Accreditation were published in 1978.
1980s	The APTA adopted a resolution that entry-level education for the physical therapist consist of a post-baccalaureate degree. The APTA became an accrediting agency for PT and PTA education. The APTA passed a new definition of physical therapy: (a) treatment by physical means; (b) the profession that is concerned with health promotion, with prevention of physical disabilities, and with rehabilitation of persons disabled by pain, disease or injury; and which is involved with evaluating patients and with treating through the use of physical therapeutic measures as opposed to medicines, surgery, or radiation. Clinical specialization: Mechanisms were put into place to recognize therapists with advanced clinical skills. The first clinical specialists were certified in cardiopulmonary physical therapy in 1985.
1990s	The Americans with Disabilities Act was signed in 1990, mandating reasonable accommodations to ensure the integration of people with disabilities. First entry-level doctorate in physical therapy (DPT) program opened at Creighton University, graduating its first class in 1996. The Balanced Budget Amendment was signed into law in August 1997, enacting widespread changes in reimbursement for Medicare patients. *Guide to Physical Therapist Practice*, a consensus document outlining patient/client management and scope of physical therapy practice, was published in 1997.
2000	Vision statement was passed by the APTA House of Delegates.

Table 1-3
APTA VISION STATEMENT FOR PHYSICAL THERAPY, 2020

Physical therapy, by 2020, will be provided by physical therapists who are doctors of physical therapy and who may be board-certified specialists. Consumers will have direct access to physical therapists in all environments for patient/client management, prevention, and wellness services. Physical therapists will be practitioners of choice in clients' health networks and will hold all privileges of autonomous practice. Physical therapists may be assisted by physical therapist assistants who are educated and licensed to provide physical therapist-directed and -supervised components of interventions.

Guided by integrity, life-long learning, and a commitment to comprehensive and accessible health programs for all people, physical therapists and physical therapist assistants will render evidence-based service throughout the continuum of care and improve quality of life for society. They will provide culturally sensitive care distinguished by trust, respect, and an appreciation for individual differences.

While fully availing themselves of new technologies, as well as basic and clinical research, physical therapists will continue to provide direct care. They will maintain active responsibility for the growth of the physical therapy profession and the health of the people it serves.[12]

sons involved in the early and more recent history of the physical therapy profession.

Vision Statement 2020

The APTA House of Delegates endorsed a vision statement (Table 1-3) that indicates a clear direction for the future of the profession of physical therapy during their June 2000 meeting.

Summary

The profession of physical therapy continues to evolve from its origins in the early 20th century. The profession currently faces challenges that will define the future role of the physical therapist in health care delivery. Clearly, this profession will continue to play an important role in health care delivery.

References

1. Cogan MI. Toward a definition of a profession. *Harvard Educational Review*. 1953;23:33-50.

2. Goode WJ. Encroachment, charlatanism and the emerging profession: psychology, medicine and sociology. *American Sociological Review*. 1960;25:902-914.

3. Pellegrino ED. What is a profession? *J Allied Health*. 1983;12:168-176.

4. Moore WE. The criteria of professionalism. In: Moore WE. *The Professions: Roles and Rules*. New York: Russell Sage Foundation; 1970:3-22.

5. *Model Practice Act Language*. Alexandria, VA: Federation of State Boards of Physical Therapy; 2002. Available from: http://www.fsbpt.org/download/MPA2002.pdf. Accessed February 6, 2005.

6. Jacobson BF. Role-model concepts before and after the formal professional socialization period. *Phys Ther*. 1980;60(2):188-193.

7. Jacobson BF. Characteristics of physical therapy role models. *Phys Ther*. 1978;58(5):560-566.

8. APTA. *APTA Background Sheet: The Physical Therapist. A Professional Profile Webpage*. Available at: http://www.apta.org/Consumer/whoareptsptas/profile. Accessed July 28, 2000.

9. APTA. *APTA Background Sheet: The Physical Therapist Assistant. A Profile Webpage*. Available at: http://www.apta.org/Consumer/whoareptsptas/Profile_A sst?id[1]=121. Accessed July 28, 2000.

10. Murphy WB. *Healing the Generations: A History of Physical Therapy & the American Physical Therapy Association*. Alexandria, Va: American Physical Therapy Association; 1995.

11. Pinkston D. Evolution of the practice of physical therapy. In: Scully RM, Barnes MR, eds. *Physical Therapy*. Philadelphia: JB Lippincott Company;1989:2-30.

12. APTA. *APTA House of Delegates endorses a vision for the future*. Available at: http://www.apta.org/news/visionstatementrelease. Accessed July 28, 2000.

PUTTING IT INTO PRACTICE

Consult your textbook and the American Physical Therapy Association website to answer the following questions about the physical therapy profession:

1. What is the APTA's toll-free (1-800) telephone number?

2. Who is the current editor of the journal *Physical Therapy*?

3. During what era did reconstruction aides work?

4. Who was the first president of the American Women's Physical Therapeutic Association?

5. What was the name of the first physical therapy professional journal?

6. What organization (outside the physical therapy profession) supervised the development and accreditation of physical therapy programs from their inception in the 1920s until the 1970s?

7. In what year did a bachelor's degree become the *minimum* entry-level educational requirement for physical therapy education?

8. What is the medical specialty name for physicians who specialize in physical medicine and rehabilitation?

9. In what year was clinical specialty certification initiated by the APTA?

10. How many clinical areas are currently available for physical therapist clinical specialist certification?

11. What is required to obtain clinical specialty certification? (choose one specialty area of interest)

12. How many accredited programs exist in your state for the educational preparation of physical therapists?

13. Which of these programs grant a master's degree? A DPT degree?

14. How many accredited programs exist in your state for the educational preparation of physical therapist assistants?

15. When and where will your state chapter conference of the APTA be held this year?

16. Access to physical therapy services without physician referral is currently legal in how many states?

17. Is it legal in your state to provide physical therapy services to a patient without a physician's referral?

18. What is the name of the current president of the APTA?

19. What is the name of the current president of your state chapter of the APTA?

20. What do the initials CSM stand for? (hint: an annual conference)

21. Which month is National Physical Therapy Month?

22. Name one section of the APTA.

23. In what year were standards for utilization of the physical therapist assistant and standards for physical therapist assistant education adopted by the APTA ?

24. What disease epidemic created the initial impetus for the physical therapy profession?

25. What degree is currently the *minimum* entry-level educational requirement for physical therapy professional education?

26. What degree will you receive when you complete your professional education program (be specific as to exact name of the degree—not "master's degree")?

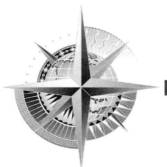

Chapter 2

The Changing World and the Future of Physical Therapy

In the past two decades, there have been widespread changes in the health care delivery system in the United States. Managed health care has changed reimbursement mechanisms and mandated widespread cost containment across all levels of care. Physical therapist role and practice parameters continue to evolve in response to these changes.

Cost Containment... Everywhere!

> *Jennifer started her new position as a graduate physical therapist and found that there were five staff members called "Patient Care Associates" who worked side-by-side with the licensed staff members in the department. She talked with one of them, who told her that he was trained on the job to perform gait training and therapeutic exercise. She wondered how his training differed from hers.*

Changing mechanisms of payment for services have forced health care organizations to develop numerous cost-containment strategies. For example, most physical therapists practice in health care environments that are largely funded by a prospective payment system (PPS). A PPS provides payment with a fixed limit or a fixed amount determined by

the diagnosis of the patient rather than by the actual time spent or individual needs of the patient.[1]

Health care providers often experience strict utilization management with increased accountability to third-party payers and health maintenance organizations. This requires an extra burden of paperwork which can be greatly simplified with use of computerized resources.

To cut costs, many health care institutions use on-the-job trained, multiskilled workers for physical therapy-related functions or reduce the time or number of treatments that patients receive. Physical therapists must therefore be able to prioritize and manage care while delegating and providing direct supervision for other members of the health care delivery team.

Cost-Effective and Efficient Outcomes

> *While sitting in his research class, John wondered why there was so little outcomes research in the physical therapy profession. Both the course instructor and the readings for the day had emphasized this point. Their guest speaker presented data that was routinely collected at their facility and indicated that they would be open to sharing this data with university researchers and students to analyze their outcomes.*

Third-party payment systems require documentation of functional outcomes of physical therapy treatment, especially in relation to costs. Physical therapists who can analyze and present data to support efficient and cost-effective patient management will have an advantage in competing for limited resources. The *Guide to Physical Therapist Practice* outlines practice patterns that are indicated for various diagnostic groups.[2]

Shift to Prevention and Wellness

The first-year physical therapy students were assigned a class project of preparing an exhibition on computer workstation ergonomics for the university health fair. They approached the project scientifically, incorporating theories of behavior change with simple, clear messages for postural evaluation and prevention of repetitive stress disorders.

As financial resources for treatment for existing illnesses and injuries have decreased, increasing attention has been shifted to health promotion, wellness, and prevention of disease and disability. Physical therapists provide not only evaluation and treatment, but also services that are aimed at preventing illness and disability. Physical therapists must have a strong background in health behavior and related health promotion strategies. More than ever before, excellent communication and patient education skills are critical.

Integrated Service Delivery

What do nurses do? What do social workers do? How does occupational therapy differ from physical therapy? When is speech pathology indicated? The case study raised all of these questions...

What services would be appropriate for an 85-year-old widow who had just returned home from a 3-week stay in a skilled nursing facility while recovering from a stroke?

As our social service and health care systems increase in complexity, physical therapists are unable to optimally meet their patients' needs without working closely with other health care professionals. Interdisciplinary case management has been associated with patients reaching higher levels of function in shorter lengths of time.[3] *Integrated service delivery* strategies involve interdisciplinary team interaction, interprofessional collaboration, and coordination between providers to provide professional services to clients and patients with multiple needs.[4] Physical therapists must have skills that foster collaboration and coordination of service delivery in addition to providing unique and specialized health care services.

Shift From Hospitals to Other Levels of Care

"Discharge planning" was a term that came up frequently in classroom discussions this semester. How does a physical therapist determine what level of care is most appropriate?

Social support   Mental status
Prior level of function   Judgment
Current functional level

Words on a screen at the front of the class. It seemed that there were so many things to consider.

Over the last several decades, patient length of stay in hospitals and rehabilitation facilities has decreased markedly with a shift from inpatient services to subacute, outpatient, and home health services.[5] Thus, patients are more likely to receive physical therapy services in a skilled nursing facility, their homes, or an outpatient center rather than in an acute hospital.

Recently, we have seen widespread cost-containment strategies at the subacute, outpatient, and home health service environments. The rules are changing rapidly in these treatment settings, necessitating that physical therapists stay informed and work closely with administrators to provide necessary patient documentation and service-related information.

Variation in Supply and Demand for Physical Therapists

When Andrea had planned on entering the physical therapy field after high school, physical therapy was forecast as one of the "hottest" professions for the future. Now it seemed like graduates were having difficulty getting full-time positions and were receiving lower salaries than they were several years ago. What happened?

Over the past two decades, there were forecasts of widespread shortages of physical therapists given their rapidly expanding roles and the growing elderly population. In contrast, many organizations have actually cut or restructured physical therapist positions in response to cost-containment initiatives.[5]

Recent increases in the number of physical therapy graduates combined with organizational staffing cuts have lead to a surplus of physical therapists in relation to available positions in some locations. This may result in lower salaries, higher case loads, and increased daily patient volume for physical therapists in some areas of the country. These changes require that physical therapists develop excellent case management skills and enter a more competitive job market with skills that will enable them to succeed in a changing health care environment.

Key Trends and Statistics that Influence Physical Therapy Practice

Physical therapists typically work with several groups of people. Changes in the number or distribution of persons with disabilities or the elderly and the prevalence of the most common public health problems change the nature of physical therapy practice. Similarly, legislation that affects access or reimbursement for physical therapy necessitates advocacy and involvement by physical therapists.

Let's look at the recent trends and legislation that have influenced the profession of physical therapy.

Josephina, a first-year physical therapy student who has been hard of hearing since childhood, sat in the first row of the classroom so that she could read the instructor's lips. She listened to the presentation about the Nagi and World Health Organization models of disablement. She wondered if her hearing problems would count as a disability.

Disability Statistics

Recent US Census estimates reflect that one in five persons in the United States has a disability and one in 10 has a severe disability.[6] This may be a chronic disease process such as heart disease, sickle cell anemia, epilepsy, or cancer; a sensory disability such as deafness, hard of hearing, or a visual impairment; a physical disability such as an amputation, paralysis, or problem with pain or movement; a learning disability such as dyslexia or attention deficit disorder; a cognitive disability such as Alzheimer's disease; or a disability related to a mental health condition. Some disabilities are not visible to the casual observer; others are obvious. Some are stable; some are progressive or intermittent in nature.

What Constitutes a Disability?

For the purposes of identification by the US Census Bureau, a person is considered to have a *disability* if he or she has difficulty performing certain functions (seeing, hearing, talking, walking, climbing stairs, lifting, and carrying), has difficulty performing activities of daily living, or has difficulty with certain social roles (doing school work for children or working at a job and around the house for adults).

"A person who is unable to perform one or more activities, or who uses an assistive device to get around, or who needs assistance from another person to perform basic activities is considered to have a severe disability."[6]

See Tables 2-1 and 2-2 for an analysis of conditions causing disability and activity limitations.

Table 2-1

CONDITIONS CAUSING DISABILITY BY BROAD INTERNATIONAL CLASSIFICATION OF DISEASES AND IMPAIRMENT CATEGORIES[9]

ICD Chapter		Number (1000s)	Percent of all Conditions
	All Conditions	61,047	100.0
	Disorders and Injuries	44,721	73.3
1	Infectious and parasitic diseases (001-139)	378	0.6
2	Neoplasms (140-239), injury, and poisoning	1628	2.7
3	Endocrine, nutritional, and metabolic diseases and immunity disorders (780-779)	3409	5.6
4	Diseases of the blood and blood-forming organs (280-289)	217	0.4
5	Mental disorders (290-316) excluding mental retardation	2035	3.3
6	Diseases of the nervous system and sense organs (320-389)	4373	7.2
7	Diseases of the circulatory system (390-459)	10,170	16.7
8	Diseases of the respiratory system (460-519)	4774	7.8
9	Diseases of the digestive system (520-579)	1728	2.8
10	Diseases of the genitourinary system (580-629)	778	1.3
12	Diseases of the skin and subcutaneous tissue (680-709)	362	0.6
13	Diseases of the musculoskeletal system and connective tissue (710-739)	10,530	17.2
14	Congenital abnormalities (740-759)	287	0.5
15-16	Certain conditions originating from the perinatal period (760-799) and symptoms, signs, ill-defined conditions (520-579)	2843	4.7
17	(800-999), not involving impairment	1205	2.0
	Impairments	16,326	26.7
	Orthopedic impairments	8608	14.1
	Learning disability and mental retardation	1575	2.6
	Visual impairments	1294	2.1
	Hearing impairments	1175	1.9
	Paralysis	1071	1.8
	Deformities	900	1.5
	Absence or loss of limb/other body part	788	1.3
	Speech impairments	545	0.9
	Other and ill-defined impairments	371	0.6

Note: Conditions in ICD Chapter 11, complications of pregnancy, childbirth, and the puerperium (630-676) are not used.

Table 2-2

MOST COMMON CONDITIONS CAUSING ACTIVITY LIMITATION[9]

Rank		Number (1000s)	Percent of all Conditions
	All Conditions	61,047	100.0
1	Heart disease (390-429)	7932	13.0
2	Deformities, orthopedic impairments, and disorders of the spine or back	7672	12.6
3	Osteoarthrosis and allied disorders (715-716)	5048	8.3
4	Orthopedic impairment of lower extremity	2817	4.6
5	Asthma (493)	2,592	4.2
6	Diabetes (250)	2,569	4.2
7	Mental disorders (290-316) excluding learning disability and mental retardation	2,035	3.3
8	Disorders of the eye (360-379)	1,577	2.6
9	Learning disability and mental retardation	1,575	2.6
10	Cancer (140-208)	1,342	2.2
11	Visual impairments	1,294	2.1
12	Orthopedic impairment of shoulder and/or upper extremities	1,196	2.0
13	Other unknown and unspecified causes	1,188	1.9
14	Hearing impairments	1,175	1.9
15	Cerebrovascular disease (430-438)	1,174	1.9

Disabilities and Employment

Who Has Jobs?

The 1994-5 Survey of Income and Program Participation (SIPP)[7] showed that only
- 22% of working-age wheelchair users
- 28% of cane, crutch, or walker users
- 26% of people unable to climb stairs
- 23% of those unable to walk three city blocks
- 27% of those unable to lift and carry 10 pounds

have jobs!

For those who do work, the chances that they will earn an equitable wage are slim. Persons with disabilities are often unemployed and live in poverty. The median monthly income for men with work disabilities averaged $1880 in 1995, according to the SIPP, which is 20% less than the $2356 earned by their counterparts without disabilities. Women with disabilities earned $1511 monthly, or 13% less than the $1737 average for women without disabilities.[8]

Legislative and Economic Aspects of Disability

> *Before beginning her physical therapy education, Nora worked part-time in the Center for Independent Living. One of the center's clients told her about his recent experience in seeking employment. He had been selected for a position that was matched perfectly with his qualifications. He wondered if he should have mentioned his need for an accessible restroom during the interview. Nora informed him that such an accommodation was his right under the provisions of the ADA.*

In the past 30 years, we have seen many legislative acts that affect the quality of life of individuals with disabilities. Table 2-3 lists a few examples of the major pieces of legislation that provide the basis for the rights of persons with disabilities in the United States.

Unfortunately, although there is legal protection in many situations, we still have a long way to go in changing public beliefs that it serves *all* people to make entrances to buildings barrier-free, to actively foster opportunities for employment for individuals with disabilities, and to provide diagnostic and treatment services to the millions of children and adults with disabilities who live in poverty.

The Aging of America

> *Alan, home on spring break, visited his elderly grandparents in their retirement community. He was amazed to read their activity calendar. He remarked, "There's more going on here than at my college. Now I see why you're never home!"*

Population aging is occurring in the United States and worldwide. The elderly population in the United States (age 65 and older) increased 11-fold from 1900 to 1994, to the present 33.2 million people. During the same period, the under-65 population grew only three-fold.[10] In 1991, the average life expectancy at birth for Americans was 75.5 years, almost double what it was in 1900. Women live an average of 79 years, while men can expect to live to age 72.[10,11]

The oldest segment of the population is growing most rapidly. In 1994, an estimated 3.5 million people were age 85 and older, representing 10% of the elderly in the United States. By the middle of the 21st century, it is projected that there will be as many people age 85 and older as there are people age 65 to 69. The projected rates of growth of the elderly population are illustrated in Figure 2-1.[11]

Further, population statistics indicate that in the coming decades, the 65+ population will be much more racially and ethnically diverse than it is today. Of the 80.1 million elderly projected for 2050, it is estimated that about 8.4 million will be black, 6.7 million will be races other than white or black, and 12.5 million will be Hispanic.[11]

New evidence shows that rates of disability and disease may be slowing among older people, suggesting that progress can be made to improve the health of people age 65+. However, with the population aging, living to very advanced age will likely mean disease and disability for increasing numbers of older Americans.

Increasing age heightens the probability of functional limitations. In one survey, 9% of people age 65 to 69 required day-to-day assistance, including help with bathing, dressing, and eating, compared with 50% for those age 85 and older. One-third of elderly women age 75 and older are functionally dependent and in need of considerable assistance.[10] The link between advancing age and increasing functional problems has enormous implications for long-term care.

Chronic conditions are prevalent among older persons. The majority of persons 70 years of age and older reported that they have arthritis, and approximately one-third reported hypertension.[11]

National Legislation with a Direct Influence on the Profession of Physical Therapy

Social Security Act of 1965

With the passage of the Social Security Act of 1965, the government began to subsidize two health care plans: the *Medicare* and *Medicaid* programs. This legislation resulted in marked changes in access to health care for the elderly and poor. For example, during the late 1950s, less than 15% of the elderly population had any health insurance. The enactment of the Medicare and Medicaid programs helped to

Table 2-3
KEY LEGISLATIVE ACTIVITY AND DISABILITY ISSUES

Legislation Affecting Persons with Disabilities

Rehabilitation Act of 1973: mandated no discrimination by federally funded agencies against workers and students with disabilities and affirmative action requirements for federally funded employers.

Americans with Disabilities Act of 1990: mandated reasonable accommodations to ensure the integration of people with disabilities in the private sector, including employment, telecommunications, transportation, and public services and accommodations.

Legislation Affecting Children with Disabilities

PL 94-142: Education for All Handicapped Children Act of 1975—mandated a free and appropriate education and the least restrictive environment (ie, mainstreaming). Annual individual educational plans (IEPs) were developed for all children with disabilities.

PL 101-476: revised provisions of PL 94-142 to include children with autism and brain injury and included training and technology provisions for education of children with disabilities.

IDEA Improvement Act of 1997: gave parents and school districts more autonomy in determining children's needs for special education services through a mediation process, further defined services available to infants and toddlers, and provided disciplinary sanctions for students who engage in criminal misconduct unrelated to disability.

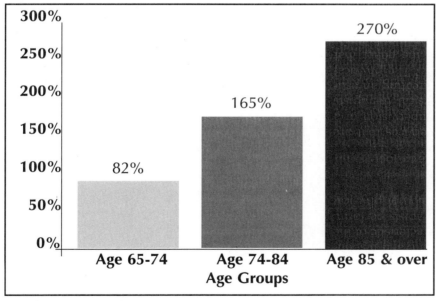

Figure 2-1. Projected percent of growth in the elderly population by age group from 1990 to 2040. Rapid rates of growth are anticipated for all segments of the elderly population, with the greatest growth occurring in those age 85 and older (adapted from National Center for Health Statistics. *Health and aging chartbook from Health, United States, 1999.* Webpage available at: http://www.cdc.gov/nchs/releases/99news/hus99.htm. Accessed June 16, 2000).

provide health insurance to nearly 85% of all Americans by 1966.[12]

To be eligible for *Medicare,* an individual must be a citizen or permanent resident of the United States who has worked and contributed to Social Security for at least 10 years and be at least 65 years of age. People under 65 are entitled to Medicare if they have been receiving Social Security benefits for 24 months or have end-stage renal disease. A person can also be eligible if their spouse has met the employment requirement.[1] *Medicaid (MediCal* in California) is a state-administered program that provides medical assistance to the poor and is financed through both state and federal taxes. Eligibility is determined by income and other requirements.

Health Care Reform—National Health Insurance Initiative Defeated

In recent decades, as health costs increased logarithmically, it became clear that a significant group of citizens had no medical insurance and were not eligible for either of these public programs. In fact, almost 20% of the US population is currently uninsured. This led to efforts in the early 1990s to create a system of national health insurance. Bitter conflicts erupted between leaders in Congress and the Clinton administration regarding the scope and content of this health care initiative.

In the mid 1990s, following the failure of national health insurance to be adopted by Congress, there was growing concern that the Medicare system would soon have no money, given the aging population demographics and escalating costs of health care. This lead to further cost containment in the Medicare system.

The Balanced Budget Amendment of 1997

Perhaps the single piece of modern-day legislation to have the greatest effect on the profession of physical therapy is the Balanced Budget Amendment of 1997. President Clinton signed HR 2015, the Balanced Budget Act of 1997, on August 5, 1997.[13]

This legislation, intended to eliminate the federal deficit, created widespread cuts in the Medicare and Medicaid systems, intended to reduce entitlement spending by $115 billion in Medicare over 5 years, and $13.6 billion in Medicaid over 5 years. The largest portion of these savings came from reduced Medicare payments to health care providers and hospitals. Hospitals were slated to lose some $40 billion in Medicare (35% of the overall cuts), while payments to managed care plans under Medicare were to be reduced by $22 billion over 5 years. Further, reductions in hospital payments, home health services, and skilled nursing facility (SNF) payments also reduced reimbursement for physical therapy services.[13]

Physical therapists were especially hard hit by the provisions of the Balanced Budget Act. The act included a provision that imposed an arbitrary annual cap of $1500 per beneficiary for combined physical therapy and speech therapy services provided by comprehensive outpatient rehabilitation facilities (CORFs), SNFs, and physicians' offices.[13] This extraordinarily low level of reimbursement fell far short of that required to provide necessary services for millions of elderly Americans. The APTA actively advocated for a moratorium on the $1500 cap until an alternate system could be put into place.

In late 1999, Congress and the White House reached an agreement on a plan to restore more than $12 billion in cuts previously made in Medicare payments. The Balanced Budget Refinement Act eliminated the $1500 caps on Medicare's coverage of physical therapy, occupational therapy, and speech pathology. It also postponed a mandated 15% reduction in payments to home health agencies and increased payments for some patients in skilled nursing facilities.[14]

The Balanced Budget Amendment of 1997 also mandated a prospective payment system for skilled nursing facilities. Changes in Medicare reimbursement schedules have resulted in widespread decreases in physical therapist staffing of skilled nursing facilities.[13]

Further, the act mandated a comprehensive assessment of adult home care patients called the Outcome and Assessment Information Set (OASIS) to measure outcomes for the purposes of quality improvement for Medicare-certified home health agencies. All of these changes have marked implications for the physical therapy profession.[13]

Summary

Changes in the health care delivery system and the changing population demographics have forced a shift in physical therapy practice. Increased accountability, variations in supply and demand for physical therapists, and changing priorities in public health will continue to influence the future of the physical therapy profession.

References

1. Kristy W. Basics of health care financing and reimbursement. In: Curtis KA, ed. *The Physical Therapist's Guide to Health Care.* Thorofare, NJ: SLACK Incorporated; 1999:13-47.

2. APTA. *Guide to Physical Therapy Practice.* Alexandria, Va: American Physical Therapy Association; 1997:viii.

3. Erickson B, Perkins M. Interdisciplinary team approach in the rehabilitation of hip and knee arthroplasties. *Am J Occup Ther.* 1994;48(5):429-441.

4. Hilton RW, Morris DJ, Wright AM. Learning to work in the health care team. *Journal of Interprofessional Care.* 1995;9(3): 267-274.

5. Lopopolo RB. The effect of hospital restructuring on the role of physical therapists in acute care. *Phys Ther.* 1997;77(9):918-932.

6. Census Brief, U.S. Department of Commerce, Economics

and Statistics Administration CENBR/97-5; December 1997: 1.

7. Disability Rights Advocates. *Disability Watch: The Status of People with Disabilities in the United States.* Available at: http://www.dsc.ucsf.edu/UCSF/pic.taf?_UserReference=F90140D74B1990AFBD2F8118&_function=search&url=BOO1X4.1. Accessed July 30, 2000

8. The income gap. In: Kaye HS, ed. *Disability Watch: The Status of People with Disabilities in the United States.* Volcano, Calif: Disability Rights Advocates; 1997. Available at: http://www.dsc.ucsf.edu/UCSF/pic.taf?_UserReferenc =F90140D74B1990AFBD2F8118&_function=search&url=BOO1X4.4. Accessed July 30, 2000.

9. *National Health Interview Survey.* Hyattsville, Md: National Center for Health Statistics; 1992.

10. National Institutes of Health Public Information Office. *Aging America Poses Unprecedented Challenge, Says New Census, Aging Institute Report.* Webpage available at: http://www.nih.gov/nia/new/press/census.htm. Accessed June 16, 2000.

11. National Center for Health Statistics. *Health and aging chartbook from Health, United States, 1999.* Webpage available at: http://www.cdc.gov/nchs/releases/99new 99news/hus99.htm. Accessed June 16, 2000

12. Relman AS. Assessment and accountability: the third revolution in medical care. *New Eng J Med.* 1988;319(18):1220-1222.

13. APTA. *The Balanced Budget Act. How It Affects Physical Therapy.* Webpage available at: http://www.apta.org/Advocacy/national/ National16. Accessed July 30, 2000.

14. APTA. *Highlights of Medicare Balanced Budget Act Refinement Acts of 1999.* Webpage available at: http://www.apta.org/Advocacy/national/BalancedBudget Refinements. Accessed July 30, 2000.

PUTTING IT INTO PRACTICE

1. Interview a person with a disability or a person over the age of 65 about his or her recent experiences in accessing health care services.

   Briefly describe the person you interviewed:

   What has been this person's experience in finding health care providers to provide services covered by his or her insurance plan?

   What has been this person's experience in finding health care providers who are able to meet his or her needs?

   What health care needs are currently unmet?

2. Interview a physical therapist who has been in practice for more than 5 years. What changes has he or she seen in the profession during that time? How has the field differed from his or her expectations before entering the profession? How has practice changed since the implementation of the Balanced Budget Amendment of 1997?

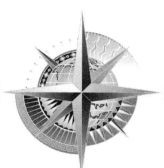

Chapter 3

The Evolving Roles of the Physical Therapist

Stephanie had expected to work in an outpatient orthopedic or sports clinic but found a better-paying job closer to home in a skilled nursing facility "health center" at a multi-level care, senior residential complex. "You're not going to work in one of those dingy nursing homes, are you?" her older sister had asked, adding, "I couldn't. Those places are so depressing." Stephanie had done some aide work at a skilled nursing facility and knew her sister was behind the times. Nonetheless, she had some reservations. Her orientation at the facility reassured her. "Wow," she commented. "This place looks like a resort! Beautiful dining room, gardens, activity areas, and skylights to brighten the interior. I'll have to bring my sister to see this."

The Future of Physical Therapy

In this world of constant change, the roles of physical therapists must inevitably also change. Physical therapists who are entering practice in the next decade will face challenges in service delivery because of the complexity of the following realities. Sensitivity to these changes is critical for all health professionals. Consider the following forces that shape the practice environment:

- The population dynamics of our country are changing markedly. The population of adults over age 65 has swelled to almost 35 million. By 2008, this figure will have risen to over 38 million.[1] Their health care needs may not be met by a Medicare system that is undergoing constant change and cost containment in an attempt to survive.

- The ethnic diversity of this population is also growing. In some states, combined nonwhite minorities currently comprise the majority of the population. Language barriers, cultural diversity, and socioeconomic challenges influence the delivery of health care services.

- Although the economy is strong, millions of our citizens continue to live in poverty and lack access to even basic medical services. More than one-fifth of the population is uninsured by any type of medical insurance program.

- There is no longer a shortage of physical therapists in some areas of the country or in some practice settings, yet the needs of the population for physical therapy services continue to increase.

- More than one-third of disability and disease in this country could be prevented by changing lifestyle habits such as diet and activity.

- Women's health issues are becoming increasingly important as heart disease, osteoporosis, and related fractures account for significant disability and untimely deaths of elderly women.

- Like most other health professions, physical therapists can no longer rely on reimbursement by third-party payment systems for their economic security. Physical therapists must explore other mechanisms of payment for their services and creative modes of service delivery to address the ever-increasing health care needs of the population.

- Heath care spending is at an all-time high and is projected to continue to rise yearly. Consumers and third-party payers continue to increase the pressure for cost-effective care. Evidence-based outcomes will continue to be the greatest source of validation for the valuable work that physical therapists do.

- Internet use has increased by over 300% in the past 3 years and by over 1000% in the past 10 years.[2] Consumers have access to health care information as never before. Physical therapists need to publicize their programs, services, and value for consumers, businesses, health care providers, and third-party payers to see and understand. Technology use by physical therapists may be the single most important mechanism to publicize the services they provide.

Consider again APTA's Vision Statement in Table 1-3. Physical therapists must embrace some of the above changes as they define their roles in the profession of physical therapy within the context of the future health care environment.

Key Roles for Physical Therapists

Physical therapists must be skilled in diagnosis and screening, evaluation and assessment, case management, consultation and delegation of treatment responsibilities to others, patient education, documentation, collaboration, and program development.

The changing health care environment requires practicing clinicians to respond to health care delivery trends and to redesign their organizational responsibilities accordingly.

Physical Therapist as Agent of Change

Helena raised her hand and contributed to the class discussion, "It seems like everything is constantly changing and it's all so complicated. I have to know how to code a patient for systems like MDS and OASIS, and no one seems to care what the best treatment is for the patient."

We have seen significant changes in the physical therapy profession and are likely to see many more in the next few years. Physical therapists must remain flexible and informed, as the present-day rules may change tomorrow, the next day, and even again next week.

But even more important than being flexible in the face of change, physical therapists must assume a proactive role as *change agents*. Rather than letting external forces dictate physical therapy practice constraints, physical therapists need to prioritize patient needs and advocate for critical services. Physical therapists must educate others regarding the legal and ethical implications of change.

On a larger scale, physical therapists must take a proactive role in organizational change processes. They must identify and communicate to others the expertise of physical therapists and determine what can and cannot be compromised in physical therapy service delivery. Physical therapists must be in control of changes in their roles and responsibilities rather than letting someone else make those decisions.

The good news is that there are many opportunities to assume new roles in the changing health care environment. Physical therapists need to be astutely aware of the past and present history of the professional role as they craft their roles for the future.

Physical Therapist as Data Analyzer and Outcomes Reporter

Ellen, during her final clinical internship, lamented to another intern, "Why do we need to do all this paperwork? Don't they know that we are more valuable actually working with the patients?"

Data. What do we really need to know? And who needs to know it? Documentation. Paper work. Evaluations. Progress reports. Discharge summaries. Outcomes.

These processes are the keys to providing evidence of the value of physical therapy services. Organized data collection, systematic analysis, and reporting of outcomes are the keys to establishing the efficacy of clinical practices and determining the best methods to deliver physical therapy service.

Physical therapists who can design systems of data collection and analyze and report the results will be able to further establish the value of physical therapy services. Computerized record keeping is an important component of any data collection system because it makes it easier to systematically collect and collate patient outcomes data.

The Physical Therapist as Program Developer

> *Yousef worked for several years on a part-time basis at the local senior center prior to entering the graduate program in physical therapy. He saw many seniors who were able to maintain an active, healthy lifestyle. He wondered how the lives of seniors might improve even more if physical therapy services could be offered just as preventive maintenance on an automobile or periodic dental cleaning by the dentist.*

Physical therapy services have traditionally been offered to address problems after the problem has already occurred. With changes in payment mechanisms, services may not be covered in traditional ways. These changes require physical therapists to look into other ways of providing services.

New program development requires that physical therapists be aware of the needs of a patient population and look at creative ways to meet those needs. It may be through a group class, a community event, a sponsored screening day, a peer network, or a telephone hotline. Innovation in program development is a key to adapting to the changing health care environment.

The Physical Therapist as Collaborator

> *Jerry sat in his first team meeting around a table with professionals from five other disciplines. He looked over his report and found that several other members who spoke before him had reported conflicting information about the patient's social support network. Perhaps this patient was not able to go home as soon as planned.*

We live in a complex world. As educational, social service, and health care systems increase in complexity, physical therapists must collaborate with other professionals to provide for the multiple needs of their patients or clients. There is evidence that outcomes improve and care is provided more efficiently when professionals use a collaborative process to plan and provide patient or client-centered services. In addition, it is important to include clients, parents, family members, and caregivers in the collaborative process to determine the best plan for each individual client.[4]

Interprofessional collaboration involves working together to reach a common goal in a supportive and mutually beneficial relationship with other team members. Collaborative team interactions include voluntary involvement, parity, and shared decision-making power among team members.[3] An awareness of organizational and group dynamics, conflict resolution strategies, leadership, and communication skills characterize effective teamwork.[4]

We are seeing a trend in academic programs to introduce opportunities for students to gain skills in teamwork and interprofessional collaboration.[5-7] Physical therapists become more valuable members of the health care team when they have strong skills in communication and collaboration.

Physical Therapist as Evaluator

> *Alberto decided to write his Professional Issues paper on physical therapy diagnosis. He interviewed practicing therapists and found that many did not feel comfortable with the idea of diagnosis.*

Diagnosis, evaluation, prognosis. Each of these terms has specific meanings to a physical therapist. The physical therapy profession has differentiated the professional role as one that is uniquely qualified to make decisions to collect and consider evaluative data to determine the need for physical therapy intervention. With decreasing resources, it becomes increasingly important that physical therapists evaluate which patients are most likely to benefit from receiving services.

Physical therapists today enter practice with specialized skills in screening and triage. Physical therapists need to determine the best use of limited resources. The questions in Table 3-1 may be helpful to ask during the screening process.

Physical Therapist as Case Manager

> *Hope heard what the clinical instructor said: "This patient will be discharged tomorrow. Where do you think he should go? What level of care is appropriate?" She wondered how to tell.*

To make this decision, physical therapists consider the patient's needs, the types of treatment environments (acute, subacute, rehabilitation, home health, outpatient), and the roles, skills, and capabilities of various personnel available to meet those needs. The case manager must be a patient advocate, educator, excellent team player, and communicator.

The discharge plan is one of the priorities for consideration when beginning a patient's evaluation. Does this patient have what it takes to be successful at the next level of care, whether that will be in an institution, outpatient clinic, or in the home?

Physical therapists who have good delegation and communication skills and use an organized follow-up system will prevent the patient from "slipping through the cracks." Unfortunately, only some health care consumers are able to survive in the current health care environment without assistance to navigate. Most patients require health care providers to be strong advocates to empower them, to educate them, to assist them in accessing the equipment, services, and referrals they need to appropriately address their health care needs.

The Physical Therapist as Educator

Vanessa sat in the front row of the classroom. She wondered, "Why do we need to spend so much time on patient education? I wanted to become a physical therapist to provide hands-on care."

Education and motivation precede the changes in behavior that lead to prevention of disability and disease. More than one-third of our population in the United States will suffer from disease or disability that can be prevented by diet and exercise. Many of

these conditions can be prevented through education and lifestyle change.

When physical therapists become effective educators, they integrate their understanding of the factors that motivate and drive health behavior with the patient's needs. Only when physical therapists use available educational technology, develop culturally and linguistically appropriate education materials, and create effective information systems can they have the maximum impact on patients.

Patients and their caregivers often need to *learn* what they must do to become independent, prevent further disability, maximize their function, reduce pain and stress, and return to work. Not to be overlooked, education *saves* money... for consumers, for their employers, and for third-party payers.

Physical Therapist as Consultant

The panel discussion at the state physical therapy conference had just begun. The first speaker said he was a consultant to a manufacturing plant. "I prevent injuries in the workplace. I save my clients thousands of dollars every year." He challenged the audience, "How can physical therapists share their expert knowledge with those who need it most?"

Consultation is a critical role for physical therapists to develop. Consultation is essentially the process of giving your opinion. This is not a new role for physical therapists. Physical therapists have been giving their opinions for years in documenting patient goals and rehabilitation potential, treatment plans, and assessments of progress. In the current health care environment, some physical therapists worry that the complexities of service delivery will be reduced to a series of "cookbook" approaches, critical pathways, and protocols. Sharing one's expertise often makes it clear that a situation is more complex than it may appear on the surface.

Physical therapists have many areas of expertise. Some physical therapists possess expert knowledge in the field of movement science and pathokinesiology, others in areas like rehabilitation and assistive technology. Still other therapists have received specialist certification in specific clinical domains: sports, orthopedics, pediatrics, geriatrics, or cardiopulmonary care. Many pursue expertise in health care administration and management.

The role of the consultant is to share one's professional expertise and to educate others. A consultant might provide an explanation of the interrelationships of pathology and functional loss, of impairment and projected outcomes, or organizational change and performance criteria. The consultant often relates known research findings to clinical or environmental problems. Consultants provide critical analysis and advanced clinical decision-making in complex situations.

Summary

Change is constant. The roles of physical therapists must change in response to the changing dynamics of the health care environment. Physical therapists who have strong leadership, case management, data analysis, and innovative program development skills will thrive in the changing health care environment.

Sensitivity to the diverse needs of the changing population, flexibility in choosing the means and methods to meet those needs and accountability in service delivery will be the hallmarks for the future physical therapist.

References

1. National Institutes of Health Public Information Office. *Aging America Poses Unprecedented Challenge, Says New Census, Aging Institute Report*. Webpage available at: http://www.nih.gov/nia/new/press/census.htm. Accessed June 16, 2000.

2. Interhemispheric Resource Center. *World Wide Internet Users*. Available at: http://www.irconline.org/bios/pdf/internet_users.pdf. Accessed July 30, 2000.

3. Erickson B, Perkins M. Interdisciplinary team approach in the rehabilitation of hip and knee arthroplasties. *Am J Occup Ther*. 1994;48(5):429-441.

4. O'Connor B. Challenges of interagency collaboration: serving a young child with severe disabilities. In: McEwen IR, ed. *Occupational and Physical Therapy in Educational Environments*. Binghamton, NY: Haworth Press, Inc; 1995.

5. Hilton RW, Morris DJ, Wright AM. Learning to work in the health care team. *Journal of Interprofessional Care*. 1995;9(3):267-274.

6. Richardson J, Edwards M. An undergraduate clinical skills laboratory developing interprofessional skills in physical and occupational therapy. *Gerontology and Geriatrics Education*. 1997;17(4):33-43.

7. MacKinnon JL, MacRae N. Fostering geriatric interdisciplinary collaboration through academic education. *Physical and Occupational Therapy in Geriatrics*. 1996:14(3):41-49.

PUTTING IT INTO PRACTICE

Physical therapists must be skilled in diagnosis and screening, evaluation and assessment, case management, consultation and delegation of treatment responsibilities to others, patient education, documentation, collaboration, and program development. Consider the evolving roles of the physical therapist and the skills needed to succeed in each role. Think of situations in which you have used these skills in the past. Explore your curriculum and identify opportunities for you to acquire these skills during your educational program. Enter this information in the appropriate boxes below.

Roles	**Skills needed to succeed in this role**	**Situations in which I've used these skills in the past**	**How to acquire these skills during my professional education program**
Change Agent			
Data Analyzer and Outcomes Reporter			
Program Developer			
Collaborator			
Evaluator			
Case Manager			
Educator			
Consultant			

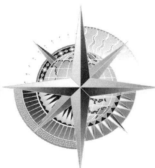

Part Two

Becoming a Physical Therapist

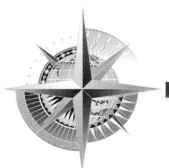

Chapter 4

Financing Physical Therapy Education

Mary, a returning student, considered pursuing physical therapy education when she became disillusioned with her career in advertising. She looked into the expenses of graduate education and realized that she would not only have to leave her current position, but would also have to pay for tuition, fees, books, and other related educational expenses. How much would it all cost?

Keith, a graduate student starting the master's program in physical therapy, waited for the financial aid counselor to return from lunch. He worried, "I have taken out so many loans... is this really worth it? How am I ever going to be able to pay all these loans back?"

Expenses for Physical Therapy Education

Depending on choice for attendance at private or public institutions, annual costs for all expenses during physical therapy education may vary from approximately $12,000 to $40,000. It is clear that a graduate student who pursues physical therapy education may end up paying over $100,000 following a 2- to 3-year course of study.

Table 4-1 lists some typical annual expenses for physical therapy education.

Financial Aid

Few students can afford to pay for graduate education without some form of education financing. There are several forms of financial aid that are available to graduate students in physical therapy. Please check with your local financial aid office for forms, deadlines, and specifics of the types of financial aid for which you qualify.

Loans

A loan is a form of financial aid that must be repaid with interest. Many students find that they must supplement their savings with government and private loans. Federal education loan programs offer lower interest rates and more flexible repayment plans than most consumer loans, making these loans a feasible way to finance your education (Table 4-2).[1]

Comparing different types of loans can be confusing. There are a number of options, including the rate of interest, how interest is calculated, and on what schedule interest is accrued. This can make a big difference in the bottom line (ie, the total you will have to pay back), even when borrowing the same principal. Table 4-3 lists some questions that students should be sure to ask when taking out a loan.

Manageable Debt

Educational debt to income ratio is the percentage of your monthly income that is required to pay your loan payment.[1] A ratio of 15% or less is optimal, the lower the better, because most graduates have other expenses such as a car payment or mortgage. Table 4-

Table 4-1
COST ESTIMATES FOR PHYSICAL THERAPY EDUCATION

	Public Institutions	Private Institutions
Tuition/fees	$2000 to $4000	$20,000 to $30,000
Books and supplies	$1000	$1000
Room and board	$5500	$5500
Uniforms and other fees	$100	$100
Personal, transportation, insurance	$2000	$2000
Annual costs	$10,600 to $12,600	$28,600 to $38,600
Cumulative costs (2 years)	$21,200 to $25,200	$57,2000 to $77,200
Cumulative costs (3 years)	$31,800 to $37,800	$85,800 to $115,800

Table 4-2
LOAN PROGRAMS FOR PHYSICAL THERAPY EDUCATION

Types of Loans[1]

Student Loans
Many students rely on federal government loans to finance their graduate education. These loans have low interest rates and do not require credit checks or collateral. Student loans also offer a variety of deferment options and extended repayment terms. *Stafford* loans and *Perkins* loans are two federal programs that are need-based and available for undergraduate and graduate students.

Parent Loans
The *Parent Loan for Undergraduate Students* (PLUS) program is available to assist parents in borrowing money to support the educational needs of their dependent children that go above and beyond the financial aid package offered by an educational institution. The debt is incurred by the parent, not the student, with these loans. Most graduate students are no longer claimed as dependents by their parents and therefore would need to seek their own loan package.

Private Loans
Private loans, also known as alternative loans, help to cover the difference between the actual cost of your education and the limited amount the government allows you to borrow in its programs. Private loans are offered by private lenders who provide different types of private loans, depending on the student's level of study.

Consolidation Loan
This loan allows the borrower to lump all of his or her loans into one loan for simplified payment.

Table 4-3

CONSIDERATIONS FOR LOAN COMPARISONS

Questions to Ask When Seeking a Loan

- Is there a loan forgiveness program? (Loan forgiveness programs, in which the borrower's loans are paid off in exchange for volunteer work or military service, offer an option for easy repayment.)

- What will my total debt be? What will my monthly loan payment be?

- How much can I afford to repay each month?

- Is interest *capitalized* (included in the loan balance) or *subsidized* (paid by the loan program while you are in school)? What are the additional costs if interest is capitalized?

- What are the terms of loan repayment/deferment? (This is especially important if you are completing a postgraduate internship after receiving your degree.)

- How does the total cost of one loan program compare to others?

Table 4-4

PLANNING FOR MANAGEABLE DEBT

(A profile of a graduate with a master's degree in physical therapy)

	Educational Debt-to-Income Ratio		
	15%	**20%**	**25%**
Maximum *Manageable* Monthly Loan Payment	$586	$782	$977
Maximum *Manageable* Debt Load	$48,320	$64,426	$77,132

Calculated for a projected annual starting salary of $46,900

4 may help you plan for manageable debt, given an average starting wage of a graduate physical therapist.

An easy loan calculator is available online at: http://www.finaid.com/calculators/

Loan Interest Rates

The lower the interest rate, the better. A student with $50,000 in total debt will pay *over three times more interest* if he or she is paying interest at credit card rates, which are often as high as 21% (Table 4-5).

The message is clear. If a student needs financial assistance to finance physical therapy education, there are many relatively low-cost loan programs available. The terms of repayment usually accommodate student situations and are *far* more manageable than credit that is available outside of student loan programs. Do not attempt to finance the costs of your education or your living expenses on credit cards. Borrow the money that you need.

How Long Will it Take to Recover the Costs of My Education?

Typical student loans are for a 10-year term (120 payments). Loan payments vary with interest rate and loan principal. You can check typical loan payment amounts in Table 4-5.

Table 4-5					
COMPARING LOAN PAYMENTS BY INTEREST RATES					
Loan Interest Rate	**8.25%**	**9.00%**	**8.25%**	**9.00%**	**21.00%**
Total debt (amount borrowed)	$30,000	$30,000	$50,000	$50,000	$50,000
Monthly payment	$368	$380	$613	$633	$1000
Total cost of loan (120 months)	$44,155	$45,603	$71,118	$76,005	$119,959
Total interest paid on loan	$14,155	$15,603	$21,118	$26,005	$69,959
Simple interest, 10-year repayment term.					

Is it Worth it?

Yes!

If you consider that your annual earning potential will increase by $15,000 to $20,000 with a graduate degree, you have covered this payment and gained some. After the first 10 years, you will have devoted a substantial portion of this salary differential to paying off your initial investment (your student loan). However, it starts to pay off after that. Over the subsequent 30 years after graduation, with step increases and career progression, this salary difference translates into a cumulative difference in salary of over $700,000. So, in 30 years, you will have paid off and gained more than 600% on your initial investment of $100,000 in your graduate education. Most investors would jump at the chance to have such an investment!

The earlier in your life that you incur these debts, the better. You will have more years of productive earning ahead of you (Table 4-6).

Grants and Scholarships

Graduate grants and fellowships are forms of aid that, unlike loans, do not need to be paid. There are thousands of scholarships available. Scholarships and grant programs usually target students with financial need who have specific educational objectives or special talents, are members of underrepresented groups, or who live in certain areas of the country.

A website to help with scholarship searching is available at http://www.fastweb.com/ib/finaid-21f

For example, in physical therapy, there is a scholarship for members of underrepresented groups (Table 4-7).

The Employment Outlook

Anna looked through the classified ads each Sunday for several weeks and saw the same two advertisements for physical therapists. Both offered part-time, temporary positions. She thought, "I hope there is more available than that." She wondered when would be the best time to start her job search.

Over the almost 80-year history of the profession, there has been a shortage of qualified physical therapists. In 1997, the Vector Workforce Study, commissioned by the APTA, shocked the profession with their predictions that there would soon be a surplus of physical therapists (Table 4-8).[3]

The study projected that the need for physical therapists would decrease overall by 3% between 1995 and 2005. It anticipated that the demand for physical therapists would be most affected by the growth of the population, long-term economic growth, the spread of the "California model" of managed care, and increases in the use of physical therapist assistants.

Simultaneously, educational programs in physical therapy have rapidly expanded their enrollments and new programs have opened.[4] The 1997 study projected a marked increase in the supply of physical therapists and physical therapist assistants during this time period (Table 4-9).

Despite the dire predictions, recent surveys have found that nationally only 3% of physical therapists who want to work are unable to find jobs.[5] However, many physical therapists are working in a combination of part-time employment situations rather than one full-time position. There have also been shifts from skilled nursing facility employment to other

Table 4-6

LIFETIME EARNING DIFFERENTIAL COMPARED WITH STUDENT LOAN COSTS

	0 to 10 years	10 to 20 years	20 to 30 years
Student loan costs* (annual total of payments)	$7032	0	0
Annual salary with graduate degree	$48,320	$60,000	$84,000
Annual salary without graduate degree	$30,000	$40,000	$45,000
Annual differential in salary with graduate degree	+$18,320	+$20,000	+$39,000
Salary differential less student loan payments	+$11,288	+$20,000	+$39,000
Additional lifetime earnings gained with graduate degree for each 10-year period	+$112,880	+$200,000	+$390,000

*Student loan payments were calculated for a total debt of $48,320 at 8.25% simple interest with repayment over a 10-year period.

Table 4-7

APTA MINORITY SCHOLARSHIP FUND[2]

The Minority Scholarship Fund was created in 1988 to assist minority students in completing their physical therapy education. There is currently more than $300,000 in the fund. Since 1988, $171,000 has been awarded to 76 physical therapist and physical therapist assistant students in their final year of physical therapy education. The awards are based on academic achievement, potential to make contributions to the profession of physical therapy, and contributions to minority services and communities.

Table 4-8

DIFFERENCES IN SUPPLY AND DEMAND FOR PHYSICAL THERAPISTS[3]

Year	Supply	Demand	Difference
1995	99,249	114,137	-14,888
2000	129,941	113,703	16,238
2005	159,523	108,575	50,948

Reprinted from Vector Research Inc. *Workforce Study*. Alexandria, Va: American Physical Therapy Association; 1997, with permission from the American Physical Therapy Association.

Table 4-9
DIFFERENCES IN SUPPLY AND DEMAND FOR PHYSICAL THERAPIST ASSISTANTS[3]

Year	Supply	Demand	Difference
1995	27,469	31,590	-4,121
2000	53,267	46,611	6,656
2005	79,108	53,843	25,265

Reprinted from Vector Research Inc. *Workforce Study*. Alexandria, Va: American Physical Therapy Association; 1997, with permission from the American Physical Therapy Association. Includes estimates of nonlicensed PTAs in states not requiring licensure.

practice settings. Check recent publications for salary figures and local job opportunities.

Summary

There are strong economic factors that support pursuing graduate education in physical therapy education. Federal and private loan programs that make graduate education accessible to all are available. In summary, even with a large school loan debt, graduate education is a good investment for the future.

References

1. *FinAid! The SmartStudent Guide to Financial Aid.* Available at: http://www.finaid.com/loans/. Accessed July 30, 2000.
2. APTA. *Mission Statement.* Department of Minority and International Affairs. Available at: http://www.apta.org/About/special_interests/minorityaffairs/dpt_minorityaffairs. Accessed July 31, 2000.
3. APTA. Vector Research Inc. *Workforce Study.* Available at: http://www.apta.org/Research/survey_stat/workforcestudy. Accessed July 31, 2000.
4. APTA. *Program Growth. Update on Program Growth in Physical Therapy Education.* Available at: http://www.apta.org/Education/ed_news/ed_news2. Accessed July 31, 2000.
5. APTA. *APTA Employment Survey Spring 2000 Executive Summary.* Available at: http://www.apta.org/Research/survey_stat/empsurveysp2000. Accessed July 31, 2000.

PUTTING IT INTO PRACTICE

1. Complete a budget and project how much financial assistance you will need to complete your professional education.

Expenses	Monthly	Annually	For Duration of Program
Rent			
Insurance			
Savings			
Other			
Tuition			
Books			
Food and beverages			
Household operations and maintenance			
Furnishings and equipment			
Clothing			
Personal allowance			
Transportation			
Medical care			
Recreation, entertainment			
Contributions, donations			
Credit card payments			
Total expenses			
Income			
Salary (after taxes)			
Scholarships			
Loans			
Graduate assistantship			
Total income			
Income less expenses			

2. When is the deadline for filing financial aid applications?

3. When is the next deadline for filing applications for scholarships?

4. When is the next deadline for filing applications for graduate assistantships?

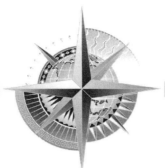

Chapter 5

A Primer on Physical Therapist Education

> It had been a busy first day of the second semester. Steve looked over the course syllabus for *Physical Therapy Interventions for the Musculoskeletal System I* and read the paragraph about the practical examination. "Students will exhibit entry-level competence in selecting, administering, and monitoring the effect of physical therapy intervention as listed below..."

Physical Therapist Education

Physical therapists promote optimal human health and function and the prevention of disability. The evolving role and changing practice environment of the physical therapist is outlined in Chapters 1, 2, and 3.

Physical therapy practice today is based on a well-developed body of scientific and clinical knowledge. Physical therapists apply knowledge from the basic, behavioral, and social sciences. Physical therapists must also demonstrate effective communication skills. Insight and sensitivity to the unique needs of diverse populations is essential to effectively maximize the client's or patient's functional potential in society.

Programs for the preparation of physical therapists must meet accreditation standards that are developed and monitored by the Commission on Accreditation in Physical Therapy Education

(CAPTE). All developing and existing programs must continuously demonstrate that they meet these standards. Physical therapist education ensures society that physical therapists have the required skills to provide high-quality health care.

Table 5-1 is a brief excerpt from the *Evaluative Criteria for Accreditation of Education Programs for the Preparation of Physical Therapists*, which outlines a few criteria for physical therapy education programs.

Let's look at the intended outcomes of physical therapy professional education.

Goals of Professional Education in Physical Therapy

Students in physical therapy professional education develop the knowledge base and skills to be capable of critical thinking, ethical practice, and provision of service to meet the changing needs of society. Students learn effective analysis and interpretation of data with which to diagnose neuromusculoskeletal movement dysfunction, make treatment-planning decisions, and predict outcomes based on sound research principles. Upon graduation, the practitioner must be prepared to assume the multidimensional roles of the master clinician, including patient care, education, consultation, and administration of physical therapy services in the broad spectrum of physical therapy practice settings and across

Table 5-1
SAMPLE ACCREDITATION STANDARD[1]

The Educational Environment
1. Professional education programs for the preparation of physical therapists must be conducted in an environment that fosters the intellectual challenge and spirit of inquiry characteristic of the community of scholars and in an environment that supports excellence in professional practice. The institutional environment must be one that ensures the opportunity for physical therapy to thrive as both an academic and professional discipline. In the optimum environment, physical therapy upholds and draws upon a tradition of scientific inquiry while contributing to the profession's body of knowledge.
2. The program faculty must demonstrate a pattern of activity that reflects a commitment to excel in meeting the expectations of the institution, the students, and the profession.
3. The academic environment must provide students with opportunities to learn from and be influenced by knowledge outside of, as well as within, physical therapy. In this environment, students become aware of multiple styles of thinking, diverse social concepts, values, and ethical behaviors that will help prepare them for identifying, redefining, and fulfilling their responsibilities to society and the profession. Of major importance is emphasis on critical thinking, ethical practice, and provision of service to meet the changing needs of society. For this environment to be realized, the missions of the institution and the education program must be compatible and mutually supportive.

Reprinted with permission from the American Physical Therapy Association.

the broad age spectrum from neonates to geriatrics.[2]

An educational program designed to allow practitioners to meet the physical therapy needs of a diverse society includes several components: physical therapists need to be open-minded, thinking individuals who are able to critically analyze ideas, understand human nature, and who have broad interests. General education helps to develop these qualities in individuals. Professional education builds on this base. The goal of professional education in physical therapy is to develop or enhance clinical competence, critical thinking, communication skills, problem-solving abilities, and the formulation of value systems consistent with the profession.

Professional education integrates physical therapy-related content with problem solving, self-awareness, and the development of professional values. There are two major components of the professional education curriculum: *clinical* and *academic* experiences. These two components are interdependent and reinforce one another. The academic setting is designed to provide the information and theory base that is integrated and expanded in the clinical setting. Clinical competence is further developed and validated in the clinical setting through a series of progressive clinical education experiences called *practicums, externships,* or *internships.* The curriculum

illustrated in Table 5-2 shows a sample of the types of courses that are included in a physical therapy professional education program.

Principles of Performance Evaluation

Physical therapy education (like all professional education programs) is focused around a set of expected outcomes or *competencies. Competency-based* education means that learning experiences and evaluation are organized around the major performance behaviors defined by specific *criteria* that must be exhibited by the students upon entry into the profession. This ensures *mastery* of the concepts, skills, and values associated with professional practice.[4,5]

This *criterion-referenced* system differs from a *norm-referenced* approach taken in many prerequisite courses in which student performance is compared to that of other students, not to a set of expected behaviors.[6,7] Most students have had the experience of being "graded on the curve." In a norm-referenced approach, student performance is measured in reference to the group average, which is based on the performance of others. This method does not assure that

Table 5-2

SAMPLE DOCTOR OF PHYSICAL THERAPY CURRICULUM

First Year—DPT1

Summer Session	Fall Semester	Spring Semester
PTS 531 (3) Gross Anatomy I	PTS 540 (3) Neuroscience I	PTS 575 (3) Clin Dec Mak I
PTS 532 (3) Gross Anatomy II	PTS 572 (4) Clin Kin & Bio	PTS 570 (3) Clin Skills
PTS 525 (2) Human Life Span	PTS 574 (3) Clin Examina	PTS 542 (3) Electrotherapy
PTS 530 (2) Foundations in PT	PTS 616 (3) Clin Research I	PTS 541 (3) Neuroscience II
	PTS 543 (1) Med-Path I	PTS 544 (1) Med-Path II

Second Year—DPT2

Summer Session	Fall (A) Semester	Spring Semester
PTS 626 (3) Ther Exer	PTS 610 (2) Clin Intern	PTS 614 (3) Neurorehab
PTS 628 (3) Musculoskel I		PTS 630 (2) Pediatrics
PTS 533 (2) Communications	Fall (B) Semester	PTS 631(2) Geriatrics
PTS 545 (1) Med-Path III	PTS 571 (3) Ther Phys	PTS 624 (3) Cardiopulmonary
	PTS 627 (3) Prosthet/Orthot	PTS 670 (2) Educ, Sup, Deleg
	PTS 546 (1) Med-Path IV	PTS 645 (2) Integument Syst
	PTS 550 (2) Pharmacology	PTS 595 (1) Elective
	PTS 606 (2) Neurolog Eval	

Third Year—DPT3

Summer Session	Fall (A) Semester	Spring (A) Semester
PTS 615 (3) Complex Patient	PTS 675 (3) Clin Dec Mak II	PTS 612 (3) Clin Internship
PTS 665 (2) Health Promotion	PTS 685 (2) Med Diag Tests	
PTS 629 (3) Spine	PTS 671 (2) Complement Ther	Spring (B) Semester
PTS 618 (3) Hlth Care Admin	PTS 617 (3) Clin Res Project	PTS 613 (3) Clin Internship
PTS 595 (1) Elective	PTS 595 (1) Elective	
	Fall (B) Semester	
	PTS 611 (2) Clin Internship	

students meet specific standards of performance, because the group average could be quite low.

Professional education uses a strict standard of performance. Society must have the assurance that health care providers will function at a high standard of care. It *would not be acceptable* for a student to receive a passing grade without mastery of the material. If that were the case, a patient's or client's well-being could be in jeopardy. In the physical therapy profession, as in all health professions, all students must demonstrate mastery and meet a predefined level of competency to pass courses and receive credit for clinical education experiences.

A student in a physical therapy program experiences many forms of performance evaluation, including exams and quizzes, practical or laboratory examinations, papers, projects, journals, and clinical evaluations. Evaluations may be used as a teaching tool (*formative evaluation*) and/or as a certification tool (*summative evaluation*).[8]

For example, in a clinical education experience, *formative evaluation* may occur during daily conferences with a clinical instructor. *Summative evaluation* occurs when evaluative comments are recorded on a final evaluation form, and student performance is graded based on accomplishment of specific *performance indicators* at that point.

Preparing for Mastery

Key elements for mastery of professional content include:

Clinical skills: Students must demonstrate competence in clinical performance skills. For example, a student must be able to safely and effectively guard a patient during an assisted transfer from a wheelchair to a bed.

Integration: This is the student's ability to access interrelated chunks of information. Students should be able to integrate content across the professional curriculum. For example, anatomical principles must be applied in clinical courses, and cardiac precautions must be integrated in the intervention of a patient with an orthopedic disorder.

Critical thinking: Problem-solving should focus on identifying problems, generating potential solutions by applying knowledge and appropriate scientific concepts, and then choosing appropriate solutions based on expected outcomes. Students should be able to incorporate scientific literature and other forms of evidence in this process. For example, a patient's poor response to a physical therapy intervention might indicate an underlying pathology that was not initially known. To make this decision, the student must understand what was expected and then generate a list of possible causes of this less than optimal response.

Metacognitive or self-regulatory skills: Students must be able to monitor their own understanding, develop strategies to address clinical problems, evaluate the relevance of accessible knowledge, and validate their decisions using sound arguments and rationale. For example, a student must recognize and appropriately respond to a request of an employer that violates ethical guidelines or legal regulations for the practice of physical therapy.

Faculty Roles and Responsibilities

Leticia sat in the orientation session and listened while the faculty members introduced themselves to the new class. She heard so many interesting things and hoped that she would one day be a faculty member herself.

There are many faculty members involved in providing physical therapy education. In addition to classroom, laboratory, and clinical instruction and student advising, faculty are often engaged in a number of research, scholarly, and service responsibilities that go far beyond their instructional responsibilities. Many academic core faculty members also stay involved in clinical practice.

The faculty in a physical therapy education program establish acceptable levels of performance within the scope of practice as defined by the profession. They facilitate student achievement of predetermined outcomes and evaluate student performance, providing feedback to the students regarding their performance.

The definitions in Table 5-3 may be helpful in identifying faculty roles and responsibilities.

Student Responsibilities

Students in a professional education program have the responsibility for their own learning. This requires that students make choices and accept the consequences of those choices. Students must solicit, provide feedback, and participate in the learning experiences that are offered. They must be self-directed and seek help when needed. They must communicate clearly, with respect for themselves and others. There are many similar behaviors that are highly valued in physical therapy students.[10,11] Table 5-4 lists qualities of successful physical therapy students.

Graduate Education

Sam read over the examination and could not find an answer that he agreed with in several questions. He went to the front of the room and had a lengthy discussion with the professor, who told him to choose "the best answer." Although the answer was marked wrong, Sam followed up during faculty office hours and eventually received credit because he was able to show references that supported his choice.

One of the greatest challenges for graduate students is to move from the comfort of the "known" and "correct answers" to a place much more consistent with reality. The illusion created by years of undergraduate coursework leaves students with the impression that knowledge is stable, unrefuted, and certain. In actuality, very little is certain, absolute fact.

This phenomenon alone shakes many student's

Table 5-3
PHYSICAL THERAPY FACULTY ROLES[1]

Program Director or Administrator: A full-time program administrator is a physical therapy educator who spends a significant part of his or her professional time devoted to enhancing the quality of the developing physical therapy education program. This individual plans and implements the academic and clinical education components of the program; demonstrates an understanding of the curriculum; and provides timely communication with the institution, profession, and other communities.

Academic Coordinator of Clinical Education or Director of Clinical Education (ACCE/DCE). The ACCE/DCE holds a faculty (academic or clinical) appointment and has the primary responsibilities to plan, coordinate, facilitate, administer, and monitor activities on behalf of the academic program and in coordination with academic and clinical faculty.

Core Faculty: Those individuals appointed to and employed primarily in the program, including the program administrator and those who report to the program administrator. Members of the core faculty typically have full-time appointments, although some part-time faculty members may be included among the core faculty. The core faculty includes physical therapists and may include others with expertise to meet specific curricular needs. The core faculty has the qualifications and experience necessary to achieve the goals of the program through educational administration, curriculum development, instructional design and delivery, and evaluation of outcomes. The core faculty is generally the group with the responsibility and authority related to the curriculum. The core faculty may hold tenured, tenure track, or nontenure track positions.

Adjunct Faculty: Individuals who have classroom and/or laboratory teaching responsibilities in the program and are not employed by the institution, though they may receive honoraria or other forms of compensation. The adjunct faculty may or may not be "appointed" to the faculty. The adjunct faculty may include, but are not limited to, guest lecturers, "contract" faculty, instructors of course modules, tutors, etc.

Clinical Education Faculty: Individuals engaged in providing the clinical education components of the program, generally referred to as either Center Coordinators of Clinical Education (CCCEs) or Clinical Instructors (CIs). While these individuals are not usually employed by the educational institution, they do agree to certain standards of behavior through contractual arrangements for their services.

Supporting Faculty: Individuals with faculty appointments in other units within the institution who teach courses that are part of the professional program (eg, faculty from a biology department who teach physiology or faculty from a school of medicine who teach pathology).

Reprinted with permission from the American Physical Therapy Association.

beliefs in the educational process. Professional education requires students to critically analyze and integrate a new and complex body of knowledge and to monitor their progress while doing so. So much about the professional education experience is overwhelming and out of the student's control.

Most students find the volume of work overwhelming, time and financial resources inadequate, and may question, "Why have I chosen to do this?" The ambiguity and demands in professional education create a dynamic that interferes with student progress and creates frustration and dissatisfaction. You may be saying, "So that's why I feel this way!"

Graduate school faculty may inadvertently add to this problem by asking students for their opinions and requiring that student judgments be sound and supported by evidence that may be scarce. Faculty who facilitate student growth often find themselves in the position of "not giving the answers," but instead pushing students to be accountable for their

Table 5-4

QUALITIES OF SUCCESSFUL PHYSICAL THERAPY STUDENTS

- Professional competence
- Critical thinking
- Self-direction
- Self-evaluation
- Self-reliance
- Sensitivity
- Clear communication
- Respect for self and others
- Lifelong learning
- Self-confidence
- Creativity
- Responsibility
- Accountability
- Caring
- Curiosity

choices, to find their own answers, and to create new ways of thinking about old problems. Again, this can be frustrating for students who are more accustomed to faculty members who assume roles of authority and pass on their truths to students who are only too happy to write them down.

Table 5-5 is the contribution of a graduate student in an entry-level physical therapist education program experiencing such conflicts. She wrote these words to try to confront many of the beliefs that were interfering with her participation in the professional education program. Her words have helped many students to examine their beliefs and experiences.[12]

Graduate Students as Workers

Students sometimes assume roles in an educational program as well. The following opportunities may be available in physical therapy educational programs.

Graduate Assistants/Teaching Assistants

These are graduate students, usually at an advanced stage in their education, who work closely with faculty to assist in providing instruction, laboratory experiences, helping with course administra-

tion, and assisting students with mastery of course content. Graduate assistants are usually paid by the university and must work a prescribed number of hours per week. Teaching assistants may have student contact, most often in discussion sessions or laboratory experiences.

Research Assistants

Research assistants are often hired by individual faculty to assist with ongoing research. Tasks might involve library research, data collection, data entry, or assisting with data analysis and presentation.

More on Graduate Education

Philosophy of Graduate Education

Some of the key differences between undergraduate and graduate education are listed. Take a look at the guidelines in Table 5-6, which further indicate student responsibilities.

Student Responsibility, Self-Direction

Graduate students are expected to be self-directed and take responsibility for their actions. The students are responsible for informing faculty members when and if they will not be in class. The student is responsible for making any special arrangements for missed classes, exams, or late papers.

Table 5-5

THOUGHTS ON STUDENT TOLERANCE OF AMBIGUITY, A LEARNING EXPERIENCE[12]

Graduate education represents a gateway transition from general, rudimentary knowledge and skills into more specialized, advanced training along a chosen career path. As with any progressive process, the essence of graduate education is developmental change, like learning to walk; and, as in learning to walk, zealous as it may be, there is risk, frustration, and uncertainty.

Uncertainty of meaning, significance, or attitude that may result in intellectual or emotional tension between two or more logically incompatible points of view is called ambiguity, from the French, "ambigere," to wander about, waiver, or dispute. It is mystery arising from a vague knowledge or understanding that has multiple interpretations.

Ambiguity often involves doubt, confusion, inconsistency, unpredictability, as well as change. The challenge of ambiguity in graduate education is reflected in the many choices, conflicting opinions, double entendres, unstable definitions, understatements, oversights, and general absences of clarity that confront students daily. The goal is growth and insight; the hazard is feeling confused, overwhelmed, and out of control.

Tolerance of ambiguity implies coping with choice and uncertainty. It employs strategies that help maintain psycho-emotional equilibrium and includes cognitive techniques that bring thinking and action in line with reality, counteracting irrational beliefs and assumptions that may have no basis in truth.

Why tolerate ambiguity? Why put up with the confusion and tension of multiple conflicting interpretations rather than demand to know what the heck is going on, and why, and how to deal with it? Sometimes it's reasonable not to passively accept sloppy communication or double meanings, but by considering a broader, perhaps more rational view of what it's all about, the student begins to accept (if not comprehend) not only undefined external events, perplexing people, and unfamiliar pressures, but inner personal truths and strengths as well as hurts, fears, and hang-ups triggered by stress and change.

"Real-world" integration of self and others involves letting go of ultimate control.

Ambiguity negates control; there is no direct control possible in an ambiguous situation. Expectations become irrelevant. New, more sophisticated ways of thinking must replace dualistic—right vs. wrong—thought. Anxiety about uncertainty is unproductive, stressful, and symptomatic of grappling for control.

Tolerating ambiguity, on the other hand, facilitates learning, adapting, seeing both sides, getting along, and getting the job done. It is integral to stress management, to becoming a professional, and to the process of graduate education itself.

Many irrational beliefs may occur to you as a student. Beware: habitual patterns of thinking often conflict with a world view conducive to change and to adaptation to graduate education.

Autonomy and Choice

Graduate students are expected to make choices, and identify and follow their interests. The student is expected to work with autonomy and independence, asking for feedback and help as needed.

Responsibility for Self in All Situations with Colleagues, Patients, and Families

In addition to being a responsible student, the student in physical therapist education is likely to also be responsible for the well-being of others during clinical learning experiences or research. It is critical that students practice in compliance with all laws, regulations, and ethical guidelines, understanding that their actions reflect not only themselves but also the academic program, the clinical institution, and the profession of physical therapy.

Relationships with Academic and Clinical Faculty

Both academic and clinical faculty play a key role in student development. Get to know the faculty. Establish good working relationships with both academic and clinical faculty members. Seek their guidance and assistance as needed.

Table 5-6
EXPECTATIONS OF GRADUATE STUDENTS[13]

1. Come to class: You cannot learn physical therapy from a book. This is a hands-on profession. Classes require your participation. Your ultimate obligation to your patients requires that you learn as much as you can.

2. Dress appropriately: Professional attire is required when involved with patients, clinical sites, and/or guest speakers. Your self-presentation is critical to your reception by patients, faculty, and colleagues.

3. Prepare for and participate in class: Read the assigned material. Your instructors will assume that you have completed the material and may not cover it in class. Remember that your questions help your classmates as much as they do you, but also remember that you need to direct questions toward areas of confusion rather than a general lack of knowledge.

4. Keep up: Budget your time for studying so that you do not fall behind. Prioritize and stay aware of multiple commitments. Organize your class and assignment schedule on a calendar you carry with you.

5. Be active: Participate in meetings, special events, committees. Be willing to volunteer and work with members of the department on special projects, work-study opportunities, etc.

6. Give feedback: Give your opinions, compliments, and criticisms in a responsible way. You may make individual appointments with faculty to make your views known.

7. Communicate: Leave phone messages with faculty if you will miss class. If you are having personal or family difficulties, communicate this before it causes you to miss class or assignments. Also develop good communication with classmates, friends, and family.

8. Be prompt: Arrive at class, meetings, clinical sites on time. This is not only common courtesy, but also a benefit to you and your patients.

9. Stay healthy and take care of yourself: Watch diet, sleep, exercise. Practice stress management techniques. Identify and use your support system.

10. Be courteous: Even under times of stress, try to be courteous.

11. Be responsible for yourself: You are an adult and expected to manage your own life. Handle your problems in a responsible manner.

Recognize that faculty roles in professional education make it inadvisable to have social relationships with students. This is especially important in clinical education, in which you may be working closely with a clinical instructor for 40 to 50 hours per week. Table 5-7 addresses some typical questions that students have in establishing good working relationships with faculty.

Computer Competence

Graduate students are expected to be computer literate and have the latest software applications to ensure compatibility with colleagues. The resources of the Internet, government agencies, medical data bases, and even your university library are available without leaving home. An increasing number of assignments and educational experiences are available "online." Check with your institution regarding their recommendations for computer specifications. Use electronic communications and make sure that your skills are up-to-date.

Information Competence

What used to be "going to the library" has become a navigational task by computer. Knowing where to look and how to search are critical skills that will determine your success in research to a large extent. Critically analyzing sources is a further concern. See Chapter 17 on Information Competence.

Grades

Graduate education requires that students maintain a grade point average (GPA) of 3.0 or better. For many students accustomed to being at the top of the class in undergraduate courses, graduate education often involves the added stress of being in classes

Table 5-7

INTERACTION WITH FACULTY IN PHYSICAL THERAPIST EDUCATION[13]

1. Address academic faculty using "Professor" or "Doctor" as his or her title unless invited to use a first name. Ask how a faculty member would like to be addressed.

2. Schedule appointments with both academic and clinical faculty. Leave voice or e-mail messages and give faculty an opportunity to call you back. Don't expect immediate attention at times that are convenient for you to drop in. Observe academic faculty office hours and realize that you may also have access to faculty by appointment at other times.

3. Both academic and clinical faculty members are busy people with multiple responsibilities. Give the faculty member the opportunity to hear your concern, interest, or problem with the time and attention that it deserves. Don't put off talking about a problem; small concerns often mushroom and escalate in a short period of time.

4. Communicate directly with faculty, not through another faculty member, staff member, or student. Faculty members may not get the message. They also may not disclose key information to other students or faculty out of respect for your privacy and confidentiality.

with an entire class of students who have been at the top of the class. Although competition is discouraged in most graduate programs, sometimes old habits are hard to break. Although students must maintain the minimum GPA, many students put additional pressure on themselves to "be the best." This causes extra stress. Student effort is better directed in supporting and receiving support from colleagues in study groups and communication with professors.

Clinical Education

Clinical education is a critical component of physical therapist education. Most educational programs include 18 to 24 weeks of clinical education experience during the educational process. These experiences are courses in the physical therapy curriculum for which students enroll, pay tuition, and receive academic credit. The trend is toward even longer postgraduate internships. Clinical faculty members provide direct supervision of students during clinical education experiences. Clinical faculty are usually employees of the facilities to which the students are assigned. The academic institution makes the clinical assignment of students to learning experiences, provides the administration of the clinical education course, and assigns the final grade. It is a joint responsibility of clinical and academic faculty to ensure that clinical learning experiences are high quality and effective learning experiences for the student.

The Academic Coordinator of Clinical Education (ACCE) is the person on the academic faculty who arranges clinical education assignments. There are many factors that enter into the assignment of students to clinical learning experiences, including availability during a given time period, type of facility, past experience of the student, interests of the student, level of the student, and geographical location. In most cases, students have input into the choice, but few students get their first choice in all cases. Students should check with the ACCE regarding policies and procedures for selecting and assigning clinical education sites.

In general, students cannot arrange their own clinical learning experiences. There are many considerations in selecting a clinical learning site. Clinical facilities are evaluated by a number of criteria before becoming involved in the clinical training of student physical therapists. Academic institutions contract with the clinical institution or organization to provide clinical training of student physical therapists. These are legal agreements that cover issues such as liability and malpractice, in addition to outlining the responsibilities of the academic institution, the student, and the clinical facility before, during, and after the clinical learning experience. Months of paperwork and negotiations often go into establishing an agreement between an academic institution and a clinical learning facility.

Clinical performance is measured by a specific instrument. Many programs for physical therapist education are using the Clinical Performance Instrument (CPI). The CPI defines 24 key behaviors, such as "Demonstrates professional behavior during interaction with others," and then gives sample behaviors that illustrate the key behavior. Each educational program establishes the level of performance required on clinical performance during each clinical learning experience. Clinical experiences are often graded on a credit/no credit basis. See Chapter 7 for more information on clinical performance evaluation.

Culminating Experience/Comprehensive Examinations

Graduate education requires a way to measure that you have comprehensive mastery of the material presented during your educational experience. Every program has either a comprehensive written or oral examination, a public presentation, or other means of demonstrating your mastery of the content of your graduate school education. Check with your program for specific requirements.

Summary

Graduate education presents many challenges that differ from the educational experience of most undergraduate programs. Physical therapist professional education requires demonstration of mastery of content and demonstration of acceptable clinical performance. Every program has slightly different requirements; acquaint yourself with the specifics of your program.

References

1. APTA. *Evaluative Criteria for Accreditation of Education Programs for the Preparation of Physical Therapists.* Available at: http://www.apta.org/Education/accreditation/evaluativecriteria_pt. Accessed June 22, 2000.

2. California State University, Fresno. *Department of Physical Therapy, 2000-2001 General Catalog.* Available at: http://wwwcatalog.admin.csufresno.edu/current/physther.html. Accessed July 31, 2000.

3. University of Miami. *DPT Curriculum* webpage. Available at http://www.miami.edu/physical-therapy/courses.htm; Accessed January 5, 2001.

4. Davis CM, Anderson MJ, Jagger D. Competency: the what, why, and how of it. *Phys Ther.* 1979;59(9):1088-94.

5. May BJ. Competency based education: general concepts. *J Allied Health.* 1979;8(3):166-71.

6. May BJ. Competency based evaluation of student performance. *J Allied Health.* 1978;7(3):232-7.

7. May BJ. Evaluation in a competency-based educational system. *Phys Ther.* 1977;57(1):28-33.

8. Bloom BS, Hastings ST, Madeus AF. *Handbook of Formative and Summative Evaluation of Student Learning.* New York, NY: McGraw-Hill Inc; 1971.

9. APTA. *Model Position Description for the Academic Coordinator/Director of Clinical Education.* Available at: http://www.apta.org/Education/clinical_edu/model_position. Accessed June 22, 2000.

10. Hayes KW, Huber G, Rogers J, Sanders B. Behaviors that cause clinical instructors to question the clinical competence of physical therapist students. *Phys Ther.* 1999;79:653-671.

11. May WW, Morgan BJ, Lemke JC, et al. Model for ability-based assessment in physical therapy education. *Journal of Physical Therapy Education.* 1995;9(1):3-6.

12. Buettell C. *Thoughts on Student Tolerance of Ambiguity, A Learning Experience.* Unpublished manuscript. California State University, Fresno; 1997.

13. Curtis KA. *Responsibilities of Graduate Students.* California State University Fresno, Department of Physical Therapy, Course Syllabus, PH TH 120: Professional Orientation; 1996.

PUTTING IT INTO PRACTICE

1. What is the name and title of the program director or administrator of your professional education program?

2. What is (are) the name(s) and title(s) of the academic coordinator(s) of clinical education in your professional education program?

3. What comprehensive examinations are required in your professional education program to demonstrate your mastery of your graduate work? At what point in your course of study will you complete these requirements?

4. How many weeks of clinical education are included *during* your professional education program? During which quarters or semesters?

5. How many weeks of clinical education are required *after graduating from* your professional education program? What are the approximate dates of this experience?

6. What are the minimal performance standards you must meet to successfully complete your professional education program?

7. Outline the names and course numbers of the courses you will take each semester in your professional program, starting with the current semester.

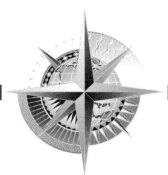

Chapter 6

Professional Behavior

Professional Conduct

> Julie waited in the second row for the anatomy professor to enter the room. The professor started the lecture by handing out a paper outlining rules of professional conduct for the anatomy lab. She wondered about the people who had now become "cadavers" and what they wanted for their bodies. She knew that she could learn so much from their generosity.

What is professional conduct? Perhaps one of the first places that physical therapy students are exposed to a code of professional conduct is in the anatomy laboratory when they begin to work with human cadavers. Both legal and ethical issues govern the handling of human anatomical materials. Consider the guidelines in Table 6-1, excerpted from an anatomy syllabus. These guidelines provide clear expectations of student conduct in relation to conduct in and around the anatomy laboratory.

Professional behavior includes such attributes as dependability, professional presentation, initiative, empathy, cooperation, organization, clinical reasoning, participation in supervision, and verbal and written communication. Review these definitions in Table 6-2.

A core of knowledge and skills is required for success in the physical therapy profession. These *generic abilities* include attributes, characteristics, and behaviors that may not be explicitly taught in the professional education curriculum.[3] These abilities are defined in Table 6-3.

Codes of Student Behavior

Acceptable behavior is defined for students in similar ways by many professions and disciplines. Academic institutions publish student codes of conduct. The underlying principles are usually similar (Table 6-4).

Students who join professional associations may also be bound by the codes of conduct of the professional organization. The American Physical Therapy Association defines guidelines for professional conduct of its members by the *Code of Ethics* and *Guide for Professional Conduct* in Appendix B. The student code of conduct in Table 6-5 refers to and includes the *Code of Ethics* and *Guide for Professional Conduct*.

Professional Appearance

You have only a few seconds to make a first impression. The way that you appear may determine whether patients and clients trust you, feel that they will be safe with you, disclose confidential information, or even consent to receiving services. Even though it seems unfair, it even influences whether

Table 6-1

SAMPLE GUIDELINES FOR PROFESSIONAL CONDUCT

Students will be expected to adhere to the following rules while in the laboratory:

1. Any student not wearing a laboratory coat or jacket will not be allowed to remain in the dissecting room.

2. Students registered for the course and authorized persons are the only people allowed in the dissecting room. Relatives, spouses, and friends are absolutely not allowed access to the dissecting room.

3. The dissecting room will be open during the scheduled laboratory periods and at various other times to be arranged. Other times may be arranged upon the approval of the instructors.

4. There is to be no smoking or eating in the laboratory at any time. No food or drinks are allowed in the gross anatomy laboratory or in the adjacent hallway. No smoking is permitted in these areas. Do not store food in the lockers in the lab.

5. Any tissue removed from the cadavers (eg, skin, fat) must be placed in the appropriate container (designated "Human Tissue Only"), which is separate from the refuse (eg, paper, gloves) container. Used scalpel blades are to be placed in special containers for that purpose.

6. Parts of cadavers are never to be removed from the laboratory. Major parts, organs, and limbs are to be kept as a unit with the remains of the cadaver.

7. Disarticulated bones are available for study in the computer lab. Keep them as free of grease as possible. Bones are fragile. Do not handle carelessly or drop them. When handling skulls, be extremely careful not to drop them. Handle the articulated skeletons with care. They, too, are fragile and though they move freely, they should not be forced.

8. While dissecting, be careful not to drop fragments or grease on the floor area around your table. Clean up any spills thoroughly and promptly before they get tracked around or someone slips and falls.

9. Keep the top of the dissecting table around the cadaver clear of debris. Wipe it clean at the end of the dissection period.

10. Models, specimens, etc. are not to be removed from the laboratory without the permission of the instructors.

11. Some materials may be checked out overnight by groups of students with permission of the instructors.

Professional conduct is mandatory! Destruction of laboratory materials, tampering with other peoples' work, or other inappropriate behavior will result in dismissal from the course and may result in other penalties imposed by the Director of Physical Therapy. Cadavers must be treated with respect and professionalism at all times! No anatomical specimens may be removed from the laboratory! To do so is illegal and unprofessional. Failure to abide by these rules will result in dismissal from the course and may result in other penalties imposed by the Director of Physical Therapy Program.

1. No photographs are to be taken in the gross anatomy laboratory.

2. Cadavers should be covered on the dissection tables with the lids closed when not being studied.

3. Be sure to hook (lock) the lift apparatus on the dissection table securely when you raise your cadaver to study it.

continued

Table 6-1, continued

4. Rubber gloves should be worn during dissection; however, lab coats and gloves should not be worn outside the gross anatomy laboratory.

5. Students who do not wear eyeglasses may want to consider buying inexpensive safety glasses to protect against splashes.

6. The outside doors to the laboratory must remain closed at all times.

7. Handle scalpels and other sharp instruments with care! Do not use them to point and put them down when you are not actually dissecting with them.

Reprinted from Jamali M. Course syllabus. *PT 3514 Laboratory for Gross Anatomy.* Arkansas State University, College of Nursing & Health Professions. Available at: http://www.clt.astate.edu/mjamali/pt3514.htm. Accessed June 25, 2000.

Table 6-2

PROFESSIONAL BEHAVIORS

Professional Behavior	Examples
Dependability	Completing tasks on schedule, being reliable, and following through with commitments and responsibilities.
Professional presentation	Appropriate dress, body posture, and affect; positive attitude.
Initiative	Self-starting projects and tasks, including own learning; functions as a change agent.
Empathy	Sensitivity to feelings, ideas, and opinions of others.
Cooperation	Working effectively with others; group cohesiveness, actively participating in region, state, and/or national groups.
Organization	Prioritizing self and tasks, managing time to meet commitments.
Clinical reasoning	Analyzing, interpreting information and research; demonstrating ethical decision-making skills.
Supervisory process	Receives and gives meaningful feedback; operates within the scope of one's own skills; demonstrates clinical and professional leadership.
Verbal and written communication	Clear, concise communication of ideas and opinions; teaching skills; writing reports for research and publication.

Reprinted with permission from Kasar J, Clark EN. *Developing Professional Behaviors.* Thorofare, NJ: SLACK Incorporated; 2000:20.

Table 6-3
GENERIC ABILITIES IMPORTANT TO PHYSICAL THERAPY

Generic Ability	Definition
Commitment to learning	The ability to self-assess, self-correct, and self-direct; to identify needs and sources of learning; and to continually seek out new knowledge and understanding.
Interpersonal skills	The ability to interact effectively with patients, families, colleagues, other health care professionals, and the community, and to deal effectively with cultural and ethnic diversity issues.
Communication skills	The ability to communicate effectively (ie, speaking, body language, reading, writing, listening) for varied audiences and purposes.
Effective use of time and resources	The ability to obtain the maximum benefit from a minimum investment of time and resources.
Use of constructive feedback	The ability to identify sources of and seek out feedback and to effectively use and provide feedback for improving personal interaction.
Problem solving	The ability to recognize and define problems, analyze data, develop and implement solutions, and evaluate outcomes.
Professionalism	The ability to exhibit appropriate professional conduct and to represent the profession effectively.
Responsibility	The ability to fulfill commitments and to be accountable for actions and outcomes.
Critical thinking	The ability to question logically; to identify, generate, and evaluate elements of logical argument; to recognize and differentiate facts, illusions, assumptions, and hidden assumptions; and to distinguish the relevant from the irrelevant.
Stress management	The ability to identify sources of stress and to develop effective coping behaviors.

Reprinted with permission from May WW, Morgan BJ, Lemke JC, et al. Model for ability-based assessment in physical therapy education. *Journal of Physical Therapy Education.* 1995;9(1):3-6.

It had been a rough morning. Janet forgot that today was dress code day—a guest speaker was coming to her Orthopedics class. She was the only student in class in cut-off jeans and sandals. Should she stay for the lecture or go home and change? She felt embarrassed as she tried to hide in the far corner of the classroom.

other professionals will respect your opinion. It may influence whether you land a job or get a raise.

Although the standard "university uniform" may be jeans with an old T-shirt or sweatshirt, professional dress requires attention to not only what you wear, but personal hygiene, hair, nails, and identification. Take a look at the sample dress code in Table 6-6.

Table 6-4

SAMPLE ELEMENTS OF PROFESSIONAL BEHAVIOR GUIDELINES

1. Respect for the rights of all individuals without regard to position, race, age, gender, handicap, national origin, religion, or sexual orientation, including compliance with laws prohibiting activities such as sexual harassment, Title IV of the Civil Rights Act of 1964, and Title IX of the Education Amendments of 1972.

2. Appropriate handling of information, records, or examination materials.

3. Respect for patients' confidentiality, privacy, modesty, and safety.

4. Proper appearance and conduct (professional appearance, speech, and behavior, including wearing identification badges, appropriate dress for professional activities, and exemplary personal hygiene).

5. Compliance with all existing laws, policies, and regulations.

6. Respect for property and instructional material.

Language and Conversations

> *The student physical therapist listserv had been up and running for a few months. Mark posted an ethnic joke poking fun at a common accent. May (a fellow student) was irate. She wrote on the listserv, "I don't think that joke is funny, nor do I think it belongs on a listserv that represents our university or our future profession." What do you think? Is May overreacting?*

Although Mark's intention was not to offend May or behave in an irresponsible way, his communication does not show sensitivity to others. The ensuing discussion after this event certainly created ample opportunity to explore cultural biases and establish proper conduct for Internet use.

The language we use is another example of professional behavior. Whether speaking or writing, make an effort to use professional language and use judgment as to whether a topic of conversation, joke, or random thought that flies by is appropriate for the context.

Also, be careful of what you write. A patient's medical record is a legal document. Your documentation must be clear and reflect the physical therapy care provided.

Confidentiality

> *The instructor for the Physical Therapy Administration class gave an example of a problem employee without using the employee's name or making any reference to a facility or point in time. Martha thought the situation sounded vaguely familiar and she knew that the instructor was a district supervisor of the same company for which she worked. She went to work the next afternoon and asked her fellow employees at the clinic about the case the instructor used. They gossiped about the details of why a former colleague was fired. Who has breached confidentiality here?*

Student physical therapists frequently have access to confidential information about clients and patients. They may also have access to confidential information about colleagues, supervisees, students, and faculty. Using good judgment requires thinking about the reasons why someone would need to know information.

In Martha's situation, even if she could identify the employee and situation with certainty, it serves no legitimate purpose for her to discuss the case with her colleagues. Avoid discussions of a colleague's situation or a patient's diagnosis, personal life, or other details even in private, unless it relates to caregiving and only with persons involved in the patient's care. Avoid patient-related communication in public places. The person next to you on the elevator may be the patient's family member or attorney.

Table 6-5

SAMPLE PHYSICAL THERAPY STUDENT CODE OF CONDUCT INCORPORATING APTA CODE OF ETHICS[4]

The Physical Therapy Department expects that students enrolled in the Master of Physical Therapy program will conduct themselves in a manner that is consistent with their future professional aspirations in the physical therapy field. To that end, the following expectations reflect qualities such as professional presentation, collegial respect, and accountability to California State University codes of student conduct as well as published professional (physical therapy) legal and ethical codes in all interactions with academic and clinical faculty, academic or clinical staff, colleagues, patients, family, and research subjects.

1. Students will observe published codes of dress and appearance as requested by academic or clinical faculty and staff, including proper clothing to permit practice of evaluation and treatment techniques in laboratory sessions. Students should assume professional dress requirements for any engagement, laboratory, or clinical experience off campus, and for any class which involves patients or outside speakers.

2. Students will arrive on time or early to scheduled classes, laboratories, or clinical assignments and will not interrupt classes or treatments in session. It is the student's responsibility to make up for material missed due to absence and to notify academic and/or clinical faculty members regardless of the reason for the absence.

3. Students will notify the designated academic or clinical faculty or staff member regarding their anticipated late arrival or absence prior to the scheduled session.

4. Students will not bring guests into the university or clinical setting unless previously cleared with the designated faculty member.

5. Students will not bring children or pets into a university classroom or clinical setting.

6. Students will use appropriate, courteous, and respectful communication whether by electronic mail (individually and on department-sponsored listservs), by letter, voicemail, telephone, or in face-to-face communication with academic and clinical faculty, academic or clinical staff, colleagues, patients, family, and research subjects.

7. Students will observe appropriate codes of conduct per the APTA Guide to Professional Conduct and Physical Therapy Practice Act (California Business and Professions Code, Chapter 5.7 Physical Therapy), and Regulations of the Physical Therapy Examining Committee (California Code of Regulations, Title 16, Division 13.2. Physical Therapy Examining Committee of the Board of Medical Quality Assurance) in all interactions with academic and clinical faculty, staff, students, employers, patients, families, and research subjects. This expectation will also include conduct in off-campus personal or employment situations in which the student may potentially be in violation of these codes of conduct.

8. Students will observe the Codes Governing Student Conduct of California State University (Sections 41301 to 41303, inclusive in Article 1, Subchapter 3, Chapter 5, Title 5, California Administrative Code; Education Code Sections 66017, 69810 through 69813 inclusive; and Penal Code Sections 626 through 626.4 inclusive), which establish grounds for expulsion, suspension, and probation of students.

Reprinted with permission from California State University, Fresno, Department of Physical Therapy.

Table 6-6
SAMPLE DRESS CODE[5]

Purpose

To provide guidelines for proper attire, while placing responsibility on the student to maintain professionalism at all times.

General Appearance

Clothing

- Dress should be neat, clean, practical, safe, avoiding extremes of fashion, and appropriate to staff duties and work area.
- No blue jeans, faded denim of any color, or sweat pants.
- Shirts should have appropriate neckline (ie, not too low), be plain or simple, and conservative colors.
- Shorts, if worn, should be no shorter than 4 inches above the knee.

Footwear

- Socks (or pantyhose) should be worn with shoes.
- Shoes to be well maintained and closed toe; casual shoes may be worn.
- Sneakers if in good condition.
- No sandals or clogs.

Accessories

- Jewelry should be minimal, smooth surface rings, watches, and small earrings.
- Conservative make-up.

Miscellaneous

- Hair—clean; long hair appropriately tied back.
- Nails—clipped and cleaned; brightly colored nail polish not recommended.
- Hygiene—all students should be clean with no discernable body odor. The use of fragrances and colognes is prohibited.
- Name tags to be worn at all times.

Students will be expected to adhere to the dress code policy of the facility/agency to which they are assigned for placement if it is different from the school's student dress code policy.

Approved by the Clinical Education Committee—Division of Physical Therapy, September 1998

Reprinted with permission from http://www.umanitoba.ca/faculties/medicine/units/medrehab/pt

---

Keep in mind that students may have access to privileged information because of their student physical therapist status. Respect that privilege and do not abuse it.

Personal Space, Privacy, and Modesty

With Other Students

Be aware that our concept of personal space is *cul-ture-specific*. We feel uncomfortable being touched on certain body parts or having people stand too close. Those limits may vary widely among your classmates.

There are many situations in professional education where you will be working within the personal space of another student. Show sensitivity to issues of privacy and modesty. Your colleagues permit you to touch them. It is not your right. Be sure that you ask your colleague first and inform him or her, just as you would a client or patient.

Allow instructors, students, and colleagues an opportunity to assist you in performing laboratory exercises that make you feel uncomfortable. If you

> *The cardiopulmonary lab assistant finished her demon-stration of breath sounds assessment. Students put their stethoscopes to their ears and began listening to each other's chests. Susie instructed Bob to breathe deeply as she placed her stethoscope first on his bronchi and then his lower airways. When she was done they traded places. Bob listened at her trachea and then excused himself to get a drink of water. He returned with Sandra, one of the older students. "Uh, Susie," he explained, "I thought I'd have Sandra show me how to do this. I'm a little uncomfortable with the, uh, area we're covering today." Sandra suggested Bob ask Susie to pull her sports bra to the side slightly so he could listen to her lungs. The rest went smoothly.*

have objections to others touching or practicing on you, inform the instructor or laboratory assistant. There are solutions that will meet everyone's needs.

With Patients and Clients

Physical therapy evaluation and treatment procedures often involve examining and treating body parts that go beyond normal social boundaries. Be clear that you are in a professional role as a physical therapist, and in that role you are accorded certain privileges. You also have professional responsibilities to preserve patient dignity and privacy.

Also be clear that your role is not possible unless you perform a detailed and thorough assessment that involves inspection, palpation, auscultation, and movement.

Be sure to observe draping guidelines and expose only those areas necessary for treatment. Be sure to inform patients and clients as to what you intend to do and the purpose of the procedure. Obtain consent before beginning. If you feel uncomfortable, ask another staff member to stay in the treatment area with you.

Sexual Harassment

> *Johanna finished the ultrasound treatment to the patient's upper thigh area. As she turned to put away the machine, the patient grabbed her hand and pressed it to his crotch and said, "Now that's more like it." What should Johanna do or say?*

The best approach is to be direct, simple, and clear. A statement such as, "Let go of my hand right now. Don't do that again. Is that clear?" would indicate the unacceptable behavior. She should request a

change in therapists if she continues to feel uncomfortable working with this patient.

Sexual harassment, unwanted sexual attention, comments, or overt sexual behavior is never appropriate, yet it is fairly common in physical therapy.[6-8] Whether the source of sexual harassment is patients or clients, other students, faculty or clinical staff, deal with it directly. Indicate that it is unwanted and inappropriate. Do not keep it to yourself. Take action. Talk with a faculty member, supervisor, or clinical director about the proper channels for action.

Remain professional. Define unacceptable behavior clearly. Document the incident in writing through whatever procedures are appropriate in the university or clinical facility.

Summary

Professional behavior takes many forms, including dependability, professional presentation, initiative, empathy, cooperation, organization, clinical reasoning, participation in supervision, and verbal and written communication. Codes of conduct define limits and boundaries of professional behavior.

Students must observe standards for professional behavior, presentation and attire, language, confidentiality, and modesty. All students who are members of the APTA must observe the standards of conduct described in the *Guidelines for Professional Conduct*. Students should check university policies for other regulations that govern student conduct.

References

1. Jamali M. *Course Syllabus. PT 3514 Laboratory for Gross Anatomy.* Arkansas State University, College of Nursing & Health Professions. Available at: http://www.clt.astate.edu/mjamali/pt3514.htm. Accessed June 25, 2000.

2. Kasar J, Clark EN. *Developing Professional Behaviors.* Thorofare, NJ: SLACK Incorporated; 2000:7-20.

3. May WW, Morgan BJ, Lemke JC, et al. Model for ability-based assessment in physical therapy education. *Journal of Physical Therapy Education.* 1995;9(1).

4. Student Manual, Department of Physical Therapy. *Professional Behavior Policy: Student Code of Conduct.* Fresno, Calif: California State University, Fresno; 2000.

5. Physical Therapy University of Manitoba School of Medical Rehabilitation. *Physical Therapy Dress Code.* Available at: http://www.umanitoba.ca/faculties/medicine/units/medrehab/pt/. Accessed July 30, 2000.

6. O'Sullivan V, Weerakoon P. Inappropriate sexual behaviours of patients towards practicing physiotherapists: a

study using qualitative methods. *Physiother Res Int.* 1999;4(1):28-42.

7. deMayo RA. Patient sexual behaviors and sexual harassment: a national survey of physical therapists. *Phys Ther.* 1997;77(7):739-744.

8. McComas J, Hebert C, Giacomin C, Kaplan D, Dulberg C. Experiences of student and practicing physical therapists with inappropriate patient sexual behavior. *Phys Ther.* 1993;73(11):762-770.

PUTTING IT INTO PRACTICE

1. Locate and make a copy of the pages of your student manual or catalog that refer to student conduct. What aspects of conduct are covered by these policies? What are the consequences for failure to observe these standards of conduct?

2. How are students in your professional education program expected to dress for the following:

    Daily classroom activities?

    Guest speakers?

    Laboratories?

    Clinical experiences?

3. Suppose you find out that one of your classmates has been working as a physical therapy aide, often unsupervised, in a local physical therapy practice. You are aware that this practice is a violation of both state law and the APTA Code of Ethics. How would you handle the situation?

4. Why is it important that student physical therapists observe professional behavior standards? What are the ramifications of violations of these standards for the following:

    The student?

    His/her classmates?

    The academic program or clinical faculty?

    The university?

    The profession?

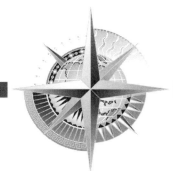

Chapter 7

Student Performance Evaluation

Evaluations in the Professional Curriculum

> Patricia waited outside the classroom for her first practical examination. She wondered, "Am I really ready for this?" She had practiced for hours the night before on her roommate, but still she worried about this new experience. The door opened. A classmate left the room and didn't look upset. She thought, "OK, I'm going to be fine."

Most evaluations in the professional curriculum are tied into a general purpose, explained in Chapter 5, to ensure that students demonstrate mastery of specific knowledge, attitudes, and skills, and meet predefined standards of performance.

There are several types of performance evaluations during the physical therapist professional education experience, including written and practical examinations, assessment centers, writing evaluations, presentation ratings, and clinical performance evaluations.

Written Examinations

Most students are experienced with written examinations through a long series of high school and undergraduate college experiences. There are many strategies that are valuable for succeeding on written examinations.

Forced-choice questions on written examinations are most commonly of three types: *multiple-choice, true-false,* and *matching*.

Constructed answers include three common types as well: *fill in the blank, short-answer,* and *essay*.

Multiple-Choice Examinations

A multiple-choice question has a *stem* and multiple *options*. Successful test-takers pay attention to some specific characteristics in these two components of the question that may provide clues that increase the examinee's chances of selecting the correct answer. It may also help to eliminate potential poor choices.

A skin graft in the left axilla makes palpation of this muscle difficult in the posterior fold:
  A. pectoralis minor
  B. rhomboids
  C. latissimus dorsi
  D. coracobrachialis

To answer this question, we need to know surface anatomy and which muscle groups are palpable in the posterior axillary fold. Because A and D are both in the anterior thorax and B does not cross the axilla, we can eliminate all choices *except* C, which is the correct answer.

Unless there is a penalty for guessing, always guess. Even if there is a penalty for guessing, it is to your advantage to guess if you can reduce your choices from four to two by a process of eliminating implausible options. Table 7-1 gives some tips for success on multiple-choice exams.

True-False Questions

Because there are only two options, you have a 50% chance of being correct on a true-false question. Unless there is a penalty for guessing, it is always to your advantage to guess.

Read carefully. Watch for specific determiners (eg, always, never, only) and the direction of the statement (eg, not, unable). These words will often exclude an answer or be overlooked by a test-taker in a hurry.

> T   F   The only people not at risk for HIV infection are married men and women.

Matching Questions

With matching questions, it is always important to read directions carefully. Know where you will place the correct answer and find out how many times an option can be selected. Eliminate the incorrect responses first, then work with the rest.

Place the number of the correct term in Column B that represents each abbreviation in Column A. You may use each item only once. Consider the context and the likelihood that one of two possibilities is incorrect.

a. LOL	1. Taking care of business
b. TCB	2. Two geese in the forest
c. TGIF	3. Little old lady
d. PI	4. Postal inspector
	5. Totally courageous boss
	6. Thank goodness it's Friday
	7. Private investigator
	8. Lots of luck

Fill in the Blank

Be careful to read the question carefully and to match your answer to the question that is asked. Be sure that your answer fits grammatically (the part of speech: neurological vs. neurology) and the same level of complexity or classification of terms.

> In a multiple-choice question, there is a *stem* and multiple_____.

First, by reading the sentence, we know that this should be a noun and it should be plural. So, we can narrow down the response to *answers* or *choices*, or if we recall the specific terminology used earlier in this chapter, we would of course respond *options*.

Short-Answer Questions

Short-answer questions allow a two- to three-sentence response to a directed question. Read the question carefully. Respond directly in line with the question asked. Be specific, clear, and concise. Number the responses if appropriate. If asked, give a simple rationale for your answer.

> Give three characteristics of a lower motor neuron lesion.
> Response: Three characteristics of lower motor neuron lesions are:
> 1. flaccid muscle paralysis
> 2. absent deep tendon reflexes
> 3. hypotonicity in response to passive movement

Essays

Essays are longer samples of timed writing that indicate your ability to organize your thoughts and respond to a more complex issue. Be sure to read the question carefully.

Essay questions often ask for responses that compare key features of one phenomenon with another. They may ask for arguments in favor or arguments against a particular stance. They sometimes ask for a response and then a rationale for that response.

Help the reader understand your answer. Organize your responses to the question in the same order as the question is asked. Use subtitles to organize your response where appropriate. See the following example of an essay question.

Instructions

Answer the following questions. Organize your response (you may use scrap paper to do this). Be clear and concise. Be sure you answer all parts of the question. Write legibly and in the available space. Illegible answers cannot be graded.

Question

In the managed care era, several trends have occurred which affect the role of the physical therapist. Indicators forecast further downsizing of health care institutions and a shift to prospective payment systems. Why is evidence-based practice an attractive alternative in this changing health care environment? Describe three problems that the physical therapy profession may face in using this practice model. Your response?

Table 7-1

STRATEGIES FOR ANSWERING MULTIPLE-CHOICE QUESTIONS[1]

Read the stem carefully:

1. Identify key words in the stem that indicate negative direction (eg, not, except, never, unacceptable, unrelated, least). Look for answers to eliminate that would answer the opposite question.

    The **least** likely to succeed on a multiple-choice test will be:
    a. the student who studies only class notes
    b. the student who does not study until the night before the test
    c. the student who prepares a little every day
    d. the student who does not read the questions

2. Identify key words in the stem that indicate value, rank, or priority (eg, first, initially, best, most). Rank the options you would think are most wrong and work backward.

    The **most** important reason to learn test-taking strategies is:
    a. to succeed in college and other testing situations
    b. to increase your intelligence
    c. to receive scholarships and grants
    d. to prevent depression from poor grades

3. Identify clues in the stem (look for a similar phrase in the answer).
    The term dysuria denotes:
    a. glucose in the blood
    b. difficulty speaking
    c. pain on urination
    d. voiding at night

Examine the options. There are clues that will help you eliminate incorrect answers (also known as the distracters):

4. Look for specific determiners in options (eg, just, always, never, all, every, none, only).
    These terms place limits on statements that would be considered correct. You can usually eliminate answers with a specific determiner unless they illustrate a law or principle that is very important. In the example below, a and b use specific determiners.

    When taking your pulse during exercise:
    a. never count for less than 10 seconds
    b. always start when the second hand is on the 3,6, 9, or 12
    c. be careful not to use your thumb
    d. find the carotid pulse just below your collarbone

5. Identify opposites in options: One of them can be correct or both can be eliminated. In the example below, b and d can be eliminated because neither is correct and they are opposites.

    In relation to the average child, a hyperactive child is:
    a. easily taught in a large class
    b. nonviolent except when provoked
    c. difficult to focus on a task
    d. often abusive to other children

continued

Table 7-1, continued

6.   Identify equally plausible/unique options. If there are two items that are no better or worse than the other option, you can usually eliminate both. In the example below, a and c are similar and thus neither are correct.

If your computer screen does not illuminate when you turn on the computer, the first thing you should do is:
a. turn the power off and on again quickly
b. check the brightness controls of the monitor
c. shut it off; wait 30 seconds, then turn it on again
d. hit the monitor gently on the side

7.   Identify duplicate facts in an option.
When an option contains two or more facts that are identical and you can identify one part as being correct, you can usually eliminate two options that are distracters. In the example below, the only two answers with a "typical college student" age group are a and c. Therefore, b and d can be eliminated.

The most common age groups on campus (including all students, faculty, and staff) are:
a. 21 to 25 and 45 to 50
b. 16 to 20 and 31 to 35
c. 21 to 25 and 56 to 60
d. 36 to 40 and 51 to 55

First re-read the question. Outline your response. There are two questions asked in the above question. This essay is asking you to consider evidence-based practice *within a defined context.*

A well-written essay would start with an introductory paragraph defining evidence-based practice, then answer the first question. The responses to the first question must be in reference to the described trend of downsizing of health care institutions and shift to prospective payment systems. Why is evidence-based practice especially important under these conditions?

Then, the responses to the second question could consist of three paragraphs to describe three problems that may arise as physical therapists attempt to use evidence-based practice. The final paragraph should be a summary statement addressing the value of evidence-based practice.

Use subtitles such as *Evidence-Based Practice, Problems,* or *Summary* to organize your response and make it easier for the reader to identify your responses to various parts of the question. Use words like *first, further,* and *finally* to help the reader define where your points begin and end.

Writing Assignments

Types of writing assessments and styles are covered in Chapter 8. Writing is evaluated and graded in the context of the purpose of the assignment. There are some desirable characteristics of all types of writing, including clarity, topic development, and correct grammar and spelling.

It is often helpful for students to assess their own writing and that of their peers prior to turning in assignments. The scoring criteria in Table 7-2 may be of value in reviewing your work.

Presentations

Strategies for preparing projects and presentations are covered in Chapter 8. Performance during a class presentation is often graded. Students are usually graded on content, style, quality of presentation, and evidence of having met the objectives of the assigned project. Look at the sample assignment and evaluation form in Table 7-3 for evaluating a presentation.

Table 7-2

SCORING CRITERIA FOR GRADUATE WRITING[2]

Rating Criteria for Outstanding = 5

- Vocabulary is precise, varied, and vivid. Uses language aptly, sometimes even eloquently. Sentences are economical and effective. Meaning is conveyed effectively.
- Only acceptable, readily identifiable abbreviations are used or a legend is included.
- Shows a clear understanding of writing and topic development. Organization is appropriate to writing assignment and contains clear introduction, development of ideas, and conclusion.
- Transition from one idea to another is smooth and provides reader with clear understanding that topic is changing.
- Active voice and parts of speech are used correctly with only rare errors that do not disrupt communication.
- Uses people-first, nonsexist language.
- Bibliographic sources are properly cited, including Internet sources.
- Not necessarily error-free, but the few errors or imperfections are outweighed by other excellent qualities.

Rating Criteria for Acceptable = 3

- Vocabulary is adequate for professional level. Meaning is conveyed but breaks down at times.
- Only acceptable, readily identifiable abbreviations are used or a legend is included.
- Shows a good understanding of writing and topic development. Topics and rationale are organized logically, but some parts of the sample may not be fully developed.
- Some transition of ideas is evident.
- Meaning is conveyed but breaks down at times.
- Mechanical errors in punctuation and spelling are present but do not disrupt communication of the message.
- Uses people-first, nonsexist language.
- Bibliographic sources are properly cited, including Internet sources.

Rating Criteria for Unacceptable = 1

- Vocabulary is simple; imprecise use of language.
- Organization may be extremely simple or there may be evidence of disorganization.
- There are few transitional markers or repetitive transitional markers.
- Meaning is frequently not clear.
- Numerous mechanical errors in spelling, punctuation, or grammar affect communication.
- Shows some understanding of writing and topic development.
- Uses nonsexist and people-first language usually.
- Bibliographic sources are properly cited.

Rating Criteria = 0

- Vocabulary is limited and repetitious.
- Sample is extremely limited in length or incomprehensible.
- No transitional markers.
- Meaning is unclear.
- Mechanical errors cause serious disruption in communication.
- Language is frequently sexist or not people-first in its orientation.
- Bibliographic sources are improperly cited.

Reprinted with permission from Duttarer J. *Scoring Rubric: Graduate Writing Requirement. Department of Physical Therapy.* Fresno, Calif: California State University; 1999.

Table 7-3
SAMPLE ASSIGNMENT AND ASSESSMENT CRITERIA FOR SEMINAR PRESENTATION[3]

Assignment

1. Your team should decide who will present the various aspects of the chosen issue. The objective of this assignment is to give the class strategies and skills they can use in physical therapy practice to deal with various aspects of the managed care environment. You will conduct an indepth investigation of the topic, explore the relevant aspects of the issue to the delivery of health care or health care policy, and identify aspects of the issue that relate specifically to physical therapy practice to provide a thorough foundation for class discussion. In your investigation, you should explore the history and current status of the issue in the delivery system, as well as seek practical examples of how practicing physical therapists have chosen to deal with the issue, whether effective or ineffective.

    You are expected to use ALL of the following sources to develop your presentation:

    1. Current literature (professional journals and publications related to physical therapy and the rehabilitation industry, health care administration publications, popular newspapers and magazines).

    2. Published positions by the APTA (both nationally and in your state's chapter) relating to your issue.

    3. Specific examples of strategies utilized by physical therapists practicing in local health care institutions, including job descriptions, administrative policies or procedures, reports, surveys, forms or documentation, personal interview data.

    4. You will have one hour to present your topic and related issues to the group. As part of your presentation, you will include a "Case Scenario" (typed and in sufficient numbers to distribute to the class) in a physical therapy practice setting, lead the group through an analysis of the situation and help the class to generate strategies to handle the situation. They should explore the best professional way to handle the scenario if it occurred in their practice or as though they were a consumer of health care (eg, You are working in a skilled nursing facility. You want to monitor the effectiveness of your services in treating total hip patients).

    5. You may use any reasonable instructional strategy that you believe will present all aspects of the issue and will facilitate participation of the group in analysis of the scenario.

    6. Your group will be evaluated on the criteria presented on the next page.

continued

Peer evaluation is also very important. Table 7-4 is an example of a peer evaluation form that can be completed by the audience during a class presentation.

Practical Examinations or Performance Assessments

Practical examinations are commonly used in courses that cover physical therapy skills. They are usually case-based and require the student to read a case and then simulate physical therapy performance with another classmate or standardized patient.

A *standardized patient* is a paid volunteer who plays the role of the patient for the purpose of examining students. Standardized patients are usually trained and may have real diagnostic findings that students must identify.

During a practical examination, students are given opportunities to perform interviews and evaluative or treatment procedures.

The following example is typical of a case study you might be given during a practical examination.

Table 7-3, continued

Date:_____   Total Points:_____

Students Presenting:_____

Topic:_____

Criteria		Rating Points									
a.	Depth and thoroughness of your investigation	1	2	3	4	5					
b.	Organization and clarity of your presentation	1	2	3	4	5	6	7	8	9	10
c.	Accuracy of information presented	1	2	3	4	5	6	7	8	9	10
d.	Statement of instructional objectives	1	2	3	4	5	6	7	8	9	10
e.	Selection of appropriate instructional strategies to present information	1	2	3	4	5	6	7	8	9	10
f.	Selection of appropriate reading material for class preparation	1	2	3	4	5					
g.	Correct format of references (AMA)	1	2	3	4	5					
h.	Effective use of audiovisual materials	1	2	3	4	5					
i.	Realism of case scenario and relationship to PT practice	1	2	3	4	5	6	7	8	9	10
j.	Facilitation of group discussion of case scenario	1	2	3	4	5	6	7	8	9	10
k.	Closure and summary of issue emphasizes viable strategies	1	2	3	4	5	6	7	8	9	10
l.	Written materials are typed and free of typographical and grammatical errors	1	2	3	4	5	6	7	8	9	10

Comments:

Jeanette is a 27-year-old woman interning as a histologist who is experiencing low back pain. Her pain increases with trunk flexion. She can't remember a specific incident when her pain began. Her PMH consists of a strained erector spinae approximately 5 years ago while moving heavy boxes from a shelf to a workbench. From your interview you learn she has two children, one is 5 months old and the other is 2 years old.

Your evaluation tells you that her ROM is limited by pain to the first one-third of the range for trunk flexion. Her strength was not tested due to pain, however her lumbar curve is flattened, she has rounded shoulders, and a forward head posture. Both reflex and sensory findings are within normal limits. Her paraspinals are in spasm on the right side more than the left, from T12 to L5. She feels uncomfortable sitting lately, so she stands bending forward at the microscope, but it doesn't seem to help.

Table 7-4

PRESENTATION FEEDBACK FORM[3]

Date: _____

Subject: _____

Speaker(s): _____

1. What was most helpful or most interesting about this presentation?

2. What would you like to know more about this subject?

3. What suggestions would you make regarding this presentation?

4. What new ideas or insights have you gained from this presentation?

Grading of a practical examination is done by observation of student performance. Student performance and choices during the examination reflect critical thinking and clinical decision-making skills, as well as understanding of course content. Communication skills come into play as students must interview the patient, give instructions, and listen to what the patient says. Performance also includes a psychomotor component in that students must position themselves and the patient appropriately and demonstrate effective and safe handling skills.

Take a look at the practical examination performance evaluation criteria in Table 7-5.

Assessment Center

An assessment center, also called an *objective, structured clinical examination* (OSCE), involves the evaluation of various components of clinical competence that are measured in a series of stations.[5,6] The student progresses from station to station carrying out specified activities in a limited time frame. Student performance is graded with specific outcome measurements. It generally involves a number of different components that simulate decision-making and skills needed for clinical practice.

An example of physical therapy assessment center and the types of activities students might perform are listed in Table 7-6.

Clinical Performance Evaluation

The *Physical Therapist Clinical Performance Instrument* (CPI) is a clinical rating instrument in wide use in physical therapy clinical education. It was developed to evaluate knowledge, skills, and attitudes in 24 clinical performance criteria. Each of these criteria is accompanied by a list of sample behaviors that serve as examples of the item (see Table 7-7).[8]

The instrument uses a 10 cm rating visual analog scale on a continuum from "novice clinical perform-

Table 7-5
SAMPLE PERFORMANCE EVALUATION CRITERIA (PRACTICAL EXAMINATION)[4]

Patient Problem: _____

Problem Identification and Treatment Plan

1. Identifies and states three functional problems.	_____ 1
2. Selects appropriate treatment tactics for patient problems/goals.	_____ 4
3. Explains correct rationale for using selected treatment tactics using acceptable medical terminology.	_____ 3
4. Correctly identifies precautions related to pathology.	_____ 2

Comments:

Subtotal Problem Identification/Treatment Plan: _____ **/10**

Treatment Skills Demonstration

1. Greets and communicates with patient effectively. Explains procedures using appropriate lay terminology.	_____ 2
2. Prepares area and equipment for procedure as indicated.	_____ 1
3. Chooses appropriate equipment for treatment technique.	_____ 1
4. Positions patient effectively for safety, appropriate body mechanics, and efficiency for therapist and patient.	_____ 1
5. Adjusts/measures equipment or repositions patient appropriately.	_____ 1
6. Demonstrates appropriate safety precautions and body mechanics in skill execution.	_____ 1
7. Performs skill correctly within course specifications.	_____ 3

Comments:

Subtotal Treatment Skills Demonstration: _____ **/10**

ance" at the low end to "entry-level performance" at the high end to rate each of the 24 indicators. Both instructors and students are able to rate progress on this line. Instructors must also record narrative comments on each page of the 24-page instrument. Compare these two definitions in Table 7-8.

Summary

Student performance is evaluated at many points and through many different processes during the educational process. Students who understand the criteria on which they are being graded and practice in ways that simulate exam conditions should fare well. Sound preparation and effective use of test-tak-ing strategies are keys to success in physical therapy education. Performance evaluation serves a critical role in determining clinical competence and identifying student needs.

References

1. Curtis KA. *Test-taking, UNIV 001: University Orientation*. Fresno, Calif: California State University; 1999.

2. Duttarer J. *Scoring Rubric: Graduate Writing Requirement—Department of Physical Therapy*. Fresno, Calif: California State University; 1999.

3. Curtis, KA. *PH TH 231 Seminar in Health Care Issues. Course Syllabus*. Fresno, Calif: California State University; 1997.

Table 7-6
PHYSICAL THERAPY STUDENT ASSESSMENT CENTER[7]

Assessment Center Stations	Activity
Station one: chart review	Perform chart review of basic medical and social history information.
Station two: interview	Perform a 5-minute interview with the "patient," role-played by a faculty member.
Station three: evaluation planning	Design and prioritize evaluation procedures. Complete a written questionnaire, answering questions about the functional limitations, diagnosis and important medical problems, contraindications, and precautions for the patient. List evaluative priorities and give the rationale for choices.
Station four: evaluation performance	Perform several evaluation procedures on the patient. Procedures include surface palpation, goniometric assessment, manual muscle testing, and reflex and sensory testing. Students are rated on organization, safety, accuracy, and effectiveness in performing each evaluative procedure. Write a short note documenting evaluative findings.
Station five: treatment planning	After reviewing the physical therapy evaluative findings, establish functional goals and a treatment plan directed toward meeting those goals. Identify contraindications or precautions considered in the treatment planning process.
Station six: treatment performance	Present a treatment plan and explain rationale. Perform a selected part of the treatment plan on the patient. The students are rated on their ability to explain and demonstrate their instructions to the patient, to adjust equipment, to prepare the treatment area, to exhibit proper body mechanics, to take appropriate precautions for patient safety, and to apply treatment skills.

4. Curtis KA. *Competency Check Form, PT 570, Clinical Skills*. Miami, Fla: University of Miami; 1993.

5. Harden RM, Gleeson FA. Assessment of clinical competence using an objective structured clinical examination (OSCE). *Medical Education.* 1979;13:41-54.

6. Deusinger SS, Sindelar B, Stritter FT. Assessment center: a model for professional development and education. *Phys Ther.* 1986;66:1119-1123.

7. Curtis KA, Haston L. *Basic Physical Therapy Skills Assessment Center: Evaluation Alternative for Entry-Level Physical Therapy Students*. Miami, Fla: University of Miami; 1994.

8. APTA. *Physical Therapy Clinical Performance Instrument*. Alexandria, Va: American Physical Therapy Association; 1997:11, 29-30.

Table 7-7

PERFORMANCE CRITERIA AND SAMPLE BEHAVIORS FROM THE CLINICAL PERFORMANCE INSTRUMENT[8]

Performs a physical therapy patient examination.

Sample Behaviors

a. Selects reliable and valid physical therapy examination methods relevant to the chief compliant, results of screening, and history of the patient.

b. Obtains accurate information by performing the selected examination methods.

c. Adjusts examination according to patient response.

d. Performs examination, minimizing risk to the patient, self, and others involved in the delivery of the patient's care.

e. Performs physical therapy examination procedures in a technically competent manner.

Reprinted with permission from the American Physical Therapy Association.

Table 7-8

DESCRIPTIONS OF NOVICE AND ENTRY-LEVEL PERFORMANCE[8]

Novice clinical performance	A physical therapist student who provides quality care only with uncomplicated patients and a high degree of supervision. Without close supervision, the student's performance and clinical decision making are inconsistent and require constant monitoring and feedback. This is typically a student who is inexperienced in clinical practice or who performs as though he or she has had limited or no opportunity to apply academic knowledge or clinical skills.
Entry-level performance	A physical therapist clinician performing at entry-level utilizes critical thinking to make independent decisions concerning patient needs and provides quality care with simple or complex patients in a variety of clinical environments. The physical therapist clinician at the professional level needs no guidance or supervision except when addressing new or complex problems.

Reprinted with permission from the American Physical Therapy Association.

PUTTING IT INTO PRACTICE

1. Survey your course syllabi for the current semester. Write the dates of all quizzes, written examinations, practical examinations, and assignments due on your daily planning calendar.

2. On what dates do you have multiple examinations or assignments due?

3. Record the results of any tests or assignments you have completed thus far on your syllabus.

4. What clinical performance rating system is used in your curriculum?

5. If you were given the choice of an examination or a project as a means to evaluate your performance, which would you choose? Why?

6. Most successful students are fairly accurate in their self-assessment of their skills and knowledge. What opportunities in the past have you had to evaluate your own performance?

    What opportunities do you or will you have in the professional education program to perform self-assessment?

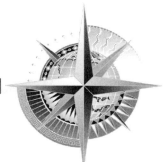

Chapter 8

Professional Presentations, Papers, and Projects

Professional Presentations

> Sara noticed on the course outline that a group case presentation was required during the 12th week of the class. She worried, "I've never been a good public speaker, but even worse, what if I end up in a group with someone who doesn't do the work?"

Professional presentations, papers, and projects are common requirements during the educational process. Later in one's professional life, they form the basis for communication between disciplines, for starting new programs or research projects, and for contributing to the base of scientific knowledge. Knowing how to effectively communicate your ideas, information, and research findings is an important skill.

Types of Presentations

There are many opportunities to present information to colleagues, professors, clinical instructors, and others. Each type of presentation may have a different purpose and therefore have different requirements.

In-Class

Students in university classes often must do indi-vidual or group presentations as part of the requirements of a course. These presentations are usually focused on a specific topic, issue, or content related to the course. These presentations are usually short (15 to 30 minutes) and focused, with specific objectives and expected outcomes. The audience is usually fellow classmates and the course instructor. These types of presentations are usually graded using specific criteria (see Table 7-3).

In-Service (Clinical) Presentations

Many students are requested to do in-service presentations as part of their clinical education experiences. The focus of these presentations is often left to the student's choice, with input from the clinical instructor. Usually, the purpose is to provide education and to demonstrate understanding and application of clinical information. In-service presentations tend to be scheduled in 30- to 60-minute periods, often during a lunch or staff meeting time. The audience is usually the clinical staff, other students, and clinical instructors.

Examinations

Presentations are also done for the purpose of a clinical or academic examination. A student might be required to present a case study, research findings, or other original work. A student in these cases is often required to meet specific criteria, address certain issues or questions, and respond appropriately to questions. The audience may be one or more faculty members either with or without fellow students.

Research

Research presentations are done for several purposes, depending on the location and audience. These types of presentations might be done to demonstrate successful completion of a project to an academic review committee, to share research findings with other investigators and colleagues at a scientific congress, and to add to the base of scientific knowledge underlying the profession of physical therapy.

Designing a Presentation

In designing a presentation, it will be helpful for you to consider the following issues:

Purpose and Objectives

State the purpose and intended outcomes of your presentation. For example, your purpose might be to present your research findings in a simple, understandable way.

Objectives are what you hope that your audience will know, feel, or be able to do following your presentation. These intended outcomes give your presentation a direction and help you to measure whether or not you have achieved your intended outcome. If your objectives are specific and measurable, it will be easier to tell if you have achieved them than if they are more general and vague.

Compare these two objectives:
- Participants will understand and appreciate the causes and results of the inflammatory process.
- Participants will be able to define inflammation, infection, edema, and induration, and differentiate the etiology and tissue pathology of each of these four processes.

Which is more measurable and more clear? Which describes an outcome? Objectives are as much for the presenter as they are for the audience. They keep you on track and help define the content you will present and path you will take.

Audience

Who is your audience? Are they colleagues or consumers? Do they have the same background, or do they differ in levels of education and specific previous exposure to the subject matter? What are their needs with respect to the subject matter? What vocabulary do they use? Should your presentation be in lay language or use professional terminology?

Needs Assessment

A needs assessment determines your audience's background and present level of knowledge. This might be accomplished by an informal questionnaire to a few representative members of the group, brief interviews, or more extensive surveys. Do not fall into the trap of assuming that all members of the audience have the same background, or that this background is similar to that of the presenter. Remember that in preparing to do a presentation, you are probably becoming far more knowledgeable than your audience.

Subject Content

The subject content that is presented should be related to the intended outcomes of the presentation. The subject content should be organized in an outline or list form as you develop the presentation. Try to simplify, condense, and summarize material for your audience.

Define terms before using complicated or technical terminology. Be sure to introduce sections of your presentation and make it clear when you are moving from one section to the next. Use simple subtitles, advanced organizers, and other techniques that will keep your audience with you.

Presentation Activities

Select an appropriate presentation technique and/or learning activity. The descriptions in Tables 8-1 to 8-3 should help you to differentiate what presentation techniques may be most appropriate. Consider the value of lecture, question and answer, demonstration, discussion, and experiential techniques to present the material. Although lecture is frequently the chosen mode, other activities may actually be far more effective in presenting material and accomplishing your objectives.

Reinforce and supplement your presentation with visual aids and written handout materials. Make your materials complement, but not duplicate, your presentation. Never read your written materials verbatim to the audience.

Instructional Media

Do not overlook the importance of media in adding to your presentation. A PowerPoint (Microsoft, Redmond, Wash) presentation, a short

Table 8-1
SIMPLE PRESENTATION TECHNIQUES[1]

Lecture

We have all experienced lecture in our formal education. It is most useful when the leader wants to transmit information that the participants do not have. Lectures are best when they are:

- Short (less than 5 minutes of monologue at a time)
- Simple (building on what participants know)
- Visually interesting (so participants can see concepts and ideas)
- Participative (involving participants via questions)

A mini-lecture is helpful to introduce the topic and provide a brief description of the problem and important background material. Participants should be involved as soon as possible to maintain their interest and attention.

Questions

The leader can insert questions in the lecture to stimulate and involve the participants. Asking for agreement/disagreement or for common experiences of participants is an easy way to begin. For example, the leader may ask, "How many of you have experienced this?" or "Does this sound familiar? I see a few of you nodding your heads."

Demonstration

Lecture can often be enhanced with demonstration of skills or techniques. Demonstration is best followed by practice and a return demonstration. When demonstrating, the leader should be sure that participants can see the demonstration. The leader should take care to illustrate and identify the key points of the demonstrated skill.

Table 8-2
DISCUSSION TECHNIQUES[1]

Discussion provides for participant sharing of knowledge, experience, and skills on the subject. Holding a discussion helps the leader to take advantage of the combined background that the participants bring to the group. Discussion is a valuable method to generate many ideas and give participants new approaches to a common problem.

Brainstorming

Brainstorming is a useful technique to generate many ideas in a short period of time. A question is asked and participant responses are recorded on a flip chart or board for all to see. It is important that the leader record responses and refrain from evaluation of responses until the group runs out of ideas.

Question and Answer

This technique is useful to involve participants and diverge from straight lecture. The instructor asks a question and then calls on an individual participant to answer the question. The leader should have a predetermined list of questions and follow-up questions to ask, which are tied into the lecture material.

Case Study

This provides a means for participants to analyze a case and apply the techniques and principles of the learning experience to it. The case provides a situation to be discussed. The leader should have a list of discussion questions prepared in advance. Participants should be encouraged to share experiences that help in making the jump from the case to their own experiences.

continued

Table 8-2, continued

Fishbowl Discussion

A small group of four or five representatives are chosen to sit either in front or in the center of the larger group. This is particularly valuable in focusing the group on their reaction to a particular exercise or experience. At the end of the fishbowl discussion, all participants have had the same experience, either directly or vicariously.

Panel Discussion

The panel discussion takes place in front of a larger group, with questions initially directed to the panelists by the leader or facilitator. Panelists typically represent different points of view or may come from different occupational groups or specialty areas.

Table 8-3
EXPERIENTIAL PRESENTATION TECHNIQUES[1]

Experiential Techniques
This term applies to a variety of techniques that allow the participant to **experience** what you want to teach rather than just studying or talking about it. Learning occurs via the reactions and emotions participants experience while they participate in the exercise. The leader has a key role in helping participants to analyze their experiences and relate them to the objectives of the learning experience.

Role Playing
- Role playing is helpful in providing an opportunity to practice a new process or skill and in illustrating different perspectives that one takes on in a "role." It is not "play acting," as it is intended to simulate reality. Role playing provides a realistic look at the participant's behavior, emotions, and experience in a "real" situation.
- Role playing is most successful when participants are given a loosely defined situation, a role to play, and an attitude or position to take. The role play should be followed up with discussion by participants and observers. This discussion should help to relate the experience to the skills, concepts, or ideas that it was intended to illustrate and support.

Games and Simulations
Games and simulations are carefully structured learning activities that assist participants in exploring their group working relationships and responses to a variety of situations. The value of using simulations is that if a mistake is made, no one is hurt. Games and simulations must have contingencies built-in for the decisions and actions that participants take. For instance, if a participant makes a decision to proceed with a particular action, there must be feedback that indicates the consequences of that choice. Therefore, the rules and results must be carefully defined.

Videotaping
This is time-consuming but quite valuable as an experiential learning tool. When videotape is used, it is essential that participants have sufficient time to observe and analyze their performance with instructor feedback.

Table 8-4
TYPES OF INSTRUCTIONAL MEDIA

Overhead projector transparencies: Useful to project words, charts, graphs, and cartoons; can be easily made on photocopy machine; lights stay on; instructor can write or draw on transparency.
Slides: Photographs, charts, graphs, words, and different colors are all possible; lights must be off; easy to control and advance.
Computer-generated images/LCD projector: Can be used to present computer-generated materials and video onto a large screen; more versatile than slides because video and special effects can be incorporated into a computer program. However, be careful of technical difficulties and incompatible versions of software and media.
Videotape: Able to demonstrate complex interactions and movement with both visual images and sound; often must be edited and cued for effective presentation.
Audiotape: Excellent for instruction or review with accompanying written materials.

Table 8-5
GENERAL GUIDELINES FOR USING INSTRUCTIONAL MEDIA[2]

1. Keep it simple. For word slides or overhead transparencies, use no more than seven lines of text.
2. Make sure that the projected image is visible from all areas of the room.
3. If you cannot see it well, do not use it (ie, do not use tiny figures on charts). If showing a table, use no more than three rows and columns of figures. Fewer will be more understandable.
4. Use media to enhance your presentation, but be sure to explain adequately.
5. Allow the audience to see and read before you talk. Pause slightly before speaking.
6. Use titles. A title on a slide or transparency helps the audience to absorb and organize the material.
7. Ensure that volume and visibility are adequate for a videotape presentation. You may want to darken the room.
8. Be prepared! Check out all equipment and your media *before* beginning your presentation.

video, and/or photographs or diagrams may help to improve understanding and keep your audience's attention. See Tables 8-4 and 8-5, which describe types of media and guidelines for presentation.

Also, think in advance about reading materials that you can recommend to complement or augment your presentation.

Equipment and Facilities

Reserve the equipment you will need. Double-check on the availability of equipment and support personnel at the presentation site. Some of the following equipment may be helpful to your presentation:

- Overhead projector (for overhead transparencies)
- LCD projector and laptop computer (for computer-generated images and video)
- Slide projector
- Videocassette player
- Microphone

Evaluation

Evaluations are done for many purposes. They serve as a form of feedback for the presenter and as validation of learning or achievement for the participants.

Table 8-6

EVALUATION TECHNIQUES

1. Paper and pencil test, survey, or reaction
2. Performance evaluation of participants
3. Behavioral observations of participants
4. Participant self-evaluation

Speakers should seek audience involvement to assess whether or not their objectives have been met and to review the effectiveness of each phase of the presentation. Evaluations can take many forms. Consider the list in Table 8-6 and determine what evaluation techniques you might choose. Some sample evaluation forms are shown in Chapter 7.

Papers and Writing Assignments

There are many writing assignments that you will be involved with in the course of the professional education process. It is important that you understand the purpose, guidelines, and parameters of each assignment. Some of the more common types of papers follow.

Review of the Literature

A review of the literature is a systematic and thorough compilation and summary of published research on a particular topic. It is important when writing this type of paper to narrow the topic enough to allow for thorough and relevant coverage of published sources. This type of paper may serve as the basis for an introduction to a research proposal or may be publishable as a review article on a particular subject.

Case Report

A case report or case study is an indepth report of an example of a phenomenon. Usually, case reports involve the application of theoretical or research-based information to clinical or administrative examples. For example, one might write a case report to present the unique management of a patient or development of a new administrative structure to address institutional downsizing. A case report usually presents a chronological series of events and often describes the effect of an intervention or change over time.

Research Abstract

Research abstracts are short summaries of a larger article. They typically include the key elements of purpose, subjects, instruments, methods, results, and conclusions. Many articles have abstracts that precede the article. Abstracts are indexed in databases such as MEDLINE and serve as a preview to help you determine if the article meets your needs.

Research Critique

Critiques are discussions of the strengths and limitations of published research articles. Critiques require that the writer has a background in the subject matter and previous research in the area and in research methodologies. A critique generally follows a prescribed format, commenting on issues such as the relevance and importance of the study, the sampling technique, the validity and reliability of instrumentation, the variables measured, the statistical analyses chosen, and the generalizability of the reported findings. Some journals (eg, *Physical Therapy*) often publish a peer-reviewed "discussion" following a research article.

Position Paper

A position paper is often focused around a controversial issue. This type of paper requires that the writer succinctly summarize the issue, provide relevant arguments from several positions, and then choose a particular stance. It is important that this type of writing focus on the establishment of an argument and position using sound rationale and acknowledging consideration of alternative points of view.

Reaction Paper

A reaction paper is a more personal account of an event or experience than any of the previous types of writing. The writer should use first person voice (eg, "I found...") when describing the experience. A reaction paper usually involves the application of theoretical or research-based findings to a real-life experience. For example, students might write a reaction paper after visiting a hospice facility and discuss their observations and feelings about the experience in relation to assigned readings.

Patient-Related Documentation

There are numerous opportunities in the professional education program to practice writing patient-related evaluations, progress notes, and discharge summaries. Be clear and concise, and use professional terminology where appropriate. Be careful not to use excessive or nonstandard abbreviations, and avoid professional jargon. Consider who will be reading this documentation, and keep in mind that insurance claims reviewers and even physicians often do not understand abbreviations like TTG (toe-touch gait), VC (verbal cueing), or SBA (stand-by assist).

The Writing Process

Drafts and Revisions

Good writers always go through numerous drafts while developing their ideas, the structure of the paper, and the proper grammar, spelling, and syntax. It often helps to have a colleague read and review your work. Be sure to use computer-based spellchecking and grammar assists. Avoidable errors detract from your work and make it appear that you have not invested much effort.

What is the Point?

Understanding the purpose of writing is important in determining what you write. Be sure to identify the focus and theme of each paragraph and check to make sure that you are communicating your ideas effectively.

Avoid Common Writing Errors

Take a look at Table 8-7 for common writing errors. Have you made some of these common errors?

Professional language

Be aware that you must choose the language style that is appropriate for the type of writing and reader. As a rule of thumb, most professional writing requires professional language. Be critical of your writing and watch the terminology you use.

> *Both Janet and Ed prepared reviews of the same article they had read. Janet took a casual, friendly approach and concluded her review as follows: "This was a totally cool article that I think everybody ought to read. I learned lots of neat stuff about how to get patients to do their exercises and I really liked all the pictures of people working out and that kind of thing." Ed took a more professional approach: "This article presents relevant new research that clinicians may find useful for their orthopedic patients. The authors conclude that social support is a necessary component of patient compliance."*

Terminology and Definitions

It is a good idea to start every technical writing piece with basic definitions of the terminology you are using. A few introductory sentences should suffice as you introduce each new topic in your paper.

Plagiarism and Copyright Infringement

Plagiarism involves misrepresenting the work of another, whether published or unpublished, as one's own work. This can be as simple as using phrases of other authors without proper citation. To avoid plagiarism, always cite your sources.

Be sure that you are citing the original source. The original source is that of the author(s) whose work is being described. Do not cite the article or book in which you read about another study. Look at the reference list at the end of the piece and find the original source. Find the original paper and read it for yourself. Your citation should always be the original source, not another author who has cited this source in his or her work.

Copyright infringement involves copying published material, whether text, illustrations, or photographs, without permission. Be careful: even copying a photograph from an Internet site into a PowerPoint presentation is a copyright infringement. Always ask permission from the copyright owner before incorporating someone else's work into your writing or presentation (copyright infringement applies even if the sources are properly referenced).

Review the laws regarding plagiarism and copyright infringement in Chapter 12.

Referencing Styles

Instructions for a paper or other writing assignment should designate which referencing style to use. Common styles for professional writing in the health fields include *American Medical Association (AMA)* and *American Psychological Association (APA)*

Table 8-7
COMMON WRITING ERRORS[3]

Goal	Incorrect	Correct
Make sure that subjects and verbs agree.	Mary is more capable than him.	Mary is more capable than he is.
Avoid using nouns as verbs.	This change will impact the way we do things.	The impact of this change will be significant.
Make pronouns and subject agree. Watch out for the words *they* or *them* when referring to one person.	The patient called to complain that I could not see them this afternoon.	The patient called to complain that I could not see him this afternoon.
Only use apostrophes to indicate possession or a contraction, not a plural (except for the word *it*).	Charles voice is very loud.	Charles' voice is very loud.
	The CD's and disks were very expensive.	The CDs and disks were very expensive.
	I found it's cord under the bed.	I found its cord under the bed.
Don't confuse affect and effect.	The affect is not known. How can I effect this outcome?	The effect is not known. How can I affect this outcome?
Don't split infinitives.	He lifted the patient to slightly move the sheet.	He lifted the patient to move the sheet slightly.
Start sentences with words other than *hopefully* or *basically*.	Hopefully, I will hear about the scholarship this week.	I hope to hear about the scholarship this week.
Use people-first language.	Disabled people need more job opportunities.	People with disabilities need more job opportunities.
Use the active voice wherever possible.	John was selected for the job.	The search committee selected John for the job.

Adapted from http://www.soyouwanna.com/site/syws/wrerrors/wrerrors.html

styles. Your library should have references available that detail these reference styles.

The journal *Physical Therapy* uses AMA style. Table 8-8 shows a sample of how references look for journal articles, books, book chapters, online journals, and websites using AMA style.

Peer Review

Peer review is a process that occurs throughout professional writing. It involves a subject matter expert or colleague reviewing your submitted writing. Following peer review, authors have the option to revise their work. Table 8-9 shows a very simple peer review form that students can use to review the work of their colleagues.

Although it may not always be easy to hear criticism of your writing, peer review is a valuable process. Through this process, writers benefit from having someone else with a similar background critically read their work, and reviewers often become better writers as well.

In general, peer-reviewed professional writing receives the highest credibility and distinction in publication. Peer-reviewed journals serve as the original sources of our scientific knowledge and as a vehicle for communicating new knowledge.

Table 8-8

REFERENCING USING AMA STYLE[4,5]

Follow AMA style (eg, *Journal of the American Medical Association; Physical Therapy*). Double-space citations in your list of references. References should be numbered in the order of their citation in the text. When citing references in the text, the numerals appear outside periods and commas and inside colons and semicolons. When more than two references are cited at a given place in the text, use hyphens to join the first and last numbers of a closed series; use commas without space to separate other parts of a multiple citation (eg, As reported previously,[1,3-8,19]).

Some common examples follow:

1. Journal articles (up to six authors):

Doe JF, Roe JP III, Coe RT Jr, Loe JT Sr, Poe EA, Voe AE. How to write a research proposal. *JAMA*. 1981;244:76-97.

2. In the case of more than six authors:

Doe JF, Roe JP III, Coe RT, et al. How to write a research proposal. *JAMA*. 1981;244:76-97.

3. In the case of a journal article that does not have consecutive pages throughout the volume (the month or the day of the issue is preferable to the issue number):

Doe JF, Roe JP III, Coe RT Jr, Loe JT Sr, Poe EA, Voe AE. How to write a research proposal. *Sci Am*. November 1981;244:76-97.

4. In the case of a journal article published in a supplement:

Gordon AS. Standards for cardiopulmonary resuscitation (CPR) and emergency cardiac care (ECC). *JAMA*. 1974;277(Suppl):833-868.

5. In the case of abstracts:

Pailard M, Resnick N. Natural history of nosocomial urinary incontinence. *Gerontologist*. 1981;24:212. Abstract.

6. Books:

Spencer H. *Pathology of the Lung*. 3rd ed. Elmsford, NY: Pergamon Press Inc; 1976:46-51.

7. Books with an editor:

Gray H; Goss CM, ed. *Gray's Anatomy of the Human Body*. 29th ed. Philadelphia, Pa: Lea and Febiger; 1973:1206. (Note Gray is author and Goss is editor)

8. Chapter or section of a book:

Schulman JL. Immunology of influenza. In: Kilbourne RD, ed. *The Influenza Viruses and Influenza*. Orlando, Fla: Academic Press Inc; 1975:373-393.

9. Online journals:

Roach KE, Ally D, Finnerty B, et al. The relationship between duration of physical therapy services in the acute care setting and change in functional status in patients with lower-extremity orthopedic problems. *Phys Ther*. [serial online] 1998;78:19-24. Available from: American Physical Therapy Association, Alexandria, Va. Accessed July 20, 2000.

10. Online websites:

Health Sciences Libraries University of Washington. *The AMA Style Guide page*. Available at: http://healthlinks.washington.edu/hsl/styleguides/ama.html. Accessed August 2, 2000. (Note: The title of the journal, book, or website should be in italics, however if this type style is unavailable, you may substitute it with underline)

Adapted with permission from Iverson C, Flanagin A, Fontanarosa PB, eds. *American Medical Association Manual of Style: A Guide for Authors and Editors*. 9th ed. Philadelphia, Pa: Lippincott, Williams and Wilkins; 1997.

Table 8-9

SAMPLE OF SIMPLE CRITERIA FOR STUDENT PEER-REVIEWED WRITING[7]

Follows stated instructions for content of paper.

Rating criteria:

_____Not done, major areas of content missing.

_____Done to a limited extent; could be improved in quality or quantity of content.

_____Exceptionally well done, organized, and complete.

Writer takes a position and develops that position.

Rating criteria:

_____Not done, superficial, and limited in development of position.

_____Done to a limited extent, some examples given, but writer's position is not clearly explained or supported in all areas.

_____ Exceptionally well-developed, complete, good examples which illustrate the points made.

Expression is clear and concise, and language is professional.

Rating criteria:

_____Not done, uses terminology incorrectly, or uses broad generalizations.

_____ Done to a limited extent, possible alternatives in terminology or sentence structure, some generalizations.

_____ Exceptionally well-done, uses first-person voice where appropriate, wide range of appropriate terminology, meaning is clear.

Paper is without typographical and grammatical errors.

Rating criteria:

_____ >5 errors

_____ 3 to 5 errors

_____ 0 errors

Projects

Class Projects

Projects take many forms. Many courses in the professional curriculum require individual or group projects that encourage students to apply course material in a meaningful learning experience. This might be through a service learning project such as doing volunteer work at a community center. It might involve researching a clinical topic or doing an indepth case study of a patient or client.

Research Projects

The research requirements in entry-level physical therapy education vary from program to program. Students may be expected to complete original research, or they may be expected to participate in faculty projects.

In a *faculty-directed research* model, students follow the research interests of faculty who have ongoing projects. Whether or not research belongs in the entry-level curriculum has been the subject of considerable debate over the years.[6] The prevailing argument is that in a busy entry-level professional curriculum, there is often neither the time nor the supervisory resources to have individual students initiate research. Student research efforts using this model contribute to a meaningful body of work developed over a longer period of time.

Collaborative Projects

Group projects allow students to collaborate to complete a project. This model is, in reality, how most work in the real world is done. Students may have an opportunity to work with other student physical therapists or with students from other disciplines.

Collaborative projects are excellent learning experiences for the real world. How does one create a collaborative project? The organization of group members for completion of a project can be simplified by breaking down the steps of the project and then assigning responsibilities and timelines for completion. The worksheet in Table 8-10 provides a sample of a project management worksheet for student research.

Summary

Professional presentations, papers, and projects are required throughout the educational process. Students can learn and implement effective strategies to complete these requirements. The skills acquired in the preparation of presentations, papers, and collaborative projects are essential for future practice.

References

1. Curtis KA. *Training Programs for Clinical Instructors*. Los Angeles, Calif: Health Directions; 1988.
2. Curtis KA. *PH TH231 Seminar in Health Care Issues Course syllabus*. Fresno, Calif: California State University; 1997.
3. *Soyouwanna.com. So You Wanna Avoid Common Writing Errors?* Available at: http://www.soyouwanna.com/site/syws/wrerrors/wrerrors.html. Accessed August 2, 2000.
4. Iverson C, Flanagin A, Fontanarosa PB, eds. *American Medical Association Manual of Style: A Guide for Authors and Editors*. 9th ed. Philadelphia, Pa: Lippincott, Williams and Wilkins; 1997.
5. Health Sciences Libraries University of Washington. *The AMA Style Guide page*. Available at: http://healthlinks.washington.edu/hsl/styleguides/ama.html. Accessed August 2, 2000.
6. Crane LD, Kroll P, Curtis KA, et al. More support for student research. *Phys Ther*. 1992;72(8):608-609.
7. Curtis KA. *Peer-Reviewed Grading Form, PHTH 142 Concepts in Patient Compliance: Course Syllabus*. Fresno, Calif: California State University; 1998.
8. Curtis KA. *Project Worksheet, Student Research Manual*. Fresno, Calif: California State University; 1999.

Table 8-10

SAMPLE STUDENT RESEARCH PROJECT MANAGEMENT WORKSHEET[8]

Project Management Worksheet Student Research		Personnel Names				
	Timeline	1	2	3	4	5
1. Literature search						
Library search						
Organization of references						
Procurement of references						
Assignment of reading						
Storage and organization						
2. Writing proposal						
Preliminary drafts						
Final draft and all forms, figures, and appendices						
3. Obtaining necessary approvals						
Filing application for human subjects committee						
Developing consent forms						
4. Logistics						
Data collection						
Printing of survey						
Mailing of survey						
Mailing postcard						
Obtaining mailing labels						
Schedule of research committee meetings						
5. Design of instruments/procedures						
Development of instrument						
Pilot testing and revisions						
6. Data analysis						
Conversion of raw data into template						
Enter from template to spreadsheet						

continued

Table 8-10, continued	Timeline	Personnel Names				
		1	**2**	**3**	**4**	**5**
Enter data into Statview						
Perform statistical analyses						
Design tables, graphs to present data						
7. Writing final paper						
Preliminary drafts						
Final paper, tables, figures, appendices						
8. Presentation for defense						
Audiovisual materials						
Handouts						
Organization of presentation						
Defense of study						
9. Presentation on campus						
Platform presentation						
A-V materials						
Delivery						

PUTTING IT INTO PRACTICE

1.   Trade papers with a colleague prior to turning in a writing assignment. Use the rating criteria on the following page to give each other feedback on your paper.

2.   Observe an instructional presentation. This could be an observation of one of your classes or a speaker in a professional conference. How would you describe the purpose, audience, needs assessment, subject content, and presentation activities involved? What instructional media was used? How was the effectiveness of the session evaluated?

Purpose

Audience

Needs Assessment

Subject Content

Presentation Activities

Media

Evaluation

Peer-Reviewed Writing

Follows stated instructions for content of paper.

Rating Criteria:

_____ Not done, major areas of content missing.

_____ Done to a limited extent, could be improved in quality or quantity of content.

_____ Exceptionally well done, organized, and complete.

Writer takes a position and develops that position.

Rating Criteria:

_____ Not done, superficial and limited in development of position.

_____ Done to a limited extent, some examples given but writer's position is not clearly explained or supported in all areas.

_____ Exceptionally well developed, complete, good examples which illustrate the points made.

Expression is clear and concise, and language is professional.

Rating Criteria:

_____ Not done, uses terminology incorrectly or uses broad generalizations.

_____ Done to a limited extent; possible alternatives in terminology or sentence structure; some generalizations.

_____ Exceptionally well done, uses first-person voice where appropriate, wide range of appropriate terminology, meaning is clear.

Paper is without typographical and grammatical errors.

Rating Criteria

_____ >5 errors

_____ 3 to 5 errors

_____ 0 errors

Comments:

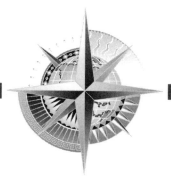

Part Three

Essentials for Success of Physical Therapy Students

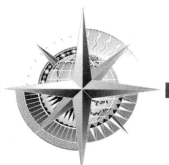

Chapter 9

Managing the Learning Process

Improving Classroom Retention and Comprehension

> *Melissa was overwhelmed. She realized during her anatomy test that she had not studied the right material. Rather than the anatomical features she had memorized, the test focused on the relationships of anatomical structures and the paralysis that would result from nerve lesions in the brachial plexus.*

Information Processing

Information processing is a cognitive science that deals with the brain's ability to sort and make sense of information. Research indicates to best increase our ability to use and retain information, we need to consider the relationship and relevance of that information. We need to consider how it relates (in similar or different ways) to past information and clarify how we will use this information.[1]

Concept Formation

We form concepts as we process information. A *concept* is the set of rules used to define the categories by which we group similar events, ideas, or objects.[1,2] We are aided in concept formation by the following strategies:

1. Use Advanced Organizers

It helps when we label and define the concept to be learned. Categorize new information and define the attributes of the concept. For example, write titles and subtitles (such as Pathology, Signs, Symptoms) frequently in your notes and in the margins of your texts. It is important to *actively* process and categorize to classify the information as you read.

Using a highlighter while you read is a *passive* technique that *does not* enhance comprehension or learning. Writing key notes in the margin or on another sheet of paper with a pencil is an *active* technique that enhances retention.

2. Give Examples and Nonexamples of the Concept

Think of examples that would be either true or false. This may be a useful way to prepare for examinations as well (eg, lower motor neuron paralysis is typically indicated by absent deep tendon reflexes and NOT by spasticity).

3. Apply the Information

Practice application of *inductive reasoning* by using examples and experiences to reach a conclusion. Make up cases and see if you can reach a diagnosis. Consider the box at the top of the following page.

Also practice *deductive reasoning* by using the diag-

> *A 29-year-old woman has a 2-week history of progressive weakness in the lower extremities, accompanied by blurred vision and diffuse sensory disturbances over the upper and lower extremities. What are likely diagnoses given this clinical picture?*

nosis to predict the findings. Consider a diagnosis and see if you can define the characteristics of a typical clinical presentation.

Consider the following:

> *The patient told the department secretary he has degenerative joint disease when calling for his initial appointment for evaluation of shoulder pain. You know that osteoarthritis is a common joint pathology resulting in shoulder pain. Given this diagnosis, what are likely causes of shoulder pain in this patient?*

As you can see from the above example, deductive reasoning involves recalling definitions and descriptions, whereas inductive reasoning involves reaching a conclusion. It may be more difficult to do inductive reasoning because there is always the possibility that you will reach an incorrect conclusion.

Improving Memory and Retention

There are many study processes that can be used to aid memory and retention of information:[1,2]

1. Pay Attention

- Attend all classes; hearing the same concepts repeatedly will assist you to establish ways of conceptualizing new information.
- Sit in a classroom location where you can easily see and hear, away from distractions that may decrease your ability to pay attention.
- Study for short periods of time and use your time productively.
- Look for indicators from the instructor that information is important.

2. Use What You've Learned in the Past

- Skim reading assignments prior to class.
- Look at figures, charts, and photographs in the text that may further illustrate this information.
- Discuss previously covered content prior to the next class.
- Record and listen to lectures while driving.

3. Look for Ways to Identify Important Information

- Identify concepts that are repeated in handouts, during lectures on the board, or in transparencies.
- Highlight and organize your further reading and review around these concepts.

4. Organize the Information

Even if the classroom presentation is not in an order that makes sense for you, try your best to impose an order in your mind and your notes. This can be done in several ways:

- Show a logical sequence from one step to another for a procedure.
- Go from simple to complex, easy to more difficult.
- Arrange historical events in chronological order.
- Cross-reference notes by source and subject matter; identify discrepancies and similarities.
- Explain your understanding to others, especially those who are learning the same material. Listen to what others explain to you and discuss differences in your understanding.

5. Categorize (Chunk) Related Information

- Develop two-dimensional grids to compare and contrast information. For example, create a table that lists pathology, signs, symptoms, treatment, and precautions across the top and diagnostic categories down the side. See if you can fill in all the boxes from your lecture and reading material.
- Think "across" courses. How will the anatomical information you are learning be important when it comes to palpating a muscle insertion during muscle testing? Look back at your notes and rediscover the relationship of information covered in past courses to your present learning.

6. Recognize and Use Opportunities for Repetition of Learning

You will have many opportunities to do this from the academic to the clinical learning situation.

- Apply the same information or principle in different situations.
- Schedule periodic reviews of previously learned concepts and skills and see if you can apply them to new situations.
- Jog your memory using drills and other memory techniques.

7. Work with a Study Group

Study groups are the single most effective way that students can improve their performance. Collaboration and group learning are very effective processes that are relevant to future practice.[2]

- Be accountable. Students stay more focused when they have partners or a group that is depending on their participation.
- Check your understanding. Information processing and retention is greatly enhanced by verbally summarizing learning in writing or in discussion.
- Share your thoughts and listen. In addition to aiding in retention, you may pick up a great idea, a new perspective, or a time-saving strategy by working with others.

Psychomotor Learning

Many skills that physical therapy students must learn involve *psychomotor learning*, requiring physical movement as well as a cognitive component. Most skills involve both cognitive and physical components such as operating machines, lifting a patient, using a computer, or examining a patient. Howard Gardner's theory of multiple intelligences suggests that different abilities can be separately developed and that there may not be such a close link between different types of abilities, such as kinesthetic and verbal abilities.[3]

Basics of Skill Learning

An understanding of the following principles will aid in psychomotor learning:

1. Avoid Trial-and-Error Learning

Once learned, a skill is not "unlearned"; it is only replaced by the learning of another skill. Therefore, it is important to avoid trial-and-error learning, which may create bad habits that later have to be corrected. Concentrate on what you are learning, solicit feedback, and correct your performance. This will prevent your having to relearn later.

2. Perfect Practice Makes Perfect Performance

Practice is required for skill acquisition. It is important that the practice be guided: Practice only makes perfect if what is being practiced is correct.[4] Learning incorrect methods can interfere with progress. Effective practice provides for knowledge of results, which reinforces and motivates future action.

3. Be Patient

Fatigue and complexity of material to be learned interfere with the speed of learning. Be patient and use all of your senses (vision, hearing, feeling) to process, learn, and practice. Schedule frequent, short practice sessions and stop when you feel fatigued.

4. Think First

Be careful when transferring learning from one situation to another. Different patient positioning or different physical environments may create a need to perform differently. Think before you act.

We all feel awkward at some times. All physical therapists are not gifted in the psychomotor domain, but most physical therapy students are able to learn how to learn the skills required for successful practice in the profession of physical therapy. The steps in Table 9-1 may aid your psychomotor learning.

Facilitating Clinical Learning

Laura reviewed her midterm CPI evaluation and read her clinical instructor's comments, "Laura seems to have difficulty with clinical problem-solving." The clinical instructor later explained that she would like to explore what is happening that prevents Laura from making the clinically appropriate decisions and plans.

First, we must acknowledge that clinical information processing uses a monumental amount of information. Students must read and digest a patient's history, interview the patient, perform tests, observe physical signs and symptoms, and select from long-term memory the appropriate clinically relevant information about differential diagnoses, philosophies of treatment, and precautions. What do we know about clinical information processing?

Novices and Experts

It may be useful to look at what differentiates *novice* from *expert* performance. Novice and expert performance tends to follow certain patterns. There is quite a bit of evidence that these types of behaviors occur across professions and/or subject matter.[5-8] Think of an area in which you have developed expertise, such as computer use or playing chess. See if these descriptions sound familiar to you:

Table 9-1
LEARNING STRATEGIES: USEFUL STEPS FOR LEARNING AND PRACTICING SKILLS[2,4]

- Write down what should be done, why, and how. How should it feel? To what should I pay attention?

- Verbalize all the necessary steps in the correct sequence as you perform them.

- Rely on all your senses for feedback. Concentrate on how it feels to perform the activity smoothly and without hesitation. Maximize your chances for success in early skill practice. When you know that you are performing correctly give yourself a chance to experience successful completion of the task.

- Break down a sequence of a complex activity into parts and perform each part of the sequence or pattern of activity well. Anticipate the next part of the sequence and prepare yourself to be in the right position and ensure that the required conditions exist for the next step. For example, it is important to maximize lifting safety by positioning the load close to the body prior to initiating the lift.

- Introduce variety to the performance of a skill. Now that you have mastered the skill on the right side of the patient, are you equally comfortable working on the left side? Can you plan for the required differences?

Novice Performance

The novice focuses primarily on objective findings, observable signs, and rules to use to make decisions. The novice's performance is governed by these rules and may lack flexibility. The novice tends to be concerned with details and may not have the experience base to be able to prioritize which information is critical and which is not. Novices tend to use systematic approaches to try to control the huge amounts of information that bombard them. Detailed assessment forms, lists of interview questions, and protocols are very comforting for a novice.

Expert Performance

The expert, on the other hand, uses a largely intuitive process, looking at the whole picture, modifying his or her approach in response to deviations from expectations. Expert performance is characterized by its fluid and flexible nature. The expert is able to simultaneously carry on a conversation and make observations. Much of this process goes on "in the expert's head" and is often not verbalized. An expert often unconsciously and automatically processes a great deal of information and arrives at a conclusion often without a systematic or organized approach to arriving at a decision. Most importantly, the expert processes information within a context, with a view that recognizes cues and vital information that change from situation to situation.[9]

Whereas novices tend to use more of a "rule-oriented" process, the expert tends to have a more holistic view. Let's look at some evidence that further defines the process.

Pattern Recognition

There is evidence that experts retain information by organizing the information in familiar patterns. Research conducted on physicians and medical students showed that physicians differed from medical students in their recall of critical information in a written text. Physicians showed significantly greater recall of critical cues and made more accurate diagnoses than did the medical students when the information was presented in a pattern that they were used to seeing (medical history-physical exam-lab findings). The recall of physicians decreased to approach the level of the medical students when the same information was presented in random order.[10]

The expert is different from the novice by his or her ability to *recognize and interpret* critical cues in *patterns of information*. Students need support in developing their thought processes to see these patterns. There are some specific steps that students can take to identify and organize the information in the environment.

Steps to Better Clinical Decision-Making

Cognitive psychologists have identified that each of the following steps aids in our information processing abilities. Students and their instructors can systematically approach the task of decision-making by using some of the following guidelines.[11]

1. Identify the Key Cues

A *cue* is something that grabs your attention. It might be a note written in a chart, an observation of a sign or symptom, or a key question that you ask in your interview with the patient. Ask yourself the following questions:

- What are the key cues I am seeing, hearing, or feeling (these may be the results of your examination and evaluation)?
- Do they differ from my instructor's view? Identify those differences.
- What cues are most critical?

Think of the intensive care unit with monitors beeping and alarms occasionally going off. To what must I pay attention to know that the patient is okay?

How do I know that a patient receiving gait training will be safe to walk by himself to the bathroom?

2. Organize and Prioritize the Cues

The next step is to organize the cues into logical units of information. This involves prioritizing information and organizing it in a way in which one is able to identify patterns (eg, identifying that arm pain that radiates to the jaw is a different phenomenon *and of greater urgency* than arm pain at a tendinous insertion of a muscle).

A problem-solving or evaluation format such as a systematic history, objective evaluation, an assessment, and an identification of problems, goals, and treatment plans serves this purpose well. The following questions may help to organize the cues:

- What subjective information that I have elicited is of the greatest concern?
- What comorbidity is of significance when I consider the patient's current status?
- What are the positive findings of the evaluative process? Are there any red flags?
- What medications may interfere with performance?
- What findings indicate the need for further follow-up?
- What information may change the approach I take (eg, prior functional status or social support at home)?

3. Identify a Pattern

The *Guide to Physical Therapist Practice* has established practice patterns for many diagnostic groups. As an initial step, it may be helpful to consider what pattern applies to the patient. This will help to guide your thinking, jog your memory, and make a well-reasoned decision regarding the intervention for the patient. The following questions may be helpful:

- What patterns of signs and symptoms do you expect with certain diagnoses (eg, hyperactive deep tendon reflexes and paralysis are consistent with an upper motor neuron lesion)?
- What would you typically recommend or do?
- What is your reasoning in using specific critical pieces of information to establish an assessment or plan for the patient?
- What is the pattern of cues that you see in this patient?

4. Identify Deviations From the Pattern

This step of the process is the most difficult because it requires constant attention to the cues in the environment and reconsideration of assumptions that you may have made. Initial impressions may lead to false conclusions unless you take this essential step. Consider this case:

> *Mr. Atkins developed acute back pain while gardening over the weekend. On Monday, he was referred to a physical therapist. In his initial evaluation, he mentioned that he has developed bladder incontinence. The physical therapist realized that this deviates from the usual symptom complex and may constitute a surgical emergency. The physical therapist made a call to the patient's physician while the patient waited. The physician sent the patient directly to the emergency room.*

This physical therapist's action lead to an immediate referral to a neurosurgeon. The patient was soon diagnosed with cauda equina syndrome and underwent a decompressive laminectomy later that evening.

Deviations from the pattern are important because they change the expected course of action. They may indicate problems, precautions, or referrals that physical therapists must make. These questions may assist you to start this process:

- What critical pieces of information do not fit the expected pattern?
- How do this patient's signs and symptoms deviate from what I might typically see?
- Are there complications, contraindications, or precautions that may result from these deviations?
- Is there a more serious problem that I need to consider?

5. Synthesize and Draw Conclusions; Integrate Information Into a Plan

The key questions here are "So what? What difference does it make that I know this information?" You may reach any of the following conclusions:

- Knowing this, I might choose one approach over another.
- Knowing this, I will have to involve the patient's caregivers in my plan.
- Knowing this, the patient may not be able to participate in the indicated duration or frequency for optimal treatment.
- Having identified symptoms that do not fit in the expected pattern, I am going to call the patient's physician for re-evaluation of his low back pain.

After developing a diagnosis and prognosis, the physical therapist designs an intervention, including a plan of care that is intended to result in expected changes in the condition.

Metacognition and Reflection

Metacognition, or an ability to monitor and alter one's process of thinking, assists in helping to refine the process of clinical reasoning. The multidimensional and complex nature of the clinical environment requires constant processing of clinical information. "Thinking about one's thinking" provides insight into attention, pattern recognition, and clinical reasoning processes.

Recent research supports the value of *reflection* during the learning process.[9,12,13] Reflection includes both consideration of the procedure and interaction involved. Evidence shows that physical therapist reasoning occurs in context, with cues and patterns of information developing different meanings in varying conditions. The knowledge base of expert physical therapists develops through reflection.[9] With increased experience and engagement in reflective processes, therapists are able to develop reasoning processes that incorporate multiple perspectives.[13]

Summary

There is ample evidence to support a systematic approach to information processing to facilitate student learning. Researchers have found that methods of clinical reasoning differ in novices and experts in predictable ways.

Principles of information processing can be applied to clinical learning to enhance clinical reasoning processes. Further, an active consideration of one's thought processes and reflection on one's experiences facilitate development of one's base of knowledge.

References

1. Curtis KA, Haston LM. *Teaching Accountable Clinical Decision Making in Physical Therapy: Integration of Entry-level Clinical Evaluation and Treatment Skills Courses.* Miami, Fla: University of Miami; 1994.

2. Graham CL. Conceptual learning processes in physical therapy students. *Phys Ther.* 1996;76:856-865.

3. Gardner H. *Frames of Mind: The Theory of Multiple Intelligences.* 10th ed. New York: Basic Books; 1993.

4. Hunter M. *Mastery Teaching.* Thousand Oaks, Calif: Corwin Press; 1994.

5. Benner P. *From Novice to Expert—Excellence and Power in Clinical Nursing Practice.* Menlo Park, Calif: Addison Wesley Publishing Co; 1984.

6. Shepard KF, Hack LM, Gwyer J, Jensen GM. Describing expert practice in physical therapy. *Qual Health Res.* 1999;9(6):746-58.

7. Jensen GM, Shepard KF, Gwyer J, Hack LM. Attribute dimensions that distinguish master and novice physical therapy clinicians in orthopedic settings. *Phys Ther.* 1992;72(10):711-22.

8. Jensen GM, Shepard KF, Hack LM. The novice versus the experienced clinician: insights into the work of the physical therapist. *Phys Ther.* 1990;70(5):314-23.

9. Jensen GM, Gwyer J, Shepard KF. Expert practice in physical therapy. *Phys Ther.* 2000;80(1):28-43.

10. Coughlin LD, Patel VL. Processing of critical information by physicians and medical students. *J Med Educ.* 1987; 62:818-828.

11. Curtis KA. *Facilitating Critical Thinking in Clinical Education.* Presented at San Joaquin Valley District Meeting, American Physical Therapy Association, May 13, 1997.

12. Cross V. Introducing physiotherapy students to the idea of reflective practice. *Med Teach.* 1993;15(4):293-307.

13. Dahlgren MA. Learning physiotherapy: students' ways of experiencing the patient encounter. *Physiother Res Int.* 1998;3(4):257-273.

PUTTING IT INTO PRACTICE

1. Select your class notes from one class period in a course you are currently taking. Reference the material to your books and reading assignments by writing notes in the margins. Note any discrepancies by asterisk. Make an appointment to talk with your instructor about any discrepancies you find or questions that arise during this activity.

2. Identify a new motor skill that you are learning. This might be performing a transfer, guarding a patient during gait training, or doing a "wheelie" in a wheelchair.

    Write down what should be done, why, and how.

    How should it feel? To what should you pay attention?

    Write down all the necessary steps in the correct sequence of performance.

3. Choose a class session to analyze. Reflect on what drew your attention during this class.

    What were the cues to which you responded?

    What was most important in the material covered or skills learned?

    Reflect on how you might apply this information. Why is it important to know?

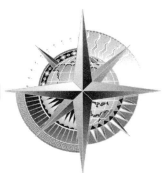

Chapter 10

Will I Do Well Enough?

Yolanda looked over her first anatomy exam as it was discussed in class. This was the first exam of the professional program. She winced as she saw the grade, "68" in bold letters at the top of the exam. "How could this have happened?" she questioned inwardly. "I have never had academic difficulty before. I have always been close to the top of the class."

Performance Anxiety

Performance anxiety is a manifestation of stress, occurring when worry and fear interferes with performance and causes distress for the performer. This can occur for musicians doing a performance, speakers giving a presentation, or students taking tests or practical examinations.[1]

The symptoms of performance anxiety are varied and can range from simple "butterflies" and mild excitement to totally debilitating panic attacks. Physical symptoms might include heart palpitations, extreme perspiration, dry mouth, shaky knees and hands, trembling voice, shortness of breath, dizziness, nausea, urinary frequency, diarrhea, and/or a sense of dread. Emotional symptoms include feeling frightened, sad, frustrated, angry, or a combination of these. Intellectually, there may be difficulty in paying attention, concentrating, and remembering.

The person experiencing performance anxiety may withdraw, feeling more isolated, have a low sense of personal effectiveness, or feel guilty or ashamed regarding the current situation. Coping strategies are often ineffective, resulting in reaction and worry rather than more effective preventative action (Table 10-1).

Research on Worry and Decreasing Performance

Research shows that anxiety resulting in worry and self-doubt interferes with information processing and memory.[1-6] Performance tests show that worry tends to divert attention and valuable cognitive processing time just when you need it most.

Therefore, in addition to not knowing what is on the test, if a student worries about it while trying to succeed on the examination, performance is likely to be even worse!

Just as the physiological, emotional, and intellectual manifestations of anxiety are varied in the moment that we feel stressed, our longer term responses to stress can also vary.

Illness

Research shows that student susceptibility to illness increases during examination periods, resulting in far greater incidences of viral and upper respiratory infections during these periods of stress.[7-10]

Table 10-1
RESPONSES TO ANXIETY[1]

Physical Symptoms
Racing pulse
Perspiration (can be extreme)
Dry mouth
Shaky knees and hands
Trembling voice
Shortness of breath
Dizziness
Nausea
Bladder and rectal pressure

Emotional Symptoms
Fear
Sadness
Frustration
Anger
Dread

Intellectual Symptoms
Difficulty paying attention
Problems with concentration
Poor memory

Similarly, persons under extreme physical stresses, such as marathon runners, show increased vulnerability to illness post-marathon.[11] There is evidence that physical exhaustion, anxiety, stress, and worry are related to compromised immune function and higher incidence of illness.

Fatigue

Overwhelming fatigue and excessive sleepiness is a common response when chronically faced with situations in which there is little sense of control over the outcome. Fatigue is a common symptom of depression as well. Fatigue interferes with attention and focus; its effects on performance are dramatic and far-reaching.

Substance Abuse

Substance abuse involves the use of external chemicals or drugs such as alcohol, legal and illegal drugs, caffeine, or tobacco. Substances are often used to numb the pain of anxiety or depression.[12-14] The performance impairment and serious health risks that accompany abuse of these substances are undesirable for anyone.

Depression and Suicide

Clinical depression can be a serious problem for students. Be aware of the symptoms and problems listed in Tables 10-2 and 10-3. Suggest that any student or colleague experiencing these symptoms seek professional help.

Identifying the Source of the Problem

Kevin had always succeeded in the past with minimal effort. His grades reflected a long history of exemplary performance in prerequisite courses. What was the problem now? As he read over the test questions, he felt like he had studied for a different test. He had a sinking feeling and felt his palms begin to sweat.

Kevin's story is common among high-ability students who have been successful in the past and face difficulties in professional education. There are a number of common problems that lead to performance difficulties on examinations.

Effort

Many students have a history of past success with less than maximal effort. In graduate education, the complexity of the material presented and the sheer volume of information one faces require different strategies to improve performance.

Study Time

Take a look at your study time. It is reasonable to expect that you will be spending 2 to 3 hours studying for each in-class hour. If you are spending this amount of time and not seeing positive results, you may be choosing the wrong information to study or

Table 10-2
SYMPTOMS OF DEPRESSION

- Persistent sad or "empty" mood.
- Feeling hopeless, helpless, worthless, pessimistic, and/or guilty.
- Substance abuse.
- Fatigue or loss of interest in ordinary activities, including sex.
- Disturbances in eating and sleeping patterns.
- Irritability, increased crying, anxiety, and panic attacks.
- Difficulty concentrating, remembering, or making decisions.
- Thoughts of suicide; suicide plans or attempts.
- Persistent physical symptoms or pains that do not respond to treatment.

Note: Not all people with depression will have all these symptoms or have them to the same degree. If a person has four or more of these symptoms, if nothing can make them go away, and if they last more than 2 weeks, a doctor or psychiatrist should be consulted.

Reprinted with permission from SA\VE—Suicide Awareness\Voices of Education, P.O. Box 24507, Minneapolis, MN 55424-0507. Phone: (612) 946-7998. http://www.save.org

Table 10-3
SUICIDAL SYMPTOMS

Danger Signs of Suicide*
- Talking about suicide.
- Statements about hopelessness, helplessness, or worthlessness.
- Preoccupation with death.
- Suddenly happier, calmer.
- Loss of interest in things one cares about.
- Visiting or calling people one cares about.
- Making arrangements; setting one's affairs in order.
- Giving things away.

*A suicidal person urgently needs to see a doctor or psychiatrist.

Reprinted with permission from SA\VE—Suicide Awareness\Voices of Education, P.O. Box 24507, Minneapolis, MN 55424-0507. Phone: (612) 946-7998. http://www.save.org

using ineffective learning strategies. See Chapter 9 to review some more effective learning strategies.

Reading Priorities

The volume of reading required will exceed your capability to read it. You must become good at skimming, reading abstracts and conclusions, and looking for key words, definitions, and other critical information. You will not be able to read all assigned reading for full comprehension and retention.

Talk with your professor about what information is most important to study. Use your class notes as a guideline. Watch for key phrases and repetitive information in your notes and books.

Use Learning Strategies

Chapter 9 presents many strategies enhanced for information processing, comprehension, and mastery of material. Put these techniques into place to assist you.

Time Management

Do you have conflicting obligations, such as work or family responsibilities? Are you using your time efficiently? Are you procrastinating? Review Chapter 11 for time management techniques.

Limited Clinical Background

Sometimes students who have had minimal contact with patients and clinical exposure lack a context in which to apply the information they are learning. This may interfere with being able to identify the most important information.

Unable to See the "Big Picture"

Are you excessively concerned with details? Many courses emphasize details and few courses pull together "the big picture." Many students find themselves studying compartments of facts and information for tests and lack opportunities to think about how this information applies to a patient's problems or physical therapy practice.

Actively ask yourself, "How am I going to use this information?" "Why is this important for me to learn?" If you or your classmates are unable to answer these questions, seek assistance from the faculty. Learning information in context will assist with retention and future application. (Review Chapter 9 for the details.)

Career Doubts

Sometimes problems with performance lead students to question whether they are well-suited for entering the profession of physical therapy. Consider why you entered this profession. If these reasons are still valid, you may want to explore what strategies you can employ to facilitate your future success.

Your future success in this field is dependent on your satisfaction and happiness doing this work. If you are having doubts, talk with an advisor, trusted faculty member, or clinical mentor. Do not brood alone with your doubts.

You are not alone, nor are you abnormal to question your choices. Questioning allows you to consider and reaffirm your choice. Even if you choose not to continue in the field of physical therapy, the reflection involved in this process is a valuable growth process.

Take Action

Let's first consider the basics of a healthy lifestyle. Are you getting sufficient rest, eating a healthy diet, and participating in regular exercise? Many students would answer no, no, and no! Examine these areas and make needed changes. Put yourself *first*.

Lifestyle Habits

Rest

Be sure that you are getting enough sleep. Fatigue interferes with both information processing and memory. Reduce caffeine intake. Do not sleep during the day, especially if you are waking up at night. If anxiety is keeping you awake, take action to address it.

Nutrition

Be sure that you consume a healthy diet that is going to give you sufficient energy for the work you are doing and prevent long-term health problems. Do not let the time pressures of professional education reduce the quality of the diet you consume. There are many alternatives to eating campus "fast-foods."

Most graduate students gain weight. In addition to high-calorie, high-fat convenience eating, insufficient exercise may also be a consideration. Don't let this add to your worries.

Exercise

Regular aerobic exercise such as walking, swimming, or biking and resistive exercise, such as lifting weights, is critical to prevent (and improve) many health problems associated with a sedentary lifestyle. Further, regular exercise habits now may protect you from common work-related injuries later. As an added bonus, there is growing evidence that supports the connection of movement and enhanced information processing.

Study Habits

Study Groups

Working in a group works! Organize a group if you are not already in one. Group work allows you to organize your study time, focus on specific class requirements and questions, and process essential information with others.

Work Harder and Increase Study Time

- Are conflicting interests reducing your study time?
- Can you study at home, or would studying in the library increase your efficiency and concentration?
- Do you need to reduce work or personal commitments?
- Can you maximize commuting time with listening to tapes of lectures or reviewing your notes?

Seek Alternative Means of Enhancing Your Knowledge Base

Are you just not getting it? Seek alternative sources. There may be computer-based resources, Internet sites, videos, and other self-directed resources that are available to augment and supplement the course material. Check with faculty, library staff, professional networks, and student resource guides.

Studying More Effectively

Review the tips in Chapter 9 on learning and information processing research. Specifically, look for the following problems in your studying strategies. Are you having difficulty:

- Prioritizing and selecting what to study?
- Identifying relationships between bits of information?
- Reading everything and not remembering anything?
- Not finding the information you need?
- Having difficulty applying information?

Remember that cognitive processing research shows us that comprehension and memory of newly acquired information is greatest if you make sense of the information, talk about it, summarize it, write it in your own words, establish a context for the new information, and apply it to real-life situations.

Reading a textbook with a highlighter in hand is a waste of your valuable time. You must do something active with what you are reading, which will enable you to relate it to something else, apply it, categorize it, or put it into context.

Monitor Your Thoughts

> *Marla lay awake in her bed worrying about the exam she took earlier that day. She discussed her answers later with her classmates and realized she had made many mistakes. She could not stop thinking about the questions she read incorrectly and worried, "What if I flunk out of school? What would I tell my parents? I've worked so hard for this."*

The thoughts that we have, especially after an unexpected failure, are related to underlying beliefs about ourselves and may increase anxiety and reduce our future expectations of success.[15] These thoughts may ruin our enjoyment of the challenges and learning experiences ahead. They may dampen feelings of success and take the fun out of sharing achievements and accomplishments with colleagues.

Chapter 9 introduces the concepts of *metacognition* and *reflection*. Take a few minutes to think about the thoughts that you frequently have. Are you guilty of "making mountains out of mole hills?" Everyone has probably had one or two nights laying awake and thinking about the "worst things that could happen." You can change the negative thought patterns that interfere with your performance. The first step is to be aware of them.

Check Table 10-4 for common habitual negative thought patterns that interfere with performance and some suggested ways of coping with these bad habits.

Use Your Resources

Faculty Involvement

Use faculty resources early and often! Ask for help as soon as you note a problem. Use faculty office hours, teaching assistants, and extra review times that are available. Be specific about your questions. Here are some good questions to start:

- What information is most important to study?

- What relationships between facts are most critical?
- Can you explain discrepancies between the reading and lecture notes? (Have specifics in mind)
- What additional resources may help my understanding?

Tutoring

Are there tutoring services available? If you need help, investigate university or department resources that might provide a tutor. Is there a graduate assistant that could spend several hours a week with you?

Focus on Clinical Applications

It may help to see a clinical application of the information. There are several strategies which may be effective:

- Study with classmates who have more diverse clinical experience. Ask them to relate their experiences and apply this information.
- Seek opportunities to spend a few hours a week with a faculty member in practice.
- Use your vacations and down time to gain some clinical experience.

Counseling Services

Investigate free counseling services through your student health center. Student concerns are their specialty. Do not let a problem get out of hand. Take action to address issues such as performance anxiety, stress, personal conflicts, and depression early and effectively.

Support Groups

There may be organized support groups for students, such as those run by a women's resource center, a re-entry center, a students with disabilities center, or a center related to specific health or mental health concerns. Support is a key factor in your success. Do not overlook the value of emotional support in improving your performance. Sometimes just knowing that others share your feelings and anxieties allows you to then focus on the tasks at hand.

Help Lines and Hotlines

Ask for help when you need it. Anonymous help lines and hotlines are available in every city across the country. They often also serve as referral centers to other resources in your university and community.

Summary

Performance anxiety and related stress is a constant concern for students in professional education. Changes in lifestyle and study habits may direct and focus your efforts more effectively. Examining and monitoring negative thought patterns can be helpful to reduce anxiety. Outside resources such as academic and emotional support services are often helpful to students experiencing worry and anxiety.

References

1. Barnes RG. Test anxiety in master's students: a comparative study. *J Nurs Educ.* 1987;26(1):12-19.
2. Garcia-Otero M, Teddlie C. The effect of knowledge of learning styles on anxiety and clinical performance of nurse anesthesiology students. *AANA J.* 1992;60(3):257-260.
3. Grinnell RM Jr, Kyte NS. Anxiety level as an indicator of academic performance during first semester of graduate work. *J Psychol.* 1979;101:199-201.
4. Ikeda M, Iwanaga M, Seiwa H. Test anxiety and working memory system. *Percept Mot Skills.* 1996;82:1223-31.
5. Onwuegbuzie AJ, Snyder CR. Relations between hope and graduate students' coping strategies for studying and examination-taking. *Psychol Rep.* 2000;86:803-806.
6. Yousseff FA, Goodrich N. Accelerated versus traditional nursing students: a comparison of stress, critical thinking ability and performance. *Int J Nurs Stud.* 1996;33(1):76-82.
7. File SE. Recent developments in anxiety, stress, and depression. *Pharmacol Biochem Behav.* 1996;54(1):3-12.
8. Leonard BE, Song C. Stress and the immune system in the etiology of anxiety and depression. *Pharmacol Biochem Behav.* 1996;54(1):299-303.
9. Stahl SM, Hauger RL. Stress: an overview of the literature with emphasis on job-related strain and intervention. *Adv Ther.* 1994;11(3):110-119.
10. Stein M, Keller SE, Schleifer SJ. Immune system: relationship to anxiety disorders. *Psychiatr Clin North Am.* 1988;11(2):349-360.
11. Peters EM. Exercise, immunology and upper respiratory tract infections. *Int J Sports Med.* 1997;18 (Suppl1):S69-77.
12. Kushner MG, Abrams K, Borchardt C. The relationship between anxiety disorders and alcohol use disorders: a review of major perspectives and findings. *Clin Psychol Rev.* 2000;20(2):149-171.
13. Roth SM. Anxiety disorders and the use and abuse of drugs. *Clin Psychiatry.* 1989;50 Suppl:30-35.
14. Pohorecky LA. The interaction of alcohol and stress. A review. *Neurosci Biobehav Rev.* 1981;5(2):209-229.
15. McKay M, Davis M, Fanning P. *Thoughts and Feelings—The Art of Cognitive Stress Intervention.* Oakland, Calif: New Harbinger Publications; 1981:17-45.

Table 10-4

COMMON NEGATIVE THOUGHT PATTERNS[15]

Pattern of Thinking	Characteristics of this Thought Pattern	A Better Way to Think	What to Say to Yourself and Others
Filtering	Magnifying the negative details, while filtering out the positive aspects of a situation.	Shift your focus. Think of strategies to cope with the problem rather than the problem itself. Focus on the positive aspects of the situation, your personal qualities, past successes, and positive events. Be realistic about the situation. If it is a one-time occurrence or a temporary problem, think of it that way.	"I am usually a very capable student; I misunderstood the instructions on this part of the exam."
Polarized thinking	All things are good or bad, perfect or a failure. There is no middle ground.	Realize that every situation is more complex than simply good or bad. There is a continuum that reflects reality. Think in terms of percentages.	"I am able to do this well 95% of the time."
Overgeneral-ization	Coming to a general conclusion based on a single incident or piece of evidence; expecting bad things to happen over and over.	Quantify rather than using words that are qualitative (terrible, horrendous, awful). How many times has this happened? Examine how much evidence you really have for your conclusion and evidence that would be against your conclusion. Throw out the conclusion until you have consistent evidence to support it. Avoid statements using words like every, all, always, none, never, everybody, and nobody. Use words, instead, like sometimes and often.	"Some of my classmates did very well on the first exam. I am succeeding in this course, even though my performance on the first exam didn't really reflect how much I know."
Mind-reading	Thinking that you know how other people feel about you and why they act the way they do without their telling you.	Check out your perceptions. Ask people what they think or feel. Be direct. Look at the evidence you have to support your conclusion and the evidence that would be against your conclusion. What are some other logical explanations?	"I'm worried because it seems like you are angry with me. Is there any truth to what I'm saying?"
Catastrophi-zing	Expecting disaster. "What if I fail this exam? What if I don't have enough money to pay my tuition next semester?"	Make an honest assessment in terms of odds or percent of probability of the event happening. Realistically look at the chances of this happening. Take constructive steps using tasks within your control to prevent future problems instead of worrying about them.	"I have had only two C's all the time I've been in college. There is a very low likelihood that I will fail now, because I'm more interested and involved in my

continued

Table 10-4, continued

Pattern of Thinking	Characteristics of this Thought Pattern	A Better Way to Think	What to Say to Yourself and Others
			studies than I have ever been." "I can apply for a loan. Even though I don't want to be in debt, it will allow me to finish my education without the added stress of compromising my studies by working too much."
Shoulds	Working from a list of strict rules about how you and other people should act. People who break the rules make you angry and you feel guilty if you break the rules.	Question any rules or expectations that include the words *should, ought,* or *must*. Realize that all action comes from personal choice. Also, there is no prescribed way to feel about a particular situation. Think of exceptions to these rules that seem to run your life. Realize what your values and opinions are and what choices you are making in your life and don't impose them on others.	"I'm choosing to spend this Sunday afternoon with my friends rather than studying."
Being right	You must be right and prove that your actions are correct. Being wrong is not acceptable to you, and you will go to any length to demonstrate your correctness.	Actively listen to what others have to say. Participate in communication by repeating what you think you've heard to verify your understanding. Defuse the immediate situation. Agree to disagree with another person. Focus on what you can learn from the other person's perspective.	"I understand your point of view. I look at the situation differently."
Blaming	Holding others responsible for your problems, or turning blame inward as an indicator of failure.	No one can be at fault for the actions and choices you have made as a responsible adult. Identify the choices you have made that have created the situation you are now in. Look at the options you now have for coping with it.	"I chose to focus on other work during the first few weeks of the semester, which has allowed me to fall behind in my reading. I will focus the next few days on catching up."

Adapted with permission from McKay M, Davis M, Fanning P. *Thoughts and Feelings—The Art of Cognitive Stress Intervention.* Oakland, Calif: New Harbinger Publications; 1981:17-45.

PUTTING IT INTO PRACTICE

1. Automatic thoughts:

Think of your experiences in the past week. Make a notation of several times that you can recall that you have experienced an unpleasant emotion, self-doubt, or negative thought. Record the thoughts that you had at the time in the second column. Refer to Table 10-4. In the third column, change your focus and enter a more positive thought.

Situation	Thoughts at the Time	A Better Way to Think

2. Evaluate habits that may alleviate performance anxiety:

Do you sleep enough each night? If not, how can you arrange your schedule to decrease fatigue?

What improvements can you make to your nutrition and diet?

What is your regular exercise schedule? If less than three times weekly, make a plan to incorporate more exercise.

Are you working in a study group with others?

Are you planning study time into your daily schedule?

Do you have adequate social and emotional support?

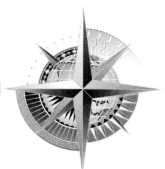

Chapter 11

Taking Control:
Self-Management Strategies

Anna looked at her daily planner and discovered that she had three written exams, two laboratory practical exams, and two papers due in the next week. She wondered, "Why don't these professors ever get together and realize that they are killing us off in this program?"

Student Role Stress

Over the years, research on the experience of physical therapy students indicates that student attitudes and behaviors are influenced by many sources of stress.[1-3] These include:

- Demanding schedule and limited time
- High workload and excessive course requirements
- High expectations of self and self-doubts
- Differing expectations of students and instructors
- Less than optimal learning environment
- Challenging student-instructor relationships
- Uncertainty in future career plans
- Financial concerns
- Unmet personal needs

Time Management

Your careful planning and budgeted use of time will be critical to your experience in physical therapy education. Skilled time managers use many effective routines (Table 11-1). There are a few strategies that students have found helpful to develop these skills.[4-6]

Spend Time Like Money—Carefully

- Realize that time is one of your most precious resources and that once it's gone, you can't have it back again. Make each moment count.
- Budget and schedule your time, including personal time for exercise, haircut, shopping, meditation, etc. Schedule that time on your calendar, treating it as you would any confirmed appointment.
- Use a "tickler file" to note important deadlines, dates, and events. Give yourself a reminder several weeks before important deadlines by writing them on the calendar. Also, write in birthdays and other personal events on your calendar. If you must do something once a year or every 6 months, make an appointment with yourself, just as the dentist does. Do not rely on your memory. There are many integrated online planners that will automatically notify you of

Table 11-1

ROUTINES OF GREAT TIME MANAGERS[4]

- Prepare a "to-do" list the night before.
- Be realistic about time allocations, including time for school, work, study, play, family, and personal matters, as well as regular time for yourself. Balance your life.
- Use a personal organizer (eg, Daytimer, Palm Pilot). You want to be able to access your schedule, telephone numbers, and key information easily. Write everything down in this one location. Keep it with you always.
- Schedule classes, study times, meetings, deadlines, and tasks in your organizer. Write them down. Do not rely on your memory. Write addresses and phone numbers in one location. Use post-it notes for one-time directions and information.
- Focus your energies on one thing at a time, for a specified period of time.
- Make yourself unavailable to others; avoid distractions.
- Change the way you do it. Organize yourself. Use a computer for tasks like banking and updating important records and addresses.
- Do it right the first time, rather than having to do and redo a task. However, be careful that you are not falling into a perfectionism trap.
- Avoid becoming side-tracked by more time-consuming details or by lower-priority requests that demand your time and talent.
- Finish what you start; there is much more satisfaction in knowing you have completed what you set out to do.
- Periodically review whether what you are doing is a good use of your time. If not, drop the activity and move onto the next scheduled task or project. Review your accomplishments at the end of the day.

upcoming events. These planners also allow you to synchronize this function with e-mail accounts, address books, calendars, and to-do lists. For example, take a look at the following website: http://planner.excite.com.

- By spending the time to organize a system, you will save more time later.

Prioritize on a Daily as Well as Long-Term Basis

- Not everything and everyone is equally important to your personal well-being.
- Determine essential information/skills you will need to succeed in the ways you spend the most time and make sure that you have access to this information (computer skills, automobile maps, library orientation). It takes less time to attend an orientation or training session than the countless hours you will spend later on trying to figure it out on your own.
- Plan and prioritize your schedule by the day, week, month, and year. Make prioritizing part of your daily routine.

Be Selective

- Spend less time on unimportant obligations and concentrate on people who really matter to you. Stop thinking that you need to know everything, be all things to all people, or absorb all the information that comes your way.
- While reading, write summarizing notes in the margins of the page or take simultaneous notes of major points and definitions. All of these activities (especially taking notes) help you to process and learn the material at the same time that you are reading it.

Learn to Say "No"

- This is a hard one for many students and practicing professionals. The habits that you develop now will stay with you throughout your life. Say yes only if you have the time or it is imperative that you become personally involved in the activity.
- Resist the urge to be a volunteer with multiple projects.

Reduce Your Standards

- Let go of perfectionism. Compromise with your-self and relax your standards on how you do things.
- Don't make it mandatory that you "know it all."
- Prioritize what is most important to know.
- Use others as resources.
- Function effectively and efficiently. Focus on the results rather than the method used to get there.

Delegate as Much as You Can

- It is often worth it to pay someone else to do it, if it will save you time. Also, it may be worth pay-ing an expert rather than spending your time learning how to do a task that can be completed in minutes by a trained person.
- Organize family members or roommates to divide household work.

Consolidate Similar Files, Things, Tasks, or Errands in One Location

- Keep class notes and projects organized in the same folder or location. Dedicate bookcase space, file drawer space, and an area of your home that will not be disturbed. It will save time in having to locate materials to begin studying.
- Organize materials in looseleaf notebooks while they are still active. Store materials from previ-ous courses in files.
- Organize computer files on separate labeled floppy disks, with a retrieval system that makes locating files easy. Back-up hard drive files on floppy disks or zip disks. If you revise a docu-ment, be sure that you save the revised file with a new date or name. Throw away all drafts when the project has been completed. Be sure to save the finished project with a name like "FINAL" and other identifying information.
- Avoid making several trips when you can do several errands in one trip, even if it means delaying action for several days. Consolidate phone calls to be returned in one sitting.

Confront Issues and Problems Early, Before They Compound

- Deal with problem people and events early on.
- Get help in courses, make appointments to talk

with faculty, and work out group project respon-sibilities at the first sign of trouble rather than waiting until the situation is irreconcilable. It will take far less time to deal with a problem in its early stages than to deal with a more serious situation.

Don't Waste Time Worrying

- Focus your energies on productive studying, constructive thoughts and discussion and review before exams.
- Cut negative thoughts off when you recognize them. Replace them with more positive images (see Table 10-4).

When You Make a Mistake, Don't Dwell on It

- Do not waste time feeling guilty about mistakes you made, things you did not do, or opportuni-ties that you let pass by.
- Try to remember that a mistake is another way to do things, no more. Avoid making the same mis-take **twice**.

Overcome Procrastination

- Make commitments for your time and stick to them.
- Do not offer excuses for why something is not done or accept that past habits are unchangeable.
- Be accountable for your time and efforts. Set deadlines and stick to them. Use the buddy sys-tem, in which a friend or colleague checks in with you to ask about your progress.
- Do a little on big projects every day. Do the worst first. Reward yourself at the end of a specific time you have spent by doing something more pleasurable. Be strict with yourself.

Make Meetings Count

- Always have an agenda and a defined objective for the meeting. Set a quitting time in advance. Keep the meeting on track if the subject wanders. Start and end on time.
- Move meetings along toward the assignment of tasks.
- Summarize decisions made, tasks assigned, and direction developed in writing, and distribute to all concerned after the meeting.

Remember That Working Hard is Not the Same as Working Smart

- Working smart involves delegation, project planning, finding new ways to do things, accepting help from others, and giving up perfectionism.
- Being "busy" is not an end in itself. Re-evaluate what you are actually accomplishing.

Financial Management

Cynthia had worked for 4 years as a health educator at a local community center. She had recently been promoted to the position of education coordinator for three centers in her district. Her job description included 30 hours per week of office work, some driving, and special events several times per month. She felt that her job would perfectly complement her physical therapy studies, and anyway, she was unwilling to give up her steady income now that she had worked her way up to an administrative position. Is this a realistic plan?

Just as you can plan for use of your time, you can plan for use of your financial resources. It is unlikely that you will have the time to work in a job that will provide for all of your school-related and living expenses. Review Chapter 4 regarding the investment that you are making and financial aid options.

Whether to Work

Many students wonder if, when, and how much they can work while in school. It is important to look carefully at how much your time is worth and whether working in a minimum wage job is a good use of your time. In addition, you must look carefully at what contacts, skills, and/or knowledge you are gaining and whether that exposure will benefit you in the long run.

For example, a physical therapy aide position in a physical therapy clinic may be quite beneficial in the long run, given the professional networks and exposure involved, even if the pay is low. An entry-level clerical position in a university office may not provide that same benefit for the same wage and time commitment.

Graduate Teaching and Research Assistantships

There are often opportunities for graduate students to receive tuition assistance in conjunction with responsibilities as a graduate, teaching, or research assistant. These opportunities often work out to benefit students; even though an hourly wage or stipend may be minimal, the combination of tuition assistance is an attractive package. Usually the work that you are doing is related to your educational objectives.

Time vs. Money

Your time may be more valuable devoted to succeeding in your studies. In Table 11-2, you can see that a student who works 15 hours per week and makes a wage of $10.00 per hour brings home less than $2000 each semester. It may be well worth taking out a loan for the same amount of money.

Budgeting

A budget is a planning tool that can both reveal problem spending areas and help fine-tune your cash flow. The mere process of gathering information to begin or maintain a budget can help you control your spending, quantify your needs for financial aid, and make plans to save, invest, or pay off debt.[7]

Basic Budget Guidelines

1. A monthly budget is often the most useful because some expenses and income items are paid less frequently; figure their annual or semi-annual amounts and then divide by 12. The goal is an estimated picture of your future cash flow.
2. List all of your income and expenses. Take a look at the budget categories in Table 11-3 to assist you.
3. As one of your regular expense items, you should include payments into a savings (or investment) account, otherwise known as paying yourself first. A good minimum savings goal is 10% of your gross income. The importance of this step cannot be stressed enough; given enough time, it can literally bring you financial independence or save you in an emergency.
4. Subtract expenses from income. You should have a positive amount remaining; this is your bottom line and cushion for unforeseen expenses. A negative bottom line is a sign that you need to work at reducing your expenses or increasing your income.

Listed in Table 11-4 are average percentages per general expense category. They are meant as guidelines and suggested maximums. Educational expenses are likely to account for 15% to 50% of a student's

Table 11-2
HOURLY WAGE CHART

Hourly Wage	Time Per Week (hours)	Semester Wages (15 weeks)	Sample Take-Home Pay*
$6.00	5	$450.00	$352.13
$6.00	10	$900.00	$704.25
$6.00	15	$1350.00	$1056.38
$7.00	5	$525.00	$410.81
$7.00	10	$1050.00	$821.63
$7.00	15	$1575.00	$1232.44
$8.00	5	$600.00	$469.50
$8.00	10	$1200.00	$939.00
$8.00	15	$1800.00	$1408.50
$9.00	5	$675.00	$528.19
$9.00	10	$1350.00	$1056.38
$9.00	15	$2025.00	$1584.56
$10.00	5	$750.00	$586.88
$10.00	10	$1500.00	$1173.75
$10.00	15	$2250.00	$1760.63

*Less FICA at 6.75% and federal taxes at 15%

Table 11-3
SAMPLE BUDGET

Expenses	Monthly	Annual	Percent of Total Income
Rent	$500.00	$6000.00	21%
Insurance	$75.00	$900.00	3%
Savings	$50.00	$600.00	2%
Tuition	$1000.00	$12,000.00	42%
Books	$83.33	$1000.00	3%
Food and beverages	$300.00	$3600.00	13%
Household operations and maintenance	$50.00	$600.00	2%
Furnishings and equipment	$50.00	$600.00	2%
Clothing	$50.00	$600.00	2%
Personal allowance	$50.00	$600.00	2%
Transportation	$50.00	$600.00	2%
Medical care	$20.00	$240.00	1%
Recreation, entertainment	$50.00	$600.00	2%
Contributions, donations	$8.33	$100.00	0.3%
Credit card payments	$30.00	$360.00	1%
Other	$10.00	$120.00	0.4%
Total expenses	$2376.67	$28,520.00	100%
Income			
Salary (after taxes)	$468.17	$5618.00	20%
Scholarships	$166.67	$2000.00	7%
Loans	$833.33	$10,000.00	35%
Graduate Assistantship	$916.67	$11,000.00	38%
Total Income	$2384.83	$28,618.00	100%
Income less expenses	$8.17	$98.00	

Table 11-4
RECOMMENDED BUDGET ALLOCATIONS[7]

Budget Category	Recommended Average Percentage of Gross Income
Housing + utilities	25% to 40%
Taxes	20%
Transportation and related costs	15%
Food	10%
Clothing	5%
Savings	10% and up
Entertainment + vacations	5%
Debt (credit cards, personal loans)	5%
Other expenses	5% and up

For an easy online home budget system go to: http://www.smilebuilder.com/budgetsheet.htm

Reprinted from http://www.smilebuilder.com/budget.htm

budget. Realistically, few students can absorb these expenses without making compromises in other areas.

Support Systems

Students often encounter barriers that can become a source of frustration, confusion, and disappointment. A strong support system serves as a powerful mediator of the stress involved in an intensive professional education system. Your family and friends can certainly provide emotional support and encouragement. They may also provide a welcome relief from the rigors of studying, writing papers, and practicing clinical techniques.

Peer Support

Peer support involves sharing experiences and reactions with those who have had or are having common experiences. Peer support can provide valuable mediation of stress experienced during the educational process and later during the transition from school to work.[8,9]

During your professional education experience, you will have opportunities to both receive and give support. It is important that you realize how powerful your support of your colleagues is in going through this process together.

Peer Support Involves:

- Discussing feelings about similar experiences and emotions
- Validating goals
- Sharing information, tips, and resources
- Participating in social and recreational activities
- Empowering your colleagues to take effective action
- Practicing skills
- Collaborating on projects

This does not mean complaining and griping with your friends. It involves listening and acknowledging the feelings and beliefs and relating your own experiences.

Providing Support Involves:

- *Empathy:* the peer supporter's understanding of the other person's feelings, experiences, and goals, and knowing how to correctly communicate this understanding to the other person(s). Being caring, sensitive, and responsive are basic in establishing a supportive relationship.
- *Respect:* the peer supporter's respect for the experience and feelings of the other person.
- *Sincerity:* the peer supporter's honesty and genuineness.
- *Trustworthiness:* a peer supporter's honesty, willingness to maintain confidentiality, and consistency.

- *Self-disclosure:* the peer supporter relates his or her own experiences and feelings.

Take Action

The Buddy System

Having a "buddy," "peer mentor," "big sister," or "big brother" is the way that many educational programs arrange for a peer support relationship to develop. If a program exists in your university, use it. If not, you may want to suggest developing one.

Rest and Relaxation

Even though the demands of the professional program are great, you can relax occasionally and participate in social activities with your classmates and future colleagues. Identifying a class "social chair" is often a way to formalize regular social events outside of class. Again, scheduling social events is as important as scheduling your exercise commitments and personal priorities.

Celebrate!

Many landmark events occur during the educational process. Important exams, first clinical experiences, papers, projects, and presentations are just a few examples. It is important to celebrate your achievements during the process and acknowledge and recognize the positive accomplishments of your classmates.

Involve Significant Others

Significant others, the people who are closest to you, are critical to your support and wellbeing while going through the program, yet they are often left out due to the tremendous demands that the professional education program places on your time, effort, and attention. Keep significant others involved as much as possible and help them to know how they can best support you.

Keep the Memories Forever

Photos, videos, and other records of the time your class has spent together will solidify the supportive experience and provide a long-lasting memory of the time you spent in your educational program. Appoint a class photographer or class historian to spearhead this effort.

Summary

Students face many sources of stress and uncertainty during the educational process. Time management, financial management, and peer support strategies are valuable and proven ways to gain a sense of control over the sometimes overwhelming demands of the educational program.

References

1. O'Meara S, Kostas T, Markland F, Previty J. Perceived academic stress in physical therapy students. *Journal of Physical Therapy Education.* 1994;8:71-75.
2. Hayward LM, Noonan AC, Shain D. Qualitative case study of physical therapist students' attitudes, motivations, and affective behaviors. *J Allied Health.* 1999;28(3):155-164.
3. Graham C, Babola K. Needs assessment of non-traditional students in physical and occupational therapy. *J Allied Health.* 1998;27(4):196-201.
4. Curtis KA. *PH TH 120 Professional Orientation.* Fresno, Calif; California State University; 1999.
5. Culp S. *Streamlining Your Life—5-point Plan for Uncomplicated Living.* Cincinnati, Ohio: Writer's Digest Books; 1991.
6. Pollar, O. *Organizing Your Workspace—A Guide to Personal Productivity.* Menlo Park, Calif: Crisp Publications, 1992.
7. Financial Planning. *The Importance of a Budget.* Webpage available at: http://www.smilebuilder.com/budget.htm. Accessed July 30, 2000.
8. Lees S, Ellis N. The design of a stress-management program for nursing personnel. *J Adv Nurs.* 1990;15(8):946-961.
9. Curtis KA. Survival training for clinical practice. *Rehab Management.* 1991;4(2):78-79.

PUTTING IT INTO PRACTICE

1.   Evaluate your personal habits in regard to time management. What changes can you make in each of the following areas that will save you time?

Time-Management Strategy	Ideas for Improvement
Writing a daily to-do list	
Keeping a current appointment book with addresses and phone numbers	
Scheduling sufficient time for personal needs, study, and exercise	
Doing things well the first time, so that they don't have to be done over again	
Lowering standards of perfectionism	
Taking notes while you are reading assignments	
Saying no	
Delegating tasks to others	
Organizing work space and study materials	
Addressing high priority tasks first	
Using an agenda for all meetings	

2.   Access the following financial planning website: http://www.smilebuilder.com/budgetsheet.htm Create a personal home budget following the guidelines presented.

3.   Evaluate your support network. How can you improve your support to others? How can you improve the support available to you?

Your Support Network	Examples of Support
To whom do you give support?	
From whom do you receive support?	
From whom do you request support?	

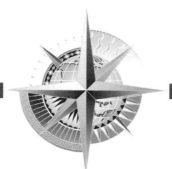

Chapter 12

Legal And Ethical Considerations For Physical Therapy Students

Lina sat in her Professional Foundations course and listened to the lecturer. She was surprised to hear that it was both illegal and unethical for physicians to supervise aides who provided physical therapy treatment in the clinic. The outpatient work injury center in which she worked for several years prior to her admission to the physical therapy program had a physical therapist on the premises only 2 days a week. Physicians, therefore, directed and supervised all physical therapy treatment activities. She wondered why they didn't know that this was illegal.

Laws, Regulations, and Ethics

There are many types of *legal* and *regulatory* influences that control health care practice. Their interpretation is usually through judicial bodies, review boards, and similar mechanisms.

In contrast, *ethical standards* deal with conduct and moral choices, which arise from professions, society, religion, and culture. Ethical dilemmas are usually resolved on the individual level.

Laws

There are four sources of *law* in the United States:[1]
1. Constitutional law. The US Constitution guarantees personal rights and liberties in the *Bill of Rights*. In general, these laws take precedence over all other laws and regulations.

2. Statutory law. *Statutes* are laws that are established through legislation at either the state or federal level. For example, physical therapy practice acts are state laws; every state's practice act is different.

3. Common law. *Common laws* are derived from judicial decisions that create legal precedent in areas that are not covered by previously enacted statutes. Previous cases provide the basis for common laws.

4. Administrative law. Administrative agencies are authorized by executive and legislative branches of government to establish and enforce *administrative law*, the rules and regulations that govern many of the daily activities of health care professionals. For example, the Centers for Medicare and Medicaid Services (CMS) is charged with establishing the regulations by which the Medicare system is administered.

Private Regulatory Authorities

In addition to the four sources of laws, private agencies such as the Joint Commission on Accreditation of Healthcare Organizations (JCAHO), establish standards to which member organizations subscribe. The American Physical Therapy Association (APTA) defines *Standards of Practice* (see Appendix D), which are acceptable standards for delivering physical therapy services. Institutional policies and procedures almost always reflect the

Table 12-1
ETHICAL PRINCIPLES AND TERMINOLOGY[4,5]

Term	Definition
Nonmaleficence	To do no harm (even if we cannot do good)
Beneficence	To promote good
Justice	To distribute benefits and burdens fairly
Autonomy	To make one's own choices
Veracity	To speak and act truthfully
Fidelity	To keep promises and commitments
Informed consent	To present benefits and risks of planned interventions to patients
Duty	Obligations that an individual has to society
Confidentiality	Keeping sensitive patient information in confidence
Paternalism	Failure to respect the autonomy of another person

standards of the regulatory agencies that monitor their service delivery.

Third-Party Payers

The organizations that provide reimbursement for health insurance plans often establish standards that require health care providers to practice in specified ways. A third-party payer creates and enforces *policy* that governs the operation of the organization. For example, third-party payers publish forms requiring specific types of information. Although this is not a statute, it is required if the provider wants payment for his or her services from the third-party payer.

Code of Ethics

Professions establish their own codes of conduct, called a *code of ethics.* You will recall from Chapter 1 that this is one of the criteria that defines a profession. Codes of ethics are specific to the particular discipline governed by the code and are enforced by the profession. A code of ethics serves several purposes described below.[2,3]

Standards for Behavior

A code of ethics provides standards for professional behavior. For example, Principle 2 of the code of ethics adopted by the APTA states: "Physical therapists comply with the laws and regulations governing the practice of physical therapy."

Protection of the Public

A code of ethics provides mechanisms for the protection of patients, clients, their families, and the public. See if you can find a principle in the APTA

Code of Ethics that protects the rights of recipients of physical therapy services.

Each of the principles in a code of ethics represents one or more of the ethical principles in Table 12-1.

APTA Code of Ethics

The APTA has jurisdiction over 70,000 member physical therapists and physical therapist assistants. The APTA *Code of Ethics* and accompanying *Guide for Professional Conduct* (Appendix B) protects the rights of patients and clients, establishes standards for professional autonomy, defines standards for professional review and reimbursement for services, and outlines professional responsibilities for members of this organization. In addition, there are disciplinary processes to submit complaints of suspected ethical violations by association members.

State Physical Therapy Practice Act

Each state has jurisdiction over the definition and legal requirements for practicing physical therapy in the state. Although all state practice acts differ, the *Model Definition of Physical Therapy for State Practice Acts* (Appendix A) provides a standard for the definition of physical therapy.

Physical Therapy:[6,7] Physical therapy is the care and services provided by and under the direction of a physical therapist.

Licensure

A physical therapist must apply for licensure in each state in which he or she will practice. Each state practice act differs. Some states do not allow practice by qualified physical therapist license applicants (new graduate physical therapists) until they have taken and passed the state licensure examination and received a license to practice. Some states offer temporary licenses, and other states define the role of a physical therapist license applicant. An online directory to state practice acts is available at: http://www.apta.org/advocacy/state/state_practice

Each of the 50 states, the District of Columbia, Puerto Rico, and the US Virgin Islands have specific requirements for licensure of physical therapists. The following website provides links to each of these 53 licensing boards:

http://www.fsbpt.org/directory.cfm

Direct Access

Direct access to physical therapy (without requiring a referral from another health care provider) is another professional practice issue that is governed by state law.

> **Direct Access:**[8] The right of the public to directly access physical therapists for evaluation, examination, and intervention. The public is best served when access is unrestricted.

Direct access to physical therapy services, physical therapist evaluation, examination, and intervention varies from state to state. In 33 states, the public may directly access physical therapists' services.

The state statutes governing direct access to physical therapy services can be classified into two categories: *omission* and *provisions*. Omission means that no referral language exists in state statute. Provision means that the public may access physical therapists in a defined manner, which may include stipulations regarding a time frame, therapist years of experience, and the nature of the patient's problems.[8]

Of these 33 states, 14 states have direct access by omission, and 19 states have direct access under provisions.[8] Download the following: http://www.apta.org/pdfs/gov_affairs/directalaws.pdf for a listing of states and check in which category your state falls.

Roles of Physical Therapy Personnel

In addition to governing the access to physical therapy, state practice acts govern the supervisory requirements of physical therapy personnel. State

---

Ellen, a licensed physical therapist in California, was delayed arriving at the office following a corporate breakfast meeting. Jeff and Sam, physical therapy aides in her private office, greeted the first patients of the day and started the patients' treatments, having them begin their therapeutic exercise programs by warming up on the treadmill in the gymnasium. Are they in violation of state law? (Check Table 12-2 to read the excerpt of the California State Practice Act that applies and make an interpretation.)

---

practice acts often define the roles of physical therapists in the supervision of physical therapist assistants, physical therapy aides, physical therapy students, and physical therapy license applicants.

Take a look at how the state law illustrated in Table 12-2 defines the number of aides allowed and nature of supervision required for a physical therapy aide.

If you answered yes to the question in the box you are absolutely correct. They are in violation of state law. There are several issues involved in this case.

First, by state law, only one aide may be engaged in patient-related tasks and under Ellen's supervision. This may already be a violation in that two aides are employed and work simultaneously. Only one may provide patient-related services under Ellen's immediate supervision.

Second, the law states that "the aide shall at all times be under the orders, direction, and immediate supervision of the physical therapist. Nothing in this section shall authorize an aide to independently perform physical therapy or any physical therapy procedure."

Finally, the law states that "the aide must be supervised by a physical therapist in the same facility as, and in proximity to, the location where the aide is performing patient-related tasks, and shall be readily available at all times to provide advice or instruction to the aide." Ellen is not in the facility. They may prepare the patients for treatment by taking them to a treatment room or prepare the treatment area before Ellen returns to the clinic, but they may not initiate treatment.

APTA Standards of Practice

The *Standards of Practice for Physical Therapy* is a document published by the APTA that defines the conditions and performance that are essential for high-quality physical therapy. The *Standards* cover conduct in compliance with legal and ethical guidelines, expectations of physical therapist role, scope of responsibilities, and administration of physical ther-

Table 12-2
SAMPLE EXCERPT FROM STATE PRACTICE ACT[9]

California Codes
Business and Professions Code
Section 2630-2640

2630. It is unlawful for any person or persons to practice, or offer to practice, physical therapy in this state for compensation received or expected, or to hold himself or herself out as a physical therapist, unless at the time of so doing the person holds a valid, unexpired, and unrevoked license issued under this chapter. Nothing in this section shall restrict the activities authorized by their licenses on the part of any persons licensed under this code or any initiative act, or the activities authorized to be performed pursuant to Article 4.5 (commencing with Section 2655) or Chapter 7.7 (commencing with Section 3500). A physical therapist licensed pursuant to this chapter may utilize the services of one aide engaged in patient-related tasks to assist the physical therapist in his or her practice of physical therapy. "Patient-related task" means a physical therapy service rendered directly to the patient by an aide, excluding nonpatient-related tasks. "Nonpatient-related task" means a task related to observation of the patient, transport of the patient, physical support only during gait or transfer training, housekeeping duties, clerical duties, and similar functions. The aide shall at all times be under the orders, direction, and immediate supervision of the physical therapist. Nothing in this section shall authorize an aide to independently perform physical therapy or any physical therapy procedure. The board shall adopt regulations that set forth the standards and requirements for the orders, direction, and immediate supervision of an aide by a physical therapist. The physical therapist shall provide continuous and immediate supervision of the aide.

The physical therapist shall be in the same facility as, and in proximity to, the location where the aide is performing patient-related tasks, and shall be readily available at all times to provide advice or instruction to the aide. When patient-related tasks are provided to a patient by an aide, the supervising physical therapist shall, at some point during the treatment day, provide direct service to the patient as treatment for the patient's condition, or to further evaluate and monitor the patient's progress, and shall correspondingly document the patient's record.

Reprinted from the State of California, Department of Consumer Affairs, Physical Therapy Board.

apy service delivery. Take a few moments to review the *Standards of Practice for Physical Therapy* in Appendix D.

Legal and Ethical Issues for Physical Therapy Students

Responsibilities as a Student Physical Therapist

The actions of student physical therapists and student physical therapist assistants are regulated by state law, the *Code of Ethics*, the *Guide for Professional Conduct*, and the Guide *for the Conduct of the Affiliate Member.*

Student Rights

The rights of students are protected under many federal and state laws. Educational institutions must establish policies to address the provisions of federal and state legislation that influence many aspects of university programs and operations. The university must also provide information regarding channels to pursue for inquiries and complaints.

There may also be specific university regulations that reflect laws requiring health immunizations and screening tests, such as rubella and measles immunizations. Following are some of these laws.

Student Privacy in Education Records

The federal Family Educational Rights and Privacy Act of 1974 established requirements designed to protect the privacy of students concerning their education records maintained by universities. This statute governs access to student records maintained by an educational institution and the terms for release of such records. The law requires that the institution must provide students access to records directly related to the student and an opportunity for a hearing to challenge such records on the grounds that they are inaccurate, misleading, or otherwise inappropriate. The law also requires the conditions under which written consent of the student be received before releasing personally identifiable data about the student. The law provides that the university is authorized to provide access to student records to campus officials, employees, and related agencies and organizations that have legitimate educational interests in such access. The policies of individual institutions should reflect compliance with this legislation.

Nondiscrimination

Gender

Title IX of the Education Amendments of 1972 and related amendments to administrative regulations prohibit discrimination on the basis of gender in education programs and activities of a university. This legislation provides equal opportunities to male and female students in all campus programs, including intercollegiate athletics.

Sexual Harassment

In addition, Title VII of the Civil Rights Act also prohibits discrimination on the basis of sex. Sexual harassment violates Section 703 of Title VII. *Sexual harassment* is defined as "the unwanted imposition of sexual attention usually in the context of a relationship of unequal power, rank, or status, as well as the use of one's position of authority in the university to bestow benefits or impose deprivations on another. Harassment can include verbal, nonverbal, and/or physical conduct that has the intent or effect of unreasonable interference with individuals' or groups' education or work performance. This may also include actions that create an intimidating, hostile, or offensive working or learning environment. Both men and women can be the victims of sexual harassment."[10]

Disability

Section 504 of the Rehabilitation Act of 1973 and related amendments and regulations and the Americans with Disabilities Act (1990) prohibit discrimination on the basis of disability in admission or access to, or treatment or employment in, a university's programs and activities. See Chapter 13 for a more detailed discussion of student rights related to disabilities.

Equal Opportunity

Most institutions publish policies regarding their commitment to equal opportunity for all, regardless of race, color, national origin, gender, age, marital status, religion, disability, or sexual preference. The provisions of Title VI of the Civil Rights Act of 1964 and the Americans with Disabilities Act address equal opportunity in employment, admissions, recruitment, financial aid, placement counseling, curricula, and housing for students.

Student Misconduct and Disciplinary Action

Sean was not a "morning person." It was difficult for him to arrive on time for his 7:30 class. In the previous class, the instructor reminded the students to review the syllabus regarding late arrivals and said that he would be closing and locking the classroom door promptly at 7:30 am so that the students in class would not be interrupted by latecomers. Sean arrived at 7:40 and saw the classroom door was closed. He knocked on the door softly. There was no response. He began to pound on the door, shouting, "Open this door! I've paid money for this class!" The instructor inside the classroom called the university police and reported that Sean was disturbing the class in session. Sean had no idea that this was student misconduct. The faculty of the physical therapy program had serious concerns about Sean's judgment and recommended that the university place him on probation.

Universities publish policies regarding student conduct. Student misconduct, on or off campus, involving any of the following activities might result in university expulsion, suspension or probation, in addition to consequences of violating state and local laws.

- Cheating and plagiarism
- Forgery or alteration of documents
- Misrepresentation or providing misinformation
- Obstructive or disruptive behavior
- Physical abuse or the threat of physical abuse
- Theft or nonaccidental destruction of property
- Unauthorized entry or use of campus property
- Sale or possession of drugs except under specific medical or research purposes

- Possession of explosives, dangerous chemicals, or deadly weapons
- Lewd, indecent, or obscene behavior on campus
- Abusive behavior toward another or hazing

The university catalog is a good place to look for a list of policies. Students in professional education programs such as physical therapy are subject to the regulations and disciplinary actions that apply to all students in the university.

Cheating, Plagiarism, and Copyright Infringement

> MaryAnne and Jerry had become good friends during their first semester. They often studied together. When they were faced with writing up their first patient case study, they worried about what to write. A student from the previous year's class gave them a model paper that the instructor had given to students the year before. They copied the goals and wrote an intervention, sampling liberally from the excellent examples on the model paper. Each student submitted the same paper, with only a different cover sheet. The instructor returned the papers a week later. They each received a zero on their paper and a note to meet with the course instructor after class. They were shocked when the instructor explained that they had cheated and this would be noted in their student record.

Professional education students must be specifically aware of issues involving academic dishonesty in actions such as cheating, plagiarism, and copyright infringement.

Cheating

Cheating occurs when students use fraudulent or deceptive means to improve a grade, obtain course credit, or gain an unearned academic advantage.[10] When in doubt, ask faculty members. Receiving old exams from members of last year's class without the professor's knowledge is cheating. Misrepresenting clinical experience on an evaluation form is cheating.

Do not tolerate cheating of any kind in academic or clinical education. Remember that ultimately, students who cheat are cheating the public, patients, and clients (ie, the consumers who will rely on their care and the profession that they are entering).

Plagiarism

Plagiarism is a serious form of academic fraud when one misrepresents work of another, whether published or unpublished, as one's own work.[11] This may involve such obvious acts as downloading term papers from the Internet, to more subtle forms of plagiarism such as using phrases of other authors without proper citation. Students sometimes do not understand that they can also plagiarize themselves by turning in work done for one class as original work for a subsequent class. To avoid plagiarism, always cite your sources.

Copyright Infringement

> Karen was concerned about the high cost of books. One book that was required for her administration class cost $25.00 and was only 300 pages long. She thought, "I could photocopy this book for only $15.00 at the office supply store that advertises photocopies for 5 cents." She thought further, "I could even make a little money if I charged my classmates $20.00 per book. That would still be better than paying the bookstore's prices."

Copyright infringement is a form of theft. Copyrights are protected by the US Constitution and by the Federal Copyright Statute; these protect the literary works in addition to artistic works, sound recordings, and computer software.[12] Copying a book, illustration, videotape or portion of a videotape, a published graph, cartoon, photograph, computer program, or sound recording without permission are all examples of copyright infringement. Be careful—even copying a photograph from an Internet site into a PowerPoint presentation is a copyright infringement. Charging admission to view a rented videotape or taped sports presentation without paying royalties is also a violation.

It is important to understand that copyrights are property rights of the author, which may be sold or transferred to another entity such as a publisher. Authors or those to whom they have transferred their copyrights hold the rights to copy, create new works, distribute, and display their works. To avoid copyright infringement, make sure that you have permission to use the work of the author.[12] Write to the author or publisher and request permission. Be aware that although many authors are happy to share their work for educational purposes, some authors and their publishers ask for a fee. You have the choice to pay the fee or not use the material. See samples of letters requesting permission to use copyrighted materials in Tables 12-3 and 12-4.

Fair Use

Libraries and copy centers can advise you regarding policies for "fair use" of copyrighted materials

Table 12-3

SAMPLE COPYRIGHT PERMISSION REQUEST

Student Name_____
Address_____
City, State, Zip Code_____

April 25, 2001

SLACK Incorporated
Attn: Permissions
6900 Grove Road
Thorofare, NJ 08086

To Whom It May Concern:

I am writing to request your permission to include the material described below in a manuscript entitled "Developing Patient Education Materials in Physical Therapy," as part of the requirements for a course in my graduate education program.

I would like to reproduce three tables relating to readability of written patient education materials from one of your publications, Johnson, *Patient Education and Practice*, 2nd Edition. The material I would like to have permission to reproduce is:

p. 51 Table 1. Sample Material
p. 52 Table 2. Gunning Fog Index Scale
p. 53 Table 3. Flesch Formula

Please advise as to whether reproduction of this material will be permitted. I will give full credit to the author and original source. If there is an additional source that I must contact for permission to use the above material, I would appreciate any information you can forward to me.

If I can answer any questions, you can reach me at (phone) or by e-mail at (e-mail address).

I will look forward to hearing from you.

Sincerely,

Student Name
Graduate Student or Student Physical Therapist
(Name of Physical Therapist Professional Education Program)
(Educational Institution)

Attachments: pp51-53, Johnson, *Patient Education and Practice*, 2nd Edition

Table 12-4

SAMPLE COPYRIGHT PERMISSION REQUEST (ONLINE MATERIALS)

Date: Fri, 28 Jul 2000 11:52:46 -0700
To: Publisher/Author or Webmaster (look for this link at bottom of a site's homepage)
           webmaster@domain.com
From: (your email address)
Subject: Permission to reproduce materials from your site
Cc: (include your faculty advisor here)

I am a graduate student at (university) studying physical therapy. I am doing a presentation on shoulder pathologies for my class, *Advanced Concepts in Orthopedic Management*, and found the diagrams on your website to be perfect.

I would like your permission to electronically reproduce this graphic and use it in a PowerPoint presentation. The material I would like to have permission to use is Histology Atlas, Shoulder Joint at the following URL: http://www.sru.edu/depts/pt/histo/shoulder1.htm

Please advise as to whether reproduction of this material will be permitted. If there is an additional source that I must contact for permission to use the above material, I would appreciate any information you can forward to me.

If I can answer any questions, you can reach me at (phone) or by e-mail at (e-mail address).

I will look forward to hearing from you.

Sincerely,

Student Name,
Graduate Student or Student Physical Therapist
(Name of Physical Therapist Professional Education Program)
(Educational Institution)

(Attach the material to the e-mail)

---

for educational and research purposes. An excellent resource on fair use exists online at http://www.fairuse.stanford.edu/

Remember, when in doubt, ask! Avoid academic dishonesty!

To avoid plagiarism, always cite your sources. To avoid copyright infringement, make sure that you have permission to use the work of the author.

Research on Human Subjects

The rights of subjects in research studies conducted by faculty, staff, and students at academic institutions are well-protected. Each institution must establish standards for the conduct of research that employs or influences humans and/or animals. All research at the university must comply with these provisions. Students should familiarize themselves with the provisions for the protection of human subjects before they undertake any research efforts as part of the academic curriculum.

Informed Consent

Students must be clear in identifying themselves as students or interns when working with patients or clients in academic, clinical, or research situations. They must also be aware that the patient or research subject has the right to refuse participation and that they must respect that right. Inform appropriate clinical or academic faculty and research principal investigators if a patient, client, or subject does not want to participate or does not want to work with a student. Do not take it personally.

Supervision During Clinical Education Experiences

Students enroll in university courses that may encompass clinical training, cooperative education, and service learning. Physical therapy students may practice the techniques and decision-making activities they are learning as part of their education while enrolled in such university courses, in compliance with state laws governing the practice of physical therapy and supervision of student physical therapists.

Regardless of the type of course, physical therapy students enrolled in university courses require the *continuous onsite supervision* of the supervising physical therapist. This means that the student cannot provide care in a single therapist clinic if the therapist is out for lunch or at a conference offsite. Similarly, the student may not visit a patient in the home to provide physical therapy services, unless supervised onsite by the physical therapist.

In summary, to provide patient-related physical therapy services, physical therapy students enrolled in university courses require the continuous onsite supervision of a supervising academic or clinical faculty member who must be a licensed physical therapist. A supervising physical therapist cannot transfer this responsibility to a physical therapist assistant, physician, or other health care provider, even for a few hours.

Student Employment Situations

Many students work in clinics on a part-time basis during school or during the summer months. Students must remember that their status as physical therapy students only extends to those situations in which they are enrolled in a university course and

the clinical staff provides instruction (and appropriate supervision) for this course.

For all other situations, unless students already hold a state license as a physical therapist assistant or other licensed health professional, they are *unlicensed personnel*, usually functioning in the capacity of a physical therapy aide, personal care attendant, or personal trainer. Be careful that you are not practicing physical therapy without a license. Know your state laws!

In addition, there are always potential violations of the APTA *Code of Ethics* and *Standards of Practice* inherent in these types of employment situations.

Working as a Physical Therapy Aide

Physical therapy aides are nonlicensed support personnel who are trained under the direction and supervision of a physical therapist. They do not independently deliver physical therapy services in any setting. Physical therapy aides do not perform evaluations, determine what they should do with a patient or client, or perform techniques that require clinical decision-making or clinical problem-solving. They do not make judgments or clinical decisions. Aides may function only with the continuous onsite supervision by the physical therapist, or in some states, by the physical therapist assistant. Chiropractors and physicians may not provide supervision for physical therapy aides who provide patient-related physical therapy services.

This means that physical therapy aides, who also happen to be physical therapy students, may not perform the evaluation and clinical decision-making activities they are learning as part of their education at any point in their education, unless it is as a part of their enrollment in a university course or university-supervised activity. Students should be wary of inadvertently practicing physical therapy without a license.

Providing Attendant Care or Home Exercise Programs

Some students also work as personal care attendants for persons with disabilities. Personal care attendants (PCAs) are unlicensed personnel as well, usually hired directly by a person who needs such services. The same issues may arise in providing personal attendant care because students can easily overstep their legal boundaries.

When a family or person with a disability hires a physical therapy student to carry out a home exercise program or personal care routine, the student must be very careful that the program was established by a licensed health care provider or professional staff caring for the patient. The PCA should carry out a program of care that could be performed by anyone. It is not the role of the PCA to make clinical judgments, modify, or progress the program. The student should be careful to refer the patient or client back to licensed health care providers for any problems or alterations to the care program.

Providing Personal Training in Health Clubs or Fitness Facilities

Students who provide consultation or advice regarding weight training or fitness must also exercise caution. Performing strength and flexibility assessments, setting training goals, and providing exercise interventions to address client needs is *not* physical therapy.

Further, personal trainers are not physical therapists and may not use the initials, "PT." Students who work as personal trainers must be very clear to disclose their limitations and role in working with clients. Practicing physical therapy without a license is a violation of state law. Be sure that you are not in violation of state law, ethical, and other published professional guidelines.

You be the judge of the following situation:

> *Joe S. responded to an advertisement in his local newspaper stating, "Busy physical therapy practice seeks physical therapy aide for afternoon and evening hours."*
>
> *He interviewed, and the employer was delighted to find out that he was a physical therapy student only months away from his graduation in the DPT program. The employer gave him his own caseload and put two new evaluations on his schedule for the next afternoon. Joe was elated at first but then wondered, "Am I practicing physical therapy without a license?" What do you think?*

When enrolled in an academic or clinical course, students are able to function with direct and immediate supervision of clinical faculty and perform tasks that are indicated by their level of education and the objectives of the clinical experience.

In employment situations in the physical therapy field while in school, unless the student holds a current state license to practice as a physical therapist or physical therapist assistant or holds another type of license, the student is restricted to a role as a physical therapy aide regardless of knowledge or skills acquired in academic or clinical courses.

Therefore, Joe should not agree to perform functions that clearly go well beyond the scope of duties of a physical therapy aide.

After Graduation

In some states, a new graduate physical therapist may work in a special status as a *physical therapist license applicant* (PTLA) or under a *temporary license* only after the requirements of licensure have been met and an application has been filed. In most cases, the PTLA or temporary licensure status is valid only until the first opportunity to take the state licensing examination. Other states do not permit practice until the license has actually been received. Most states have strict supervision requirements for personnel in this status. It is important to know the regulations of your state.

Summary

Students must be aware of ethical and legal issues involved in academic/clinical education and part-time employment situations. Federal and state laws, professional codes of ethics, and other practice guidelines must become part of the working knowledge of the physical therapy student.

References

1. Scott RW. *Promoting Legal Awareness in Physical and Occupational Therapy*. St. Louis, Mo: Mosby; 1997.
2. Scott R. *Professional Ethics: A Guide for Rehabilitation Professionals*. St. Louis, Mo: Mosby; 1998.
3. Swisher LL, Krueger-Brophy C. *Legal and Ethical Issues in Physical Therapy*. Boston, Mass: Butterworth Heinemann; 1998.
4. Kornblau BL, Starling SP. *Ethics in Rehabilitation. A Clinical Perspective*. Thorofare, NJ: SLACK Incorporated; 2000.
5. Purtilo R. *Ethical Dimensions in the Health Professions*. 3rd ed. Philadelphia, Pa: WB Saunders Co; 1999.
6. APTA. *Guide to Physical Therapist Practice*. Alexandria, Va: American Physical Therapy Association; 1999.
7. Guide to physical therapist practice: Revisions. *PT Magazine of Physical Therapy*. 1999;7(9):46-50.
8. APTA. *Direct access webpage*. Available at: http://www.apta.org/Advocacy/state/directaccess/State3. Accessed July 30, 2000.
9. Physical Therapy Practice Act, State of California Department of Consumer Affairs. *Business and Professions Code Section 2630-2640 webpage*. Available at: http://www.leginfo.ca.gov/cgi-bin/displaycode?section=bpc&group=02001-03000&file=2630-2640. Accessed July 30, 2000.

10. California State University, Fresno General Catalog 2000-2001. *Policies and Regulations website*. Available at: http://www.catalog.admin.csufresno.edu/current/policies.html. Accessed July 30, 2000.

11. University of Indiana Writing Resources. *Plagiarism. What it is and how to avoid it webpage*. Available at: http://www.indiana.edu/~wts/wts/plagiarism.html. Accessed July 30, 2000.

12. Stanford University Libraries. *Copyright and Fair Use webpage*. Available at: http://fairuse.stanford.edu. Accessed July 30, 2000.

PUTTING IT INTO PRACTICE

1. Using the ethical principles in Table 12-1, identify which of these principles are represented in each of the principles in the APTA *Code of Ethics* and *Guide for Professional Conduct* (Appendix B).

Term	Definition
Nonmaleficence	To do no harm (even if we cannot do good)
Beneficence	To promote good
Justice	To distribute benefits and burdens fairly
Autonomy	To make one's own choices
Veracity	To speak and act truthfully
Fidelity	To keep promises and commitments
Informed consent	To present benefits and risks of planned interventions to patients
Duty	Obligations that an individual has to society
Confidentiality	Keeping sensitive patient information in confidence
Paternalism	Failure to respect the autonomy of another person

Cite particular aspects of the *Guide for Professional Conduct* that apply.

Ethical Principle(s)	Principles/APTA Code of Ethics
	1. Physical therapists respect the rights and dignity of all individuals.
	2. Physical therapists comply with the laws and regulations governing the practice of physical therapy.
	3. Physical therapists accept responsibility for the exercise of sound judgment.
	4. Physical therapists maintain and promote high standards for physical therapy practice, education, and research.
	5. Physical therapists seek remuneration for their services that is deserved and reasonable.
	6. Physical therapists provide accurate information to the consumer about the profession and about those services they provide.
	7. Physical therapists accept the responsibility to protect the public and the profession from unethical, incompetent, or illegal acts.
	8. Physical therapists participate in efforts to address the health needs of the public.

2. Of these 33 states that have direct access to physical therapy, 14 states have direct access by omission, and 19 states have direct access under provisions.[8] Download the following file, http://www.apta.org/pdfs/gov_affairs/directalaws.pdf for a listing of states and find the category in which your state falls.

3.   Find your state practice act by accessing the web site: http://www.apta.org/advocacy/state/state_practice

Download provisions relating to the roles of and supervision requirements for physical therapy students, temporary licensees or license applicants, physical therapist assistants, and physical therapy aides.

Summarize those provisions below:

Role	Role Definition	Supervisory Requirements
Student Physical Therapist		
Physical Therapy License Applicant or Temporary Licensee (if this status exists)		
Physical Therapist Assistant		
Physical Therapy Aide		

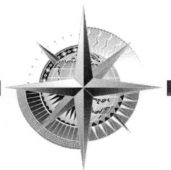

Part Four

Support for Special Student Needs

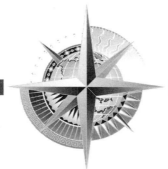

Chapter 13

Students with Disabilities

Jerome had become interested in physical therapy during his own rehabilitation after an automobile accident at age 15. Following a very serious left lower leg fracture, his surgeons performed a below-knee amputation. He wears a prosthesis and maintains an active lifestyle. In fact, he competed in football and hockey in high school and currently plays intramural basketball. He hoped that he would be able to help others with amputations in the future.

Universities and Students with Disabilities

Federal and state laws and most university policies require the university to provide reasonable accommodation in its academically related programs to students with disabilities. This applies to students in health professions education.[1-11]

University academic accommodations and support services are intended to provide students equal access by reducing the negative impact of their disabilities. The key federal legislative acts that support the rights of students with disabilities are Section 504 of the Rehabilitation Act of 1973 and the Americans with Disabilities Act (1990).

Section 504, Rehabilitation Act of 1973

The Rehabilitation Act of 1973 states that "No otherwise qualified individual with a disability in the

United States, as defined in section 706 (8) of this title, shall, solely by reason of his or her disability, be excluded from the participation in, be denied the benefits of, or be subjected to discrimination under any program or activity receiving federal financial assistance or under any program or activity conducted by any executive agency or by the United States Postal Service." Institutions of higher education are included in the definition of institutions receiving federal financial assistance.[12]

Americans with Disabilities Act

The Americans with Disabilities Act (ADA) was signed July 26, 1990. It prohibits discrimination based on disabilities in the areas of employment, public services, transportation, public accommodations, and telecommunications. It requires all affected entities (businesses) to provide reasonable accommodation to persons with disabilities.[13,14]

The ADA defines disability as "(A) a physical or mental impairment that substantially limits one or more of the major life activities of such individual; (B) a record of such impairment; or (C) being regarded as having such an impairment."[13]

What Is a Disability?

This legislation applies to persons with disabilities such as amputation, arthritis, autism, blindness,

Table 13-1
EXAMPLES OF SERVICES FOR STUDENTS WITH DISABILITIES[15]

Adaptive equipment	Disability parking	Real-time captioning
Assistive listening devices	Housing assistance	Registration assistance
Campus orientation	Interpreters	Special materials
Campus van service	Mobility assistance	Support groups
Computer lab	Peer mentoring or counseling	Test proctoring
Computer technology	Priority enrollment	Tutoring
Disability counseling	Reader	Workshops

burn injury, cancer, cerebral palsy, cystic fibrosis, deafness, head injury, heart disease, hemiplegia, hemophilia, respiratory or pulmonary dysfunction, mental retardation, mental illness, multiple sclerosis, muscular dystrophy, musculoskeletal disorders, neurological disorders (including stroke and epilepsy), paraplegia, tetraplegia and other spinal cord conditions, sickle cell anemia, specific learning disability, and end-stage renal disease. The disability must substantially limit a major life activity.[13,14] (This is not an all-inclusive list.)

What Is an Accommodation?

Accommodation refers to the provision of services that ensure equal access to a student with a disability (eg, providing extended examination time for a student who processes information more slowly than other students because of a learning disability).[13,14]

Academic accommodations and support services are determined on an individual basis. Each accommodation is based on documented functional limitations and designed to meet a student's needs without fundamentally altering the nature of the student's instructional program(s) or altering any directly related licensing requirement.

Appropriate academic accommodations may include readers, note-takers, access to adaptive technology, part-time enrollment or relaxed time frame for completion of degree requirements, substitution of coursework required for graduation, and testing accommodations.

What Are Academic Support Services?

Appropriate disability-based support services may involve services such as disability-related counseling; priority enrollment; referral to faculty, staff, campus resources, and community agencies; mobility assistance; and assistance in compensatory strategies for reading, writing, math, and basic study skills.

Campus Resources for Students with Disabilities

Most campuses provide an office that coordinates services to students with disabilities. These services focus on encouraging independence, assisting students in realizing their academic potential, and eliminating barriers to their participation in the academic environment. Services are provided in accordance with the specific documented needs of the student. Tables 13-1 and 13-2 show examples of the types of services available on university campuses for students with disabilities.

Requesting Accommodation

Student Responsibilities

The student, not the university, is responsible to

Table 13-2
EXAMPLES OF UNIVERSITY DISABILITY-SPECIFIC SERVICES[15]

Learning disability services	Disability-related counseling with a learning disability specialist, taped textbooks, extended time for tests, alternative test formats, note-takers, taped lectures, adaptive technology, tutoring, support groups, learning skills workshops, and peer counseling.
Deaf and hard-of-hearing student services	Sign language interpreters, note-takers, real-time captioning, assistive listening devices, disability-related counseling, and tutoring.
Mobility assistance program	Transportation services, orientation and mobility assistance for students with visual impairments, disability parking.
Note-taker services	For students with disabilities that limit their abilities to take notes.
Reader services	Tape-recorded assigned classroom readings.
Testing accommodations	Test-taking conditions (longer time periods, distraction-free rooms), test proctoring to ensure test security and that indicated conditions are in place.
Priority enrollment	Priority enrollment for access to certain classes.
Special materials and equipment	Written materials and textbooks in alternative formats, such as enlarged print, Braille, raised-line drawings, and tape recordings.
Technology and resources	Adaptive equipment and assistive computer technology including scanners, voice synthesizers, reading machines, voice recognition programs, large screen displays, Braille screen displays and printers.

disclose and define the student's disability and request accommodation. In other words, identifying that you have a disability and asking for accommodation are personal decisions.

If a student requests accommodations, he or she is likely to be responsible for registering with the appropriate on-campus office and making his or her specific needs for accommodation known.

Most on-campus offices for students with disabilities require that students take responsibility for providing documentation of the disability and making specific requests for reasonable accommodations and academic support services. Table 13-3 lists typical student responsibilities in requesting accommodation.

Documentation of Disabilities

Students requesting accommodations and/or support services under the ADA and/or Section 504 of the Rehabilitation Act of 1973 must provide documentation of the disability that substantially limits a major life activity. In order to accurately determine the appropriate accommodations, the documentation must be current and reflective of the adult's current functioning.[13,14]

Physical Disabilities

Documentation of physical disabilities must be based on appropriate diagnostic evaluations administered by trained and qualified (ie, certified and/or licensed) professionals (eg, medical doctors, ophthalmologists, psychologists, neuropsychologists, audiologists). Disability diagnosis categories include orthopedic disability, blind or visual impairment, deaf or hard-of-hearing, traumatic brain injury, and other health-related/systemic disabilities.

Table 13-3
SAMPLE OF STUDENT RESPONSIBILITIES IN REQUESTING ACCOMMODATION[16]

1. Supply supporting current clinical documentation in the required time frame.

2. Request accommodations and academic support services in the required time frame.

3. Confirm the adequacy of accommodations and academic support services as soon as possible and request adjustment whenever unsatisfactory conditions are encountered.

4. Approach faculty and staff in a confidential setting to discuss requested accommodations and deliver, in person, letters for request of accommodation to faculty or staff.

5. Obtain syllabi and lists of course materials for reproduction in alternate formats.

6. Adhere to deadlines established for submission of medical documentation and requests for accommodations and academic support services, preregistration, and financial aid.

Reprinted with permission from http://www.brown.edu/Student_Services/Office_of_Student_Life/dss/Student_Resp.html

The diagnostic report must include a clear diagnosis and history including secondary conditions, results of diagnostic tests, associated symptoms, medications, and functional manifestations. This must include substantial limitations to one or more major life activities and indicate the degree of severity. The report should also include recommendations and the rationale for accommodation. If the accommodation recommendations are specific to limitations in learning, an appropriate evaluation of a learning disability must also be performed. Students should always check well in advance regarding deadlines for required documentation. Late submissions may result in delays in service delivery.

Learning Disabilities

The National Joint Committee on Learning Disabilities defines the term *learning disabilities* using the following definition:[17]

The term learning disabilities refers to a heterogeneous group of disorders manifested by significant difficulties in the acquisition and use of listening, speaking, reading, writing, reasoning, or mathematical abilities. These disorders are intrinsic to the individual, presumed to be due to central nervous system dysfunction, and may occur across the life span. Problems in self-regulatory behaviors, social perception, and social interaction may exist with learning disabilities but do not by themselves constitute a learning disability. Although learning disabilities may occur concomitantly with other (disabling) conditions (eg, sensory impairment,

serious emotional disturbance) or with extrinsic influences (eg, cultural differences, insufficient or inappropriate instruction), they are not the result of these conditions or influences.

Many students with learning disabilities typically have average to superior ability, yet experience marked difficulty in one or more academic areas as a result of a significant information processing disorder. To be considered a disability that warrants accommodation, the disorder must substantially interfere with the student's participation in the educational process.

The student who requests services from a university must provide a current and comprehensive written evaluation of his/her learning disabilities. A more comprehensive discussion of the nature of this evaluation is available at the Association for Higher Education and Disability website at http://www.ahead.org/ldguide.htm

There must be clear and specific evidence and identification of the student's disability. Individual learning or processing differences do not constitute a learning disability. The determination of a learning disability is based on the following criteria:

- Educational history
- Behavioral observations
- Clearly specified and significant intracognitive and cognitive-achievement discrepancies
- Current functional limitations imposed by the learning disability in the academic setting
- Evidence that the disorder substantially interferes with the student's educational progress.[17]

Table 13-4

ESSENTIAL FUNCTIONS DEFINED BY PHYSICAL THERAPY EDUCATION PROGRAM DIRECTORS[18]

Essential Function	Percentage
Utilize appropriate verbal, nonverbal, and written communication with patients, families, and others	100
Practice in a safe, ethical, and legal manner	100
Determine the physical therapy needs of any patient with potential movement dysfunction	98
Demonstrate ability to apply universal precautions	96
Safely, reliably, and efficiently perform appropriate physical therapy procedures used to assess the function of the movement system	92
Perform treatment procedures in a manner that is appropriate to the patient's status and desired goals	90
Develop and document a plan of care for a patient with movement dysfunction	88
Recognize the psychosocial impact of dysfunction and disability and integrate the needs of the patient and family into the plan of care	88
Demonstrate responsibility for lifelong professional growth and development	88
Demonstrate management skills, including planning, organizing, supervising, delegating, and working as a member of a multidisciplinary team	81
Develop and apply programs of prevention and health promotion	79
Apply teaching/learning theories and methods in health care and community environments	75
Participate in the process of scientific inquiry	50

Reprinted with permission from the American Physical Therapy Association.

Standards of Performance in Physical Therapy Professional Education

Individual academic programs are responsible to define standards of performance and request that students inform them if they require reasonable accommodation to meet those standards.

Physical therapy professional education program directors have indicated essential functions (Table 13-4) that student physical therapists must be able to complete, with or without accommodation.[18]

Take a look at Table 13-5 for a more expanded explanation of essential functions for student physical therapists from University of Kansas Medical Center.[19]

Employment Issues for Physical Therapists with Disabilities

The ADA requires employers to make reasonable accommodation for a qualified individual with a known physical or mental disability. Examples of reasonable accommodations include job restructuring, reassignment to a vacant position, part-time or modified work schedules, assistive technology, aides, or qualified interpreters. The ADA does not require employers to make accommodations that pose an "undue hardship" (defined as significantly difficult or expensive). Tax credits are available to businesses who remove architectural barriers, target jobs for individuals with disabilities, or provide

Table 13-5

SAMPLE OF TECHNICAL STANDARDS IN PHYSICAL THERAPIST EDUCATION[19]

Physical Therapy Education
University of Kansas Medical Center

Technical Standards

Because a Master's of Science Degree in Physical Therapy signifies that the holder is eligible to sit for the American Physical Therapy National Examination and signifies that the holder is prepared for entry into the profession of physical therapy, it follows that graduates must have the knowledge and skills to function in a broad variety of clinical, private, community, or school-based situations and to render a wide spectrum of physical therapy services. Therefore, the following abilities and expectations must be met by all students admitted to the program.

It is your responsibility to notify the Admissions Committee if there is any reason why you cannot meet any of the expectations for physical therapy students described below. If there is any expectation that you cannot meet, explain in the space provided (attach additional paper if necessary). Individuals with disabilities are encouraged to apply to the program. Candidates whose response indicates that they cannot meet one or more of the expectations listed will be reviewed further by the Admissions Committee, with applicant and faculty input, to determine what reasonable accommodations might be possible to facilitate successful completion of the physical therapy curriculum, preparation for the national examination, and entry into the profession.

1. Observation: The candidate must be able to observe demonstrations and learn from experiences in the basic sciences and in the clinical physical therapy laboratory, such as accurately read dials on electrotherapeutic equipment; accurately read numbers on a goniometer; hear heart and breath sounds; assess normal and abnormal color changes in the skin; and observe pupil changes.

2. Communication: Communication includes not only speech but reading and writing. The candidate must be able to assimilate information from written sources (texts, journals, medical/school records, etc). The candidate must be able to attain, comprehend, retain, and utilize new information presented in written formats as well as produce appropriate written documentation. Candidates should be able to speak, to hear, and to observe patients in order to elicit information; describe changes in mood, activity, and posture; and perceive nonverbal communications. Candidates must be able to communicate effectively and efficiently in oral and written form with all members of the health care team. Response time to emergency/crises situations, as well as more routine communication, must be situationally appropriate.

3. Sensorimotor: Candidates must have gross motor, fine motor, and equilibrium functions reasonably required to carry out assessments (palpation, auscultation, percussion, and other diagnostic maneuvers), and to provide physical therapy intervention. A candidate should be able to execute motor movements required to provide therapeutic intervention (patient transfers, exercise, and application of electrotherapy) and emergency treatment to patients. Quick reactions are necessary not only for safety, but for one to respond therapeutically. Such actions require coordination of both gross and fine muscular movements, equilibrium, and functional use of the senses of touch and vision.

4. Intellectual, conceptual, integrative, quantitative, and problem-solving: Candidates should have cognitive abilities including measurements, calculation, reasoning, analysis, and synthesis. Problem solving, the critical skill demanded of physical therapists, requires all of these intellectual abilities. In addition, the applicant should be able to comprehend three-dimensional relationships to understand the spatial relationships of structures.

5. Judgment: The candidate will be expected to demonstrate judgment in classroom, laboratory, and clinical settings which shows an ability to make mature, sensitive, and effective decisions in the following areas: 1) relationships with supervisors, peers, and patients/clients; 2) professional behavior; 3) the effectiveness of intervention and research strategies. He/she must demonstrate an understanding of the rationale and justification for his/her performance.

continued

Table 13-5, continued

6. Behavioral and social attributes: Candidates must possess the emotional health required to utilize their intellectual abilities fully, exercise good judgment, complete all responsibilities attendant to the physical therapy diagnosis and care of patients, and the development of mature, sensitive, and effective relationships with patients and their families. Candidates must be able to tolerate physically taxing workloads and to function effectively under stress. They must be able to adapt to changing environments, to display flexibility, and to learn to function in the face of uncertain ties inherent in the clinical problems of many patients/clients. Compassion, integrity, concern for others, interpersonal communication skills, interest, and motivation are all personal qualities that are assessed during the education process.

Reprinted with permission from Kansas University Medical Center, Physical Therapy Education.

Table 13-6

DEFINITION OF ESSENTIAL FUNCTIONS[20]

Essential functions are the basic job duties that an employee must be able to perform, with or without reasonable accommodation.

Factors to consider in determining if a function is essential include:
- Whether the reason the position exists is to perform that function
- The number of other employees available to perform the function or among whom the performance of the function can be distributed
- The degree of expertise or skill required to perform the function

---

assistive technology or interpreters to workers with disabilities.[19]

Employers are required to make reasonable accommodation for qualified individuals with a disability, defined by the ADA as individuals who satisfy the job-related requirements of a position held or desired and who can perform the *essential functions* of such position, with or without reasonable accommodation (Table 13-6).

The employer identifies the job's essential functions. Job descriptions are prepared before an individual is interviewed or selected for a position giving evidence of a job's essential functions. If the individual cannot perform an essential function, even with accommodation, the individual is not considered *a qualified individual with a disability* under the law.

The employer and employee determine the type of accommodation that will enable the employee to perform the essential functions of the position. Accommodations of a personal nature (eg, a guide dog for a visually impaired employee or a wheelchair) would not be the employer's responsibility.

Clinical Education Issues

Melissa was diagnosed with multiple sclerosis during the first semester of the physical therapy program. Two years later, she was in remission; however, she often felt fatigued with physical exertion. Although she tried to conserve energy, she found herself wiped out at the end of an 8-hour clinical day. She requested an 18-week clinical assignment instead of the usual 9 weeks and requested that she attend the clinic from 8:00 am to noon daily.

University education courses are often held in distant clinical sites. Those clinical sites, through their agreements with the university, agree to make accommodations for student learning. Changes in the type of assignment, daily hours, or duration of the assignment would all be reasonable accommodations.

The student, however, is always responsible for requesting accommodations that will assist him or her to meet the essential job functions. The clinical and academic faculty are responsible to ensure that all educational conditions meet national and state laws and are in compliance with ethical guidelines for the practice of physical therapy.

Summary

Federal and state legislation mandate accommodations for students with disabilities. An understanding of the types of services available for students with disabilities and university requirements to provide those services will assist students with disabilities to successfully complete professional education in physical therapy.

References

1. Colon EJ. Identification, accommodation, and success of students with learning disabilities in nursing education programs. *J Nurs Educ*. 1997;36(8):372-377.

2. Watson PG. Nursing students with disabilities: a survey of baccalaureate nursing programs. *Prof Nurs*. 1995;11(3):147-153.

3. Helms LB, Weiler K. Disability discrimination in nursing education: an evaluation of legislation and litigation. *J Prof Nurs*. 1993;9(6):358-366.

4. Shuler SN. Nursing students with learning disabilities: guidelines for fostering success. *Nurs Forum*. 1990;25(2):15-18.

5. Shomaker TS. The Americans with Disabilities Act and family practice residency programs. *Fam Med*. 1999;31(9):622-623.

6. Losh DP, Church L. Provisions of the Americans with Disabilities Act and the development of essential job functions for family practice residents. *Fam Med*. 1999;31(9):617-621.

7. Smith JJ, Gay SB. Disabled residency candidates and federal law: implications of the Americans with Disabilities. *Act Acad Radiol*. 1998;5(3):207-210.

8. Reichgott MJ. "Without handicap:" issues of medical schools and physically disabled students. *Acad Med*. 1996;71(7):724-729.

9. Helms LB, Helms CM. Medical education and disability discrimination: the law and future implications. *Acad Med*. 1994;69(7):535-543.

10. Ward RS, Ingram DA, Mirone JA. Accommodations for students with disabilities in physical therapist and physical therapist assistant education programs: a pilot study. *J Phys Ther Educ*. 1998;12(2):16-21

11. Hendrickson S, Lyden S, Tarter C, Banaitis D, Cicirello N. Implementation of the Americans with Disabilities Act into physical therapy programs. *J Phys Ther Educ*. 1998; 12(2):9-15

12. US Department of Labor. *Section 504 Rehabilitation Act of 1973 webpage*. Available at: http://www.dol.gov /dol/oasam/public/regs/statutes/sec504.htm. Accessed August 14, 2000.

13. US Equal Opportunity Commission. *Facts about the Americans with Disabilities Act webpage*. Available at: http://www.eeoc.gov/facts/fs-ada.html. Accessed August 14, 2000.

14. Kinder DC. Americans with Disabilities Act Document Center. *The Americans with Disabilities Act: A Brief Overview webpage*. Available at: http://janweb.icdi. wvu.edu/kinder/overview.htm. Accessed August 14, 2000.

15. University of California, Los Angeles. *Office for Students with Disabilities at UCLA webpage*. Available at: http://www.saonet.ucla.edu/osd. Accessed August 14, 2000.

16. Brown University Disability Support Services. *Student's Responsibility webpage*. Available at: http://www.brown. edu/Student_Services/Office_of_Student_Life/dss/Stude nt_Resp.html. Accessed August 14, 2000.

17. Brinckerhoff LC, Shaw SF, and McGuire JM. *Promoting Postsecondary Education for Students with Learning Disabilities: A Handbook for Practitioners*. Austin, Tex: Pro-Ed; 1993;67-87.

18. Ingram D. Opinions of physical therapy education program directors on essential functions. *Phys Ther*. 1997; 77:37-45.

19. Kansas University Medical Center. *Technical Standards webpage*. Available at: http://www.kumc.edu/SAH/ pted/techstnd.html. Accessed July 12, 2000.

20. US Equal Employment Opportunity Commission. *The ADA: Your Responsibilities as an Employer webpage*. Available at: http://freeadvice.com/gov_material/eeoc-ada-responsibilities-of-employer.htm. Accessed July 12, 2000.

PUTTING IT INTO PRACTICE

1. Write down the contact information for your campus office for students with disabilities. If there is a webpage, also write down the URL address.

   Name of director:

   Campus location:

   Telephone:

   Website:

2. If you have a disability, write down any accommodations that you will request to enable you to complete your professional education in physical therapy.

   If you do not have a disability, consider the accommodations that the following students requested. From your understanding of the provisions of the ADA, discuss whether these are reasonable. Why or why not? What services might be of value to these students?

   Case A:

   Selena had been hard of hearing since early childhood. She had never experienced difficulty before in her academic work. When she received an "F" on her first pathophysiology test, she requested that the instructor prepare a written transcript of each lecture prior to the lecture so that she could read it as the instructor spoke in class.

   Case B:

   Karen's asthma was worse than usual this semester. The chemicals in the anatomy lab seemed to trigger her chemical sensitivities and cause increased shortness of breath. She requested a rebreathing mask, similar to that used by firefighters, to eliminate this as a problem.

   Case C:

   John fractured his left tibia in a roller blading accident during summer break. His cast was removed 2 weeks prior to beginning his final clinical internships. He began his first internship and found his foot swelling at the end of the day. He found it impossible to continue at the pace required in the clinic. He requested an 8-week leave of absence from the program and went to recuperate at his parents' winter home.

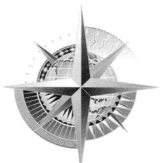

Chapter 14

English Is Not My First Language

Maria bought her books during the first week of class and was frightened by the size of the books and how small the writing was. Although she had studied English as a second language in an intensive course last semester, she was afraid that she wouldn't be able to keep up with her reading assignments.

Common Issues for Second-Language Speakers

Non-native English speakers face a double challenge in entering the profession of physical therapy. Students must not only master the professional content, but they must do so in English, comprehending and learning what they read and using this new vocabulary in written and spoken communications.

There are many strategies for that which may help the English as a second language (ESL) speaker cope with the challenges of professional education.

Professional and Lay Language

First, it is important to understand that students are learning a professional language, using medical terminology, abbreviations, and terms that have meaning only to those in the profession. Everyone who learns the language of a profession initially struggles to communicate using both "lay language" with patients and clients and "professional language" with colleagues.

Be aware that there are terms that are appropriate for use in professional communication. Other terms would not be appropriate for use in professional communication. For example, compare these statements, which both describe the same event:

Professional Language

"The patient consulted the orthopedic surgeon for treatment of his left ulna fracture."

Lay Language

"The patient went to the doctor to get a cast on his broken arm."

Reading

There are strategies that students can use to improve both their vocabulary and comprehension of reading assignments.[1] It may also help to review the active learning strategies suggested in Chapter 9.

Survey and Skim First

Determine the structure of the material. Before you read, look for the main ideas and points.

Table 14-1
READING DIFFICULT MATERIAL[2]

1. **Scan the table of contents** to get a general overview of the book's organization. Pay attention to the subtitles and descriptions that indicate the content of the chapter.

2. **Read the title page of each chapter.** You may be able to get the general idea from the first few paragraphs of the chapter.

3. **Read the conclusion at the end of the material**. It may be helpful to scan the summary for key phrases, terms, ideas, and concepts in the chapter.

4. **Look up new terms in the glossary and index.** This will give you an idea of how terms and concepts are used in the book. Use your English and medical dictionaries to assist you.

Examine how a chapter or article is organized. Look at headings and points of emphasis, often in italics or bold print. Look for summaries. Try to identify a few main ideas. Before you read thoroughly, write a sentence that expresses the main idea of what you will read.

Look for words like *first*, *second*, and *finally* to indicate a progression and sequence of topics and transitions between different ideas.

Identify Your Purpose

Why do you need to read this? Is it for the general idea or for details? You will adjust your reading strategy accordingly.

Assess Difficulty and Choose What to Read

How difficult is this material? Do you know the vocabulary? Choose a few sentences to read thoroughly. If it will be too time-consuming to read word by word, look for the sentences that start and conclude a section of text. There are some additional strategies for reading difficult material in Table 14-1.

Choose What to Read in a Systematic Way

Identify statements, definitions, and formulas that you must understand completely and remember precisely. Look for definitions, highlighted areas, and text that accompany figures, graphs, and tables. These usually summarize the major ideas and facts of a chapter. Table 14-2 lists some techniques to maximize reading speed.

Build Your Professional Vocabulary at the Same Time

Use a medical dictionary. Write down unfamiliar terms and phrases and their definitions on a separate sheet as you do your assigned reading. Review these terms later. Look for these words in your reading. Write down questions that arise as you are learning new terms. Make it a point to use these words in a new sentence or question.

Test Your Comprehension

Make up questions about the material. Write the question. Answer the question in writing. Talk about the material with others. These steps in thinking about the material after reading are the keys to remembering it.

Listening

There are many strategies that will improve your listening comprehension.[1]

Become Familiar with the Material First

Skim the assigned reading. Look for key words and ideas. These phrases will be very important in recognizing the topic being discussed and keeping up in class.

Choose a Good Seat in the Classroom

Sit in the front of the classroom. There will be

Table 14-2
IMPROVING ENGLISH READING SPEED[2]

1. **Do not define each word.** Phrases carry much more meaning than each individual word. To improve your speed, try to read a phrase in the context of a sentence, rather than word by word.

2. **Read silently.** Pronouncing each word will limit you to reading at the speed at which you can speak or whisper. You can read two to three times faster if you read silently. Pronounce only key terms as you read a passage.

3. **Do not read the same material over and over.** Focus on the main idea, not the details. Skim the material in advance, and identify key phrases in a paragraph or section. If a particular section is very difficult, then look for a section later in the chapter that you do understand. Writers often give examples to support an opening statement. Look for a restatement in a conclusion.

fewer distractions and it will be easier to hear and see. Arrive early so that you have your choice of seats.

Attend All Classes and Take Notes

Never miss a class. Take notes in the classroom and review your notes later. Organize your notes by date and keep them in one place. Do not try to write down everything the instructor says. Leave spaces in your notes so that you can add to them later.

It may be helpful as well to tape lectures and use the recording to augment and amend your notes after you have had a chance to review them.

Use Outlines and Course Syllabi

Use outlines, handouts, and other materials that the professor provides to orient you during a lecture. If you are not understanding all of it, do not worry about what you have missed. Listen and write what you can. You can fill in the details after the lecture.

Identify the Most Important Points

Listen for cues as to important points, transitions from one point to the next, repetition of points for emphasis, changes in voice inflections, or lists of a series of points. Most instructors present a few major points and several minor points in a lecture. Much of the rest of the material explains those points.

Write Down What Is on the Board

Write down *everything* that the professor writes on the board. This is a good way to prioritize the key concepts and vocabulary related to the subject.

Use All of Your Senses

Use all of your senses (seeing, hearing, feeling) to learn. Focus on visual materials and demonstrations in addition to what is in writing. Practice skills by moving and saying instructions out loud.

Eliminate Distractions

Focus 100% of your attention and concentration during lectures and while studying. Take a break when needed to revitalize and refresh your mind.

Writing

It is often very helpful to see samples of work that previous students have done. Ask the faculty member for good examples of the kind of work he or she expects.

Ask for feedback prior to submitting your final paper. Many faculty members are willing to review your written work in a draft form and give you feedback. In fact, this type of feedback is frequently the most helpful in revising your writing.

Use on-campus writing resource centers to assist you in presenting your ideas. Professional writing differs from other types of writing. Professional writing is concise, directed toward a specific purpose, and often follows a predefined format. Review Chapter 8 for examples of the requirements of different types of writing assignments.

Express Yourself

Professional writing styles use several techniques that will improve the reader's understanding of your thoughts and ideas. English writing styles change with the type of writing and purpose of the assignment. Professional writing tends to be goal-directed, concise, and clear. Writing in English for professional purposes may differ considerably from a student's past experience. Some guidelines are presented in Table 14-3. You may find it helpful to review Chapter 8 as well.

The Voice of Your Writing

The active voice is simpler and more effective in conveying your ideas. Many cultures and languages commonly use the passive voice. Consider the differences between the passive and active voices presented in Table 14-4. How does the active voice improve your understanding of what has been written?

Proofreading

Mitsumi received her paper back and it was covered with red ink. How could it be possible that she had made so many errors? She felt embarrassed and went to see the professor during office hours to discuss her grade on the paper.

Proofreading is essential for all writers. All writers make errors in their professional writing. Using the following strategies may help to find those errors.[5]

Read Very Slowly

Read out loud if possible, one word at a time. Read what is actually on the page. Proofread more than once and if possible have someone else check your work. Repeat after you have finished.

Identify Common Mistakes and Look for Them

Look for common spelling errors using a spellcheck function in your computer word-processing program. It will be more difficult, but not impossible, to find common errors in usage that are spelled correctly.

English is a complicated language with many irregularities. The grammatical errors that non-native English speakers make fall into several common categories. Be careful of the errors described in Table 14-5.

Test-Taking

Non-native English speakers face some particular challenges in taking examinations. Often, a single word may change the meaning of a question. Review Chapter 7, as test-taking strategies apply here as well. Be careful of some common problems (Table 14-6) that are particularly difficult for non-native English speakers.[8]

Cultural Adjustments for International Students

On the first day of class, Sadia was surprised when her instructor told the class to call him by his first name, Tom. She thought to herself, "I want to treat my professors with respect. I just don't feel right about doing that."

International students may find that teaching and learning methods and social customs are very different than those practiced in their home country. International students are often surprised to see differences in relationships between students and instructors and expectations of students. In addition, differing social customs such as dress, informality in relationships, and what is acceptable behavior in many academic and professional situations may differ considerably. This is a predictable and common reaction to immersion in a different culture where the behavior and values seem to be so different.

Sociologists define this as *culture shock*. Students often feel lonely, alienated, and exhausted. They may feel frustrated and angry. They may withdraw and hold back from fully participating in the new culture.[10]

Coping with Culture Shock

Coping with such feelings is essential to progress with your education. Try some of the following strategies:[10]

- **Avoid stereotyping.** Try not to stereotype the characteristics of "Americans" based on your experiences with a few individuals. Try to look at each situation as new and each individual as unique.

- **Express your feelings.** Talk about your feelings and observations with others in the same situation. Ask others if they have experienced similar feelings at some times.

Table 14-3

GUIDELINES FOR PROFESSIONAL WRITING IN ENGLISH[3,4]

Strategy	Explanation
Outline and organize your ideas before you begin writing.	Review the assignment and establish a writing outline that follows the directions of the assignment.
Provide connections between your ideas or indicate a progression of points.	Use words that indicate similarities and differences, such as *similarly*, *in contrast*, or *next*.
Give examples and evidence of the statements you make.	Follow an introductory sentence with one or two sentences that illustrate the initial idea of the paragraph. Use statistics, facts, and outside references to support the points you make.
State your purpose.	Identify the purpose of the paper in the first few paragraphs. "The purpose of this paper is to examine the evidence that supports the use of ultrasound as a therapeutic modality."
Use headings and subheadings to orient the reader.	Help the reader to follow your ideas by making brief titles to describe the sections of your paper (eg, APTA Position, Interview Findings).
Use the active voice.	Avoid passive verbs. Identify an actor for the actions you present in your sentences (see Table 14-4 for more examples).
Use appropriate language; avoid slang.	Use phrases like *many* instead of *lots of* (eg, "There are many books" instead of "There are lots of books").
Take a stand. Be clear about why you have made a decision, or have an opinion or position.	State your decision or position and the reasons and rationale that support your position. Indicate Indicate your thought processes. "I recommended the lumbar stabilization exercises because the patient has a recurrent history of low back pain and shows poor muscle strength of the lower abdominal muscles with hypermobility of the lumbar spine. I see no evidence of neurological involvement at this time."
Follow referencing styles.	If there is not a referencing style indicated in the instructions, inquire as to what style the faculty prefers that you use.
Make sure that your work is free of spelling and grammatical errors.	Use a computer spellchecker to check your work.

Table 14-4
SAMPLES OF PASSIVE AND ACTIVE VOICE

Passive Voice	Active Voice
The patient was interviewed before beginning the treatment.	The instructor interviewed the patient before beginning the treatment.
We were given the assignment on Thursday.	The professor gave us the assignment last Thursday.
The students were asked to complete a three-page questionnaire.	The students completed a three-page questionnaire.
I was told that you called yesterday.	Janet, our receptionist, told me that you called yesterday.

- **Open yourself to the experience.** Try to learn about the history and culture of the community in which you live. Think of this experience as an adventure. Focus on now, not yesterday or the future.

- **Use humor.** Maintain a sense of humor and a friendly outlook. Find amusement in your observations. You may feel better if you try to maintain a positive outlook.

- **Join the group.** Group activities which involve your classmates will be very helpful to develop the kind of friendships that will help you to overcome culture shock.

- **Relax and be patient.** This is a common reaction. Assume that these feelings will pass and do not dwell on them. You are not alone, and you will find it easier if you remind yourself that this is not permanent.

Summary

International students often face unique challenges in struggling through professional education in a second language (English). Non-native English speakers will benefit by using strategies for reading and taking notes that maximize attention to key concepts in the written material. Proofreading is an essential step in the writing process because non-native English speakers are likely to make errors that must be corrected prior to handing in the assignment. Student-instructor relationships and expectations of students may be quite different in the US higher education system. Students should take active measures to cope with culture shock so that it does not cause problems in their academic pursuits.

References

1. Carter C, Bishop J, Kravits SL. *Keys to Effective Learning*. Upper Saddle River, NJ: Prentice-Hall Inc; 1998.

2. Virginia Polytechnic Institute and State University, Cook Counseling Center. *Study Skills Self-Help Information webpage*. Available at: http://www.ucc.vt.edu/stdyhlp.html. Accessed November 7, 2001.

3. Gocsik K. *Cultural Difference and Its Impact on Rhetoric: An Overview. English as a Second Language webpage*. Available at: http://www.dartmouth.edu/~compose/tutor/problems/esl.html. Accessed August 2, 2000.

4. Holt S. *Responding to Non-Native Speakers of English*. Available at: cisw.cla.umn.edu/wac_respondingnon-nativespeakers.html. Accessed August 2, 2000.

5. Purdue University Online Writing Lab. *Proofreading Strategies webpage*. Available at: http://owl.english.purdue.edu/handouts/general/gl_proof.html/. Accessed September 3, 2000.

6. Edupass. The Smart Student Guide to Studying in the United States. *Common Usage Errors webpage*. Available at: http://www.edupass.org/english/errors.phtml. Accessed August 2, 2000.

7. Gocsik K. *Common ESL errors-The Top Ten List. English as a Second Language webpage*. Available at: http://www.dartmouth.edu/~compose/tutor/problems/esl.html. Accessed August 2, 2000.

8. University of Victoria Learning Skills Program. *Strategies for Reading Exam Questions webpage*. Available at: http://www.coun.uvic.ca/learn/program hndouts/Readexam.html. Accessed September 2000.

9. Dartmouth College. *Tips for International Students-The U.S. Classroom: A Few Guidelines webpage*. Available at: http://www.dartmouth.edu/admin/acskills/lsg/intl.html. Accessed September 3, 2000.

10. University of Wisconsin Eau Claire Counseling Services. *Cultural Differences: International Students Coping with Culture Shock webpage*. Available at: http://www.uwec.edu/admin/counsel/pubs/shock.htm. Accessed September 3, 2000.

Table 14-5

COMMON ENGLISH AS A SECOND LANGUAGE ERRORS[6,7]

Type of Error	Incorrect Form	Correct Form
Absent determiners (the, a, an)	She is good physical therapist. What is answer?	She is a good physical therapist. What is the answer?
Incorrect choice of preposition (in, on, with, over, above, below, beside)	My lab coat is stained in coffee.	My lab coat is stained with coffee.
Incorrect verb sequences, especially involving tense agreement	The patient should have recover by now.	The patient should have recovered by now.
Incorrect choice of verb to use with the infinitive	I wouldn't mind to take a vacation.	I would like to take a vacation.
Disagreement between determiners and nouns	He ate many tomato on Wednesday.	He ate many tomatoes on Wednesday.
	She identified some abnormal neurological finding yesterday.	She identified some abnormal neurological findings yesterday.
Sentence fragments	Sending the letter yesterday.	She sent the letter yesterday.
Irregular verbs, nouns, and adjectives, such as go/went/gone, drive/drove/driven, think/thought, send/sent, and child/children	He sended the report of the evaluation to the physician.	He sent the report of the evaluation to the physician.
	I thinked about that answer for a long time during the test.	I thought about that answer for a long time during the test.
Subject-verb agreement errors	The results of the test was negative.	The results of the test were negative.
Commonly confused words, such as to/too/two, except/accept, effect/affect, which/that, then/than, piece/peace	Their are to many patients.	There are too many patients.
	Everyone is turning there work in on time accept for John.	Everyone is turning in their work on time except for John.

An excellent online resource is Purdue University Online Writing Lab. *ESL Resources for Students.* Available at: http://www.owl.english.purdue.edu/handouts/esl/eslstudent.html

Table 14-6

COMMON TESTING ERRORS FOR NON-NATIVE ENGLISH SPEAKERS[8]

Error	How Is This Error Made?	Example
Missing a double negative in a question	Words like *not, lack,* or *absence* are easy to find and indicate the negative condition. It is more difficult to find whole words that indicate the negative condition, such as *illogical* or *uncertain*. Remember that these words also indicate a negative condition. Two negative words together indicate a positive condition.	Which of the following situations are NOT illegal? 1. Not having the patient sign the consent form. 2. Offering to change the dates on the insurance claim. 3. Lack of consideration of the patient's request for an appointment in the morning. 4. Leaving an unsupervised aide in the clinic while you go for lunch. To correctly answer this question, the test-taker must look for the only situation that is *not illegal,* or in other words, *legal.*
Missing a qualifying word	Single words such as *always, never, just, only,* and *except* change the meaning of a phrase (and may also indicate unlikely correct choices). Extreme words (always, never, totally) are frequently associated with incorrect answers.	A patient with a blood pressure of 90/60 will always complain of dizziness upon standing. (false) Although it is true that a patient with a blood pressure of 90/60 might feel dizzy, the word *always* is an important clue in this question.
Confusing look-alike options	Be careful to read all of the options because a phrase may be repeated in a similar way with the intent to mislead you. Be aware of details.	The most reliable sign of hypertension is: a. Resting systolic blood pressure over 90 b. Resting diastolic blood pressure over 90 c. Resting heart rate over 90 d. 90-point difference between systolic and diastolic blood pressure Don't be fooled! Look for the correct term (diastolic) that matches with the repeated value (90).

PUTTING IT INTO PRACTICE

1.   Identify a reading assignment in one of your classes. Give yourself only 5 minutes. Skim the assignment. Write down all the key words and phrases you can find in that time.

2.   Correct the following sentences:

Incorrect	Correct
I can to give her the assignment tonight.	
Many student talked to me after class today.	
I go to the clinic yesterday.	
He want more exercises to practice.	

3.   Many international students are surprised about various aspects of life in American universities. Write down an observation that was surprising to you. How have you coped with this difference? Have you changed your expectations? Do you look at this differently now?

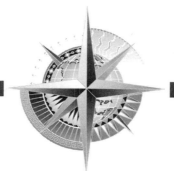

Chapter 15

Re-entry And Second-Career Students

by ChrisTina Buettell, MPT

A *re-entry student* is loosely defined as any student age 25 or older.[1] The concept of re-entering the academic arena also implies that a student has not been continuously enrolled full-time at the university level.[1,2] The term *nontraditional student* is commonly used synonymously with re-entry student but more specifically refers to students who do not fit the traditional university profile of full-time attendance, ages 18 to 22, with on-campus residency.[1,2]

A nontraditional student is alternately defined as having multiple roles and at least 1 year in a nonacademic role between high school or last college experience and present enrollment in college.[3] Frequently, nontraditional or re-entry students are beginning a second career.[4]

Second Career Decisions

Physical therapy (PT) education is gradually becoming a re-entry program. For example, in 1993, the average age for students entering the PT program at California State University was 24 years.[5] In 1998, it was 27.1 years.[5] Three developments help explain this trend.

First, the age of all students graduating from university campuses is increasing. According to the US Department of Education, approximately 46% of all college students were over the age of 24 in 1997, and "the number of nontraditional students continues to rise..."[3]

Second, as PT programs have evolved to the post-baccalaureate level, student age has increased. For example, the median age of graduate students at California State University, Fresno is 31 years, as compared to 22 years for undergraduates in all departments.[6]

Third, with a social trend toward adult career changes, the physical therapy profession offers a practical, meaningful vocation in which life experience tends to enhance applicable decision-making and communication skills. "As in most higher education today, many students in physical therapy are nontraditional; that is, they are older, second-career, and/or second-baccalaureate-degree students. In institutions in which an interview is part of the admissions process, these students may score higher because of their maturity, experience, and motivation."[7]

Younger re-entry students, ages 25 to 34, have much in common with traditional students. Many are still single and without dependents, although this is also the classic marriage-childbirth-divorce age group. Time since previous schooling is minimal, and interests and activities are broad, often involving group trips and athletic recreation.

Middle re-entry students, ages 35 to 44, are frequently in committed relationships, or have been, often have children to care for, have multiple outside interests or steady employment, and may own a home or have other major responsibilities or debts. These students often have been out of school for many years and may find it difficult to make time for classes and assignments in their already full lives.

Older re-entry students, ages 45 and over, are a distinct minority. They may have established careers, teenage or grown children, and elderly parents. They are beginning to deal with issues of aging and may have begun to consider financial planning for retirement. They are old enough to be their younger classmates' parents and have few sociohistorical bonds with students who are a generation younger. They may indeed have no other classmates their age.

Predictable Strengths and Benefits

Success and retention, the big concerns for pre-admission screening, are not big issues for most re-entry students. Re-entry students tend to be highly motivated, grounded, goal-oriented students who are eager to learn and have a sense of purpose and dedication.[1-4] Findings that nontraditional students more eagerly attend classes and do homework may suggest their higher enthusiasm for learning after time spent away from classrooms.[3] This is often their second chance, so there is no backing out. This is particularly true of older students who may feel career time running out.

Older or nontraditional students tend to see themselves as more applied and process-oriented than their concrete, task-focused, traditional classmates who may be more interested in short-term goals.[8] Other unique attributes of re-entry students may include a more serious view of education and a high value placed on positive working relationships with faculty.[8]

One study comparing nontraditional female students with housewives found that the returning students experienced greater self-respect and respect from others, a more diversified life, and less boredom.[3] Service to community, enhancement of quality of life, personal career satisfaction, and acquisition of a practical skill are reasons given by PT re-entry students for taking the leap.[4]

Can I Learn as Quickly as My Younger Classmates?

Contrary to the popular notion that adult age and cognitive abilities are inversely related, recent longitudinal studies suggest that mean cognitive performance may not significantly decline until late adulthood (age 65 and older).[9] Vocabulary increases with age, and performance on language ability tests has been shown to be more strongly associated with the subject's educational level than with his or her age.[10] Additionally, students with vast life experience have more finely tuned their social and communication skills through years of practice in diverse settings.

Helen Hislop has written about the importance of "productive dissent" and the "ability to listen to opposing perceptions in a nonjudgmental manner, to deal with different ideas with an open mind..." versus rigidity and resistance to dissent.[11] Older or multi-role students often have encountered a greater variety of people and ideas than their more youthful classmates. They also have had more time to solidify rigid beliefs, but either way they have experienced many decision-making challenges. These experiences may prepare them to accommodate for clinical ambiguity, "the uncertainty principle that intrudes into every human interaction between patient and therapist," and facilitate their development of clinical intuition.[11]

Predictable Challenges and Sacrifices

Technology and You

In spite of their many positive qualities, re-entry students can face challenges when it comes to current technology and recent schooling trends. Many did not grow up with computers as students do today. Papers were written on manual typewriters using carbon paper for copies. Library card catalogs used to consist of wooden drawers of 3x5 cards, and the index for journals was the voluminous, hardbound *Reader's Guide to Periodical Literature*.

Similarly, older students may remember using trigonometry tables and slide rules for math and chemistry classes instead of today's ubiquitous calculators. There were no websites and no computerized GRE testing. For students who completed prerequisites 10 or 15 years before re-entering, certain subjects may be distant memories. Test-taking can feel terrifying, and sitting for hours in a classroom may be unfamiliar as well as uncomfortable.

What school was like 20 years ago is not what it is like upon re-entry. Trivial, everyday procedures for most students can be traumatic at first for a re-entering student.

> *Sally received her BA in liberal arts more than 20 years ago. When she studied chemistry in a premed program, she had used a slide rule to do calculations and wrote out exam answers long hand. Sitting at her first PT prerequisite physics exam, unfamiliar calculator in hand, unfamiliar scantron upside down on her desk, wearing reading glasses for the first time, wedged between two other students, surrounded by a hundred or so younger students, feeling insecure about putting her backpack up front, Sally felt like an alien and remembers saying to herself, "This is crazy; I can't believe I'm doing this."*
>
> *Re-evaluating the stressful situation, Sally requested a different seating arrangement, practiced using her new tools, and left her backpack in her locker for the next exam. By the end of the semester she was tutoring fellow students and received an A on the final exam, but it was a rough start.*

Physical and Social Challenges

Older students may experience physical challenges, such as worsening eyesight, slower thought processing, and increased sensitivity to noise, time pressures, crowding, and bedlam. Middle-aged female students may be experiencing perimenopausal symptoms. Multirole students may resent the tedium of class meetings, birthday announcements, and busywork assignments, knowing they have a sick child at home or a long night ahead at a job.

The social scene may create additional challenges. How many 40-year-old students are living in group houses and are interested in playing the singles dating game, let alone doing it with 22-year-old classmates or hearing about it day after day between classes?

Time and Stress Management

Time and stress management are challenges for all students; re-entry students are just more experienced at coping with them. Fortunately so, because they often have less time and potentially more stress than their conventional classmates. Various studies have replicated findings that nontraditional students' complex time and role demands are sources of anxiety and tension.[3] They have more responsibilities at home, less time spent with friends and peers, and less vacation time than traditional students.[3]

Financial Needs

Starving students also can be found at all echelons, but for re-entry students, financial woes are usually more complex than just paying rent and borrowing a little more from parents. Re-entry often means job loss, which means downward mobility for adults accustomed to a steady income with health insurance and other benefits. Dependents further complicate matters, especially if they also have college expenses. Homeowners may have mortgage payments as well as maintenance and homeowner's insurance to continue to pay.

Unpredictable Struggles and Growth

Returning to full-time study can be an enormous transition. You are settled, stable, and competent in what you do. Everyone's reaction is, "You want to do what?"[12] What may have begun as an off-chance of qualifying for a long-postponed dream suddenly looms as a dire threat to financial, marital, and mental stability. There may be an overwhelming sense of "Help! I can't really do this," or "Oh my gosh, what have I gotten myself into?"

Older Students, Younger Professors

In spite of expecting skills to be a little rusty, the shock of actually sitting in a classroom with students half one's age, no chalkboard, and TV monitors beaming down from opposite corners of the room can be unsettling. Additionally, even faculty and staff are no longer similar to memories of previous school days. Whereas traditional students look up to professors as older and wiser, students who are the same age or older than their professors and have themselves been teachers, parents, or employers have a hard time submitting to the conventional faculty-student hierarchy. In their own areas of prior expertise and training, re-entry students may have specific skills superior to those of most professors. Some older students may also have more experiential wisdom than their younger professors.

High Expectations

Expectations are another pitfall. Re-entry students have been through a lot to get where they are and may be demanding, impatient, and judgmental of faculty shortcomings that are viewed as impediments to their own goals. They may feel more competitive than cooperative. In a recent study, nontraditional students reported a higher impact from bad classes or teachers than did their traditional counterparts.[3] Re-entry students may cope with these perceptions with arguments, direct confrontation of authority, refusal to follow instructions, and endless unsolicited suggestions for improvement and change.

Relationships

What about friendships? Outside of school, professors and older students with mutual friends and similar interests would be naturally inclined to socialize, but role boundaries may limit social contact. Older students may have more intragenerational common bonds with same-age professors than with classmates two decades younger, but unwritten artificial barriers create segregation. Where are the limits? Faculty may be well aware of their own roles and boundaries, but newly returning students unaccustomed to academia may find it initially confusing to differentiate between acceptable friends (classmates) and friendly authorities (professors, clinical instructors, staff).

Support Systems

At the same time re-entry students are trying to foster a support system on campus, they must redefine their support network at home and beyond. One re-entry student remarked, "The magnitude of support I've had to find boggles my mind. I don't think I'd have dared to try this if I'd known how much help I'd need."

> Alicia, a 36-year-old married mother of three, works part-time at a suburban health center near her home. Interested in furthering her education, she accepts her employer's incentive to pay tuition and fees for her to upgrade her skills. She applies and is accepted for the MPT program at the state university 25 miles away. At the new student picnic, she talks to a re-entry student in the second-year class about her concerns. "Will I be able to keep up with classes if I have children at home? It sounds great, but how difficult are the courses? My computer skills are weak. I have a 40-minute commute; I don't know how I'll manage evening classes. Can I live at home during my clinicals?"
>
> The second-year student confesses that the first year was a struggle, but she has survived. "Sure, give it a try. Do you have enough support?" The new student answers that she plans to arrange after-school child care 3 days per week, her husband is employed full-time, and she's saved a little money for books and supplies. "Not enough. You'll need more help at home, more flexibility, and campus resources. Better see a re-entry counselor."

Support is more than tacit approval and occasional child care. In addition to academic demands, some of the challenges a re-entry student may contend with include residential relocation, household role reversal, poverty, self-doubt, vacations spent barely catching up, zero recreational time, health concerns exacerbated by stress, lifestyle disruption, and relationship upheaval. Multilevel support is crucial to transcend the demoralizing realization that the best one can do is to get by one day at a time. Professional and personal support can be key to recapturing the vision that originally brought one to graduate school and to making "insurmountable hurdles become just another day's adventure."[12]

And a Midlife Crisis Too?

To add to the complexities of re-entry, middle age is often developmentally a time of reevaluation, searching, spiritual growth, midlife crisis, and/or change. This may be what inspires a second-career decision in the first place. A 45-year-old student may have a very different perspective on the meaning of his or her chosen field of study than a 23-year-old who thought PT sounded like fun and hopes it will pay well. The following re-entry student statement is typical:

> I needed to change my life. I knew I could do more, and I didn't want to get stuck where I was forever. I'd always wanted to go to grad school but money, or family, or other commitments got in the way. I finally just had to make the leap; small steps weren't getting me there, and time was running out. It was terrifying, but I'm glad I did it. I wasn't really sure it was possible after so many years and with so many obstacles, but I had to find out. I would always have wondered and regretted the missed opportunity. Some days I wake up very surprised that I'm here.

These subtle surprises create unsubtle confusion for the re-entry student who is already feeling slightly lost and overwhelmed. He or she may repeatedly think, "This is silly. This shouldn't be a problem. I'm mature and experienced. I can handle this," but when he or she gets marked down for speaking out, or laughed at for being different, or just worn out from being pulled in too many disparate directions, he or she needs help. Balogun et al suggested that identification of students at risk for burnout secondary to sociodemographic and environmental factors would allow appropriate preventive measures to be initiated.[13]

Strategies for Re-Entry Students

Professional Counseling

Competent professional counseling can make all the difference in the world. In a study of role strain of nontraditional women students, "psychological support was found to be a significant factor in feelings of satisfaction for women who were re-entering the academic world."[3] This may be related to another finding that women re-entering after an average absence of 10 years had depression symptom scores twice as high as a normative population.[3]

Re-entry students who seek campus counseling services often report they are dissatisfied with the support they receive, commenting for example, "The counselor is younger than I am and doesn't understand my problems," or "When I explained what I was dealing with, the counselor seemed overwhelmed by its complexity." Campus services are geared primarily to traditional students and often rely on counseling student interns. Finding a good fit between counselor and counselee is sometimes difficult. If dissatisfied, talk directly to the head of the counseling center or ask to see the school psychiatrist.

Financial Aid

Financial aid and scholarships can be lifelines. Talk with a financial aid counselor. Submit applications on time. Research scholarships for which you are uniquely qualified. Plan ahead; have essays and references ready well ahead of deadlines. Explore private loans from friends or relatives. Barter. Temporarily downscale; this won't last forever. Work as a student assistant to integrate earning and learning.

Use Re-Entry Program Services

Re-entry programs exist at most large universities. Consider applying to schools that can offer re-entry services, including counseling, scholarship guidance, peer support groups, quiet study areas, tutoring, speaker programs, family activities, and the support of other re-entry students. Find a few students with similar concerns; get together regularly for support and problem solving. Network with same-age, same-interest students at other schools.

Solicit the Support of the Faculty

Faculty are allies. Appreciate them, trust them, work with them. Help them think of ways to help you. Tell them what you need and what you'd like to try. Be patient. Ask to work as a student assistant or to initiate a special project of interest to you. Co-teach a class or get involved in a research project.

Collaborate with Your Classmates

Your classmates of all ages can be treasures. Find a few with whom to work closely and have fun. Seek out other returning students. Welcome opportunities to work with students unlike yourself to expand your awareness and understanding. Trade skills—help those you can, ask for help as needed. Be a good group member; do your share or more and use your maturity to help facilitate good group process and to resolve conflicts quickly and effectively. Model appropriate behavior, honesty, trustworthiness, reliability, and clear communication.

Involve Your Family and Significant Others

If you are parenting very young children, carefully evaluate whether this is the best time to return to school. Graduate school may be possible, but it will not nurture very young children! You may miss a substantial part of your child's vulnerable first years.

Family members need to play a part in your educational experience. Elicit broad support. Clearly explain to everyone the potential benefits of your promised success. Give every family member a role to play. Primary school children can help label supplies, color charts, sort laundry, and unpack groceries. Older children can help locate library and Internet materials, organize tapes, create quizzes, critique practice presentations, and assist with meals and cleaning. Establish quiet study hours. Organize routine chores for maximum efficiency, and even on the busiest days share lots of hugs.

Spouses or significant others can make it or break it for a re-entry student, especially if there are dependents involved. Household duties can eat up oceans of time but spouses are trainable, theoretically, and temporarily may enjoy the opportunity to "be in charge," to nurture their own domestic talents, and to be truly indispensible. Reassurance and pep talks may be vital, and general organizational help is essential. Assistance with typing, proofing, printing, collating, and photocopying, as well as being on-hand for deadline crunches can help preserve sanity.

Siblings, parents, or friends can help by providing loans or special gifts such as children's piano lessons, orthodontist care, soccer shoes, or summer camp. Everyone can give moral support. Invite family to special presentations and include them in your accomplishments and celebrations. Ask for what you need. Remember to express appreciation, and when you can, return the favor, or the money.

Acquire Computer Skills

Become computer literate. Beg, borrow, or buy a functional computer to use at home and be able to problem solve its idiosyncrasies. Know how to create documents and files, how to share disks and avoid viruses, and how to use the Internet. Install a separate telephone line to allow unlimited e-mailing and library searching without tying up the line for family and friends. Practice new computer skills prior to panicky deadlines. Acquaint yourself with the campus computer lab for inevitable hardware breakdowns at home. Join a users' group or find a reliable friend to help you learn and keep learning. Have faith; it is all possible.

Be an Active Learner

Assert your desire to learn. Ask questions. Question discrepancies. Follow your interests. Share your enthusiasm and thinking. Get involved in interesting projects. Initiate. Explore. Seek out like-minded individuals. Accept opportunities.

Use All Your Best Survival Strategies

Do what you need to do to succeed. Sit up front in classes, tape lectures, find a tutor, schedule time with faculty, borrow materials, buy a computer, hire child care, eat healthy snacks, wear the glasses, get comfortable. Do not waste energy worrying about not fitting in. In the long run, it will not matter and may even be an advantage.

Don't Take Yourself Too Seriously

Relax. Sure you are different, but do not dwell on it. You are probably more okay and acceptable than you imagine. Contribute your perspective; so much the better if it is unique and interesting. Be yourself. Focus on what you can do rather than what you cannot do. Smile a lot, stay sane, and do the best you can.

Be Your Best Ally

You are your own best friend and advisor. Listen to your inner self. Believe in yourself. Trust your intuition. Take care of your health—physical, mental, emotional, and spiritual. Make choices that support your success. Finally, let yourself enjoy this fantastic opportunity for which you have waited.

Summary

Re-entry students face academic, social, and family challenges as they enter physical therapy professional education. A positive attitude combined with careful planning can help to reduce some of the predictable stresses involved in juggling academic and family demands. Students may benefit from using available on-campus services such as counseling, child care, and financial aid to assist in meeting their needs.

References

1. Re-entry Program and Services webpage. California State University, Fresno. Available at: http://www.csufresno.edu/ReEntryProgram/index.htm. Accessed August 6, 2001.

2. *Return to College, A Resource and Planning Guide for California State University, Hayward Adult Students.* Hayward, Calif: California State University; 1989.

3. Dill PL, Henley TB. Stressors of college: a comparison of traditional and nontraditional students. *J Psychol.* 1998;132(1):25-32.

4. Lawrence LP. The path to PT. *PT Mag Phys Ther.* 1999;7(1):46-55.

5. Porcella G. Office of Nursing and Physical Therapy Admissions. Fresno, Calif: California State University, Fresno. Interview. June, 1998.

6. Robinson M. Office of Institutional Research, Planning and Management, Fresno, Calif: California State University, Fresno. Interview. June 1998.

7. Hayes SH, Fiebert IM, Carrol SR, Magill RN. Predictors of academic success in a physical therapy program: is there a difference between traditional and nontraditional students? *J Phys Ther Educ.* 1997;11(1):10-16.

8. Bradshaw MJ, Nugent K. Clinical learning experiences of nontraditional-age nursing students. *Nurse Educ.* 1997;22(6):40,47.

9. Finkel D, Pedersen NL, Plomin R, McClearn GE. Longitudinal and cross-sectional twin data on cognitive abilities in adulthood: the Swedish adoption/twin study of aging. *Dev Psych.* 1998;34(6):1400-1413.

10. Ardila A, Rosselli M. Spontaneous language production and aging: sex and educational effects. *Int J Neurosci.* 1996;87(1-2):71-78.

11. Hislop HJ. Clinical decision making: educational, data, and risk factors. In: Wolf SL. *Clinical Decision-Making in Physical Therapy.* Philadelphia, Pa: FA Davis Co; 1985.

12. Cole BH, Brunk Q. Six rules for computers and other stumbling blocks to obtaining an advanced degree. *J Contin Educ Nurs.* 1999;30(2):66-70.

13.   Balogun JA, Hoeverlein-Miller ES, Katz JS. Academic performance is not a viable determinant of physical therapy students' burnout. *Percept Motor Skills*. 1996;83(1):21-22.

Additional Resources

National Association of Student Personnel Administrators (NASPA). Webpage available at: http://www.naspa.org/.

Adult Learners/Commuter Students and Distance Learning Listserv. To subscribe send email to listmanager@listserv.naspa.org with "join adult-learn" in body of message (no quotes).

Joint Task Force on Student Learning. Webpage available at: http://www.naspa.org/resources/stulearn.cfm.

PUTTING IT INTO PRACTICE

1.   Write down the contact information for your campus office for re-entry students. If there is a web-page, also write down the URL address. If there is no office designated for re-entry students, call the Office of Student Affairs and inquire about available student services such as child care, women's resources, or other support systems.

Name of director:

Campus location:

Telephone:

Website:

2.   Interview another student in your class.
What did he or she do prior to entering the physical therapy professional education program?

What changes has your colleague made in his or her life since entering the program?

Who else was influenced by your colleague's decision to enter physical therapy professional education?

What emotional, academic, relationship, and/or financial stresses has this decision created?

What similarities do you recognize in your own life?

What differences have you experienced?

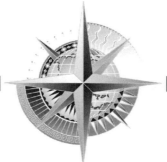

Part Five

Planting the Seeds for a Bright Future

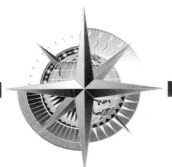

Chapter 16

Critical Thinking and Evidence-Based Practice

> *Teresa decided to do her paper on the effectiveness of magnet therapy, an alternative technique for pain management gaining considerable exposure in the medical literature. She collected articles and thought, "Even in the face of all this evidence, many people still don't believe that it works."*

Critical Thinking

Critical thinking involves the discipline, ability, and willingness to assess evidence and claims, to seek a breadth of contradicting as well as confirming information, and to make objective judgments on the basis of well-supported reasons as a guide to belief and action.[1]

It also involves an active awareness of the thinking process. *Metacognition* is the process of monitoring and considering one's thinking while in the thinking process. Awareness of choices and active involvement in determining the best way to make choices are key parts of the metacognitive process.[1]

Critical thinking requires the thinker to use a process characterized by clarity, accuracy, precision, consistency, relevance, sound empirical evidence, good reasons, depth, breadth, and fairness.

Evidence-Based Practice

> *Dr. Jenkins praised Teresa for her thoughtful and thorough analysis of the evidence supporting magnet therapy. He noted that consumers may have driven this movement. She approached Dr. Jenkins after class and asked, "I wanted to talk with you about your comment on my paper; how can I help consumers to get this information?" Dr. Jenkins suggested that she write an article for the campus newspaper summarizing the major findings reported in the literature.*

Evidence is information that tends to support something or shows that something is true, such as clinically relevant research, objective changes in function, or physical parameters. *Evidence-based practice* is the conscientious, explicit, and judicious use of current best evidence in making decisions about the care of individual patients.[2] Evidence-based practice de-emphasizes intuition, unsystematic observations of clinical experience, and the opinions of "authorities."[3] Evidence-based practice requires the critical examination of evidence from clinical research and the evaluation of clinically relevant outcomes.

Evidence-based practice involves the blending of individual clinical expertise and judgment with the best available external evidence. Thus, evidence might involve information about:

1. The accuracy and precision of diagnostic tests and screening examinations (including clinical observations)
2. The prognostic power of clinical findings
3. The efficacy and safety of therapeutic and preventive interventions[2]

The demand for evidence comes from growing consumer-driven cost-consciousness, combined with increased accountability across the health care professions. Consumers and third-party payers have largely driven this movement as information becomes more and more widely available through the Internet, television, and print media.

Types of Evidence

In describing evidence-based practice approaches, some authors have suggested several types of evidence:[1]

1. *Empirical evidence.* Empirical evidence is obtained by objective observation rather than reasoning or feeling. This is the type of evidence provided by research studies that meet currently accepted standards of design, execution, and analysis. Strong empirical evidence is derived from outcomes of experiments using rigorous controls and having clear, unequivocal outcomes.
2. *Analogical evidence.* Analogical evidence involves comparing known similarities between two systems and hypothesizing that a relationship shown to exist in one system but unknown in the other also exists in the other. For example, this type of evidence might apply the findings of animal studies to justify interventions with humans. This type of evidence is considered weaker than empirical evidence because effects are hypothesized but not tested.
3. *Anecdotal evidence.* An anecdote describes an experience in an individual or situation. A *case report* is an example of anecdotal evidence. Anecdotal evidence is considered the weakest of the three because it is difficult to repeat and difficult to draw any conclusion regarding the cause of an outcome. Even multiple case studies do not substantially add to the strength of anecdotal evidence.

Reviewing Scientific Merit

Harris suggested six criteria for review of the scientific merit of published research articles:[4]

1. The theories underlying the treatment approach are supported by valid anatomical and physiological evidence.
2. The treatment approach is designed for a specific type of patient population.
3. Potential side effects of the treatment are presented.
4. Studies from peer-reviewed journals that support the treatment's efficacy are provided.
5. Peer-reviewed studies include well-designed, randomized, controlled clinical trials or well-designed single-subject experimental studies.
6. The proponents of the treatment approach are open and willing to discuss its limitations.

We have a big problem in that not many studies of complex human phenomena, such as education or rehabilitation, meet these criteria. Even the best behavioral science research is often quasi-experimental. Further, the base of knowledge of what underlies the practice of physical therapy is vast, across disciplines and across time. Theories are often contradictory and confusing. In addition, there is the problem of how to measure, what is measurable, and what is not.

Qualitative researchers argue that there are other types of research that have scientific merit besides the randomized controlled clinical study.[5] Others contend that the complexity of the human condition is impossible to document with the requisite scientific rigor. Even if we believe it exists, we lack the tools at this point in time to measure energy flow, emotional discharge, or subtle changes in subjective well-being.[5,6]

The answer may not be in the rigid application of Harris' criteria, nor in the rejection of all but the best empirical evidence. It may lie in the approach that we take to thinking and decision-making. Training in critical thinking and making good decisions is as important as understanding the mechanisms of physiology or pathology, which underlie the approaches that we choose to take.

Evidence in Physical Therapy

Pamela Duncan was one of the first to write about evidence-based practice in physical therapy:[7]

Advances in physical therapy will be possible only if we critically evaluate our assumptions and shift our paradigm. Although scientifically based models for interventions do exist in physical therapy, the current paradigm for practice is based for the most part on expert opinion and clinical experience. It is driven by many assumptions that guide education, clinical practice, and research.[7]

This paradigm shift involves the following:

Recasting the Role of Authority

Evidence-based practice places a much lower value on "authority." Opinions offered by experts can be evaluated using available evidence. Some argue that the knowledge and skill one gains from experience can never be measured in randomized controlled studies. The key here is that the importance of what authorities offer must be appraised and evaluated in the context of underlying evidence.

Medical journals in many disciplines and specialty areas publish studies that provide such evidence. Physical therapists must look to the literature and to other disciplines in many cases for evidence supporting their practice.

Practicing by the Guide

In the absence of strong empirical evidence, we can refer to clinical practice descriptions and preferred practice patterns. *The Guide to Physical Therapist Practice* can assist practitioner and patient decisions about appropriate care for specific clinical circumstances. This document was developed by consensus, by teams of clinicians and educators without an interest in a specific treatment approach.[8] Practice descriptions assist in narrowing wide variations in practice and provide an external reference when there is disagreement regarding the benefits of various interventions.

Looking at the Context in Which Evidence Exists

Just as a physical effect may be dependent on ambient conditions of temperature, light, and humidity, the mechanisms of response to a physical therapy intervention may be dependent on complex biopsychosocial phenomena that are more difficult to measure than objective physical phenomena.

The *biopsychosocial* model integrates theory from biology, psychology, anthropology, and sociology as an explanatory theme for health and health care. This model includes issues of health and wellness, spiri-

tuality, psychoneuroimmunology, methods of coping with disability, illness or injury, ways to reduce stress, and smoking cessation.[9]

For example, many therapists would predict a better outcome for a patient with a strong social support system (such as a family) to provide care. Most therapists would also rate a patient's prognosis more favorably if he or she was functioning independently prior to an illness or injury. How are these factors measured or even considered in choosing a treatment duration or a discharge destination?

We cannot draw conclusions about the consequences of treatment decisions or the effects of an intervention without also considering evidence about the nature of the factors that may influence those outcomes. Valid, reliable, standardized assessment tools provide the best hope of quantifying the many factors that may interact to influence an outcome.

Comparing the Costs to the Benefits of Intervention

How much change in a condition can be expected? How much time and effort will it take to achieve and/or sustain that change? How expensive is the treatment compared to the potential benefit that the patient will gain? Medicine is often accused of applying technology because it exists and has some small chance of changing an outcome. It often feels better to do "something" than to do nothing.

Timing it Right

The cost-benefit issue applies on an even larger scale when it comes to prevention. It is often far less costly to provide an intervention that *prevents* a disability than to treat that disability once it has developed. It may be even less costly to provide widespread screening to identify those at greatest risk for developing a disability and then provide individual treatment to selected high-risk individuals.

The costs of providing care are usually calculated on an individual basis: the costs *to society* of *preventing* people from needing those services in the first place are unknown.

The Future

The future is clear. Physical therapists must seek evidence to justify the treatment approaches they recommend. Costly and time-consuming interventions without demonstrable effects are likely to be denied by third-party payers and refused by consumers.

In a recently published vision statement, the

Table 16-1
CLINICAL DECISION-MAKING TASKS IN PHYSICAL THERAPY[11]

1. Establish a differential diagnosis for patients across the lifespan based on evaluation of results of examinations and medical and psychosocial information.
2. Communicate or discuss diagnoses or clinical impressions with other practitioners.
3. Determine patient or client prognoses based on evaluation of results of examinations and medical and psychosocial information.
4. Collaborate with patients, clients, family members, payers, other professionals, and individuals to determine a realistic and acceptable plan of care.
5. Establish goals and functional outcomes that specify expected time duration.
6. Define achievable patient or client outcomes within available resources.
7. Deliver and manage a plan of care that complies with administrative policies and procedures of the practice environment.
8. Monitor and adjust the plan of care in response to patient or client status.

Reprinted with permission from the American Physical Therapy Association.

APTA House of Delegates addressed evidence-based care.[10] See Chapter 1 for the full statement:

> Guided by integrity, life-long learning, and a commitment to comprehensive and accessible health programs for all people, physical therapists and physical therapist assistants will *render evidence-based service* throughout the continuum of care and improve quality of life for society.

Decision-Making in Clinical Management

In what instances do physical therapists apply clinical decision-making skills? What underlies the decisions that they make? Table 16-1 lists typical tasks in physical therapy practice that involve clinical decision-making.

Chapter 9 discusses information processing and ways to improve your attention to and understanding of the wealth of information available in the clinical environment. To what you pay attention may make a tremendous difference in sifting through and processing information. Let's look at the following tasks.

Setting Goals

> *Adam listened as his professor said, "Physical therapists must set goals that are functional, realistic, measurable, and achievable within time and resource constraints..." He thought to himself, "Sounds like more paperwork."*

Who Cares and So What?

A goal "belongs" to a person who has an active interest in achieving it. Often this is the patient or client; perhaps we could also include the larger circle of family and caregivers in the group of people who care about achieving the goal. This provides the "who" of "who cares?"

The "so what" question is easy to ask. What do you want to be able to do differently? This may be sleeping through the night, being able to work an 8-hour day, or being able to get on and off the toilet or in and out of the shower independently.

Goal-setting is a complex process that on a very simple level answers the previous questions. Goal-setting determines where you are going. Just as it would be difficult to take a trip without having a destination, a goal defines a target for the therapeutic intervention. If we want to travel 20 miles, we may design a different route than if we want to travel 200 miles.

Many students and new clinicians have difficulty setting goals, especially in projecting realistic time frames for the achievement of these goals.

The process can be further demystified when consciously considering some of the following factors.

Prior Level of Function

Function is defined as one's ability to perform daily activities such as self-care, walking, climbing stairs, shopping, cooking, and working outside the home.[8] There are various scales that measure function. Most evidence in the literature indicates that a higher premorbid (pre-injury or illness) level of function is predictive of achievement of a higher level of function post-intervention.[12]

Social Support

Social support is a key factor in quality of life and speed of recovery from illness or injury. Caregivers in the home are a critical factor that influences therapist decision-making regarding discharge destination.[13]

Comorbidity

Many patients and clients have multiple medical disorders that co-exist as chronic illnesses. They may change a patient's prognosis in that a disorder such as diabetes may slow wound healing time, or heart or kidney disease may influence tolerance for activities.

Discharge Plan

Discharge destination may be a function of the efficacy of physical therapy services and may largely determine future access to physical therapy services.[12] Recommending a discharge plan is a key part of the decision-making process. Patient safety, judgment, and cognition are often just as important as the patient's physical function. Of course, social support plays a key role in discharge planning decisions.

Outcomes Assessment

Evaluating outcomes is a key activity to gather evidence of the efficacy of physical therapy intervention. First, outcome measures must meet acceptable standards of *reliability* and *validity*. *Reliable* measures minimize testing error from one tester to another or from one test to a repeated test in the future. *Valid* measures represent a true measure of the phenomenon that they are intended to assess.

On the simplest level, outcomes are the measure of whether you have reached your destination (ie, the goal). From a more complex perspective, we can look at how effectively we have used our time or resources. In other words, what did it *cost* in time or resources to reach the goal?

Efficiency

Suppose my goal is to reach a destination 20 miles away. I can travel on country roads or on the freeway to this destination.

How much time does it take to travel 20 miles on narrow winding country roads compared to driving the same distance on the freeway? I can travel 20 miles in 1 hour on the country road. In comparison, I can drive 20 miles in less than 20 minutes on the freeway.

The distance divided by the time it takes is a measure of *efficiency*.

How efficient is a physical therapy intervention? Use the example above. It takes *less time* to accomplish the same goal using a *highly efficient* treatment.

Low Efficiency	High Efficiency
$\frac{20\ miles}{1\ hour}$ = 20 mph	$\frac{20\ miles}{20\ mins}$ = 1 mile/minute or 60 mph

Value

How many gallons of gasoline will it take to travel 20 miles? If I have a motor home, it may take as many as 5 gallons of gas to travel 20 miles. A new compact car may use less than a gallon.

Low Value	High Value
$\frac{20\ miles}{5\ gallons}$ = 4 miles/gallon	$\frac{20\ miles}{.66\ gallons}$ = 30 miles/gallon

How cost-effective is a physical therapy intervention? Using the example above, it takes *fewer resources* to accomplish the same goal using a *high value* treatment.

Value x Efficiency

Continuing with the same example, we could take the same motor home on country roads or on the freeway. There are four possible methods to reach the outcome.

1. Choosing to drive the motor home on country roads to our destination wastes time and resources.
2. Choosing to drive the motor home on the freeway may save time but still is at a high cost.
3. Choosing the compact car and driving on country roads will save gas, but it still takes a long time.
4. The obvious best choice: choosing the compact car and driving on the freeway will save both time and resources.

	Low Efficiency	High Efficiency
Low Value	1. Takes a long time, costs more money **The Worst Option**	2. Time saved may be offset by high costs
High Value	3. Money saved may be offset by time lost	4. Takes short time, costs less money **The Best Option**

Clinical Applications

With the current emphasis on accountability and cost effectiveness, why would we employ a method that takes a long time and costs more money? Good question.

Evaluating the value and efficiency of the treatments we provide are keys to understanding the best choices we can make. Just as we may regret missing the scenery of the country road or the comfort of the motor home by making these choices, we must make some hard decisions regarding the best use of limited time and resources to provide health care.

Although this is a very simple example, it is easy to understand the principles of using evidence to support our treatment decisions. Various clinical tools provide quantifiable measures of function, balance, strength, or quality of life. We can easily measure the duration or frequency of treatment and its associated costs and do simple division to determine the efficiency and the value of physical therapy treatment provided.

With this information, we can make informed decisions and we can choose to compromise when we need to take a detour or stop on our path to reaching the destination.

Building Questions

To find evidence, we must ask the right question. The Centre for Evidence-Based Medicine has created a model for building questions.[14] By systematically approaching the clinical questions of greatest importance to us, we have an opportunity to both evaluate existing evidence and collect data to answer those questions for which no evidence currently exists. Review the process presented in the figure located in the Putting It Into Practice section on page 168.

Summary

Evidence-based practice requires a critical analysis of treatment goals and related outcomes. The types of evidence offered may influence our evaluation of the scientific merit of a particular study or approach. Qualitative researchers argue against using strict criteria to evaluate evidence supporting the practice of physical therapy because complex biopsychosocial phenomena influence the ways we think about the causes and effects we observe. Valid and reliable methods of measuring outcomes and the associated costs in time and resources allow us to analyze the efficiency and value of physical therapy intervention.

References

1. Gay JM. *General Terms for Epidemiology & Evidence-based Medicine, Clinical Epidemiology & Evidence-Based Medicine Glossary.* College of Veterinary Medicine. Washington State University. Available at: http://www.vetmed.wsu.edu/courses-jmgay/GlossClinEpiEBM.htm#. Accessed July 8, 2000.

2. Sacket DL, Rosenberg WMC, Gray JAM, Haynes RB, Richardson WS. Evidence based medicine: what it is and what it isn't. *BMJ.* 1996;312:71-72.

3. Lindberg DA, Hart YM, Sackett DL, et al. Evidence-Based Medicine Working Group. Evidence-based medicine: a new approach to teaching the practice of medicine. *JAMA.* 1992;268:2420-2425.

4. Harris SR. How should treatments be critiqued for scientific merit? *Phys Ther.* 1996;76:175-181.

5. Berger D, Davis CM. What constitutes evidence? *Phys Ther.* 1996;76(9):1011-1012,1014-1015.

6. Dorko B, Spielholz NI. Outside of science: where are the data? *PT-Magazine of Physical Therapy.* 1997;5(3):60-64.

7. Duncan PW. Evidence-based practice: a new model for physical therapy. *PT-Magazine of Physical Therapy.* 1996;4(12):44-48.

8. APTA. *Guide to Physical Therapist Practice.* 2nd ed. Alexandria, Va: American Physical Therapy Association; 2001.

9. Bernard LC, Krupat E. *Health Psychology: Biopsychosocial Factors in Health and Illness.* London: Harcourt Brace; 1994.

10. APTA House of Delegates endorses a vision for the future [press release]. Available at: http://www.apta.org/news/visionstatementrelease. Accessed Sept. 3, 2000.

11. APTA. *Evaluative Criteria for Accreditation of Education Programs for the Preparation of Physical Therapists.* Available at: http://www.apta.org/Education/accreditation/evaluativecriteria_pt. Accessed June 22, 2000.

12. Roach KE, Ally D, Finnerty B, et al. The relationship between duration of physical therapy services in the acute care setting and change in functional status in patients with lower-extremity orthopedic problems. *Phys Ther.* 1998;78:19-24.

13. Curtis KA, Crawford M, Johnson H, et al. The influence of perceived prior level of function and social support on physical therapist projections of patient functional outcomes [abstract]. *Proceedings of the 12th International Congress of the World Confederation for Physical Therapy*. Bethesda, Md: APTA; 1995:125.

14. Center for Evidence Based Medicine. *Focusing Clinical Questions Web Page*. Available at: http://www.cebm.jr2.ox.ac.uk/docs/focusquest.html. Accessed September 3, 2000.

PUTTING IT INTO PRACTICE

1. Refer to this website at the Centre for Evidence-Based Medicine:
    http://cebm.jr2.ox.ac.uk/docs/focusquest.html

    Using the chart below as an example, build a question by writing about a physical therapy problem.

	1 **Patient or Problem**	**2** **Intervention** (a cause, prognostic factor, treatment, etc)	**3** **Comparison Intervention** (if necessary)	**4** **Outcomes**
Tips for Building	Starting with your patient, ask "How would I describe a group of patients similar to mine?" Balance precision with brevity	Ask "Which main intervention am I considering?" Be specific	Ask "Which is the main alternative to compare with the intervention?" Again, be specific	Ask "Which can I hope to accomplish?" or "What could this exposure really affect?" Again, be specific
Example	"In patients with heart failure from dilated cardiomyopathy who are in sinus rhythm..."	"...Would adding anticoagulation with warfarin to standard heart failure therapy..."	"...When compared with standard therapy alone..."	"...Lead to lower mortality or morbidity from thromboembolism. Is this enough to be worth the increased risk of bleeding?"

Reprinted with permission from the Centre for Evidence-Based Medicine.

Problem	Intervention	Comparison	Outcomes

2. Review a few pages of one of your current textbooks. What statements provide evidence to support the proposed intervention or recommended technique?

    What type of evidence supports most of the information presented in your textbooks?

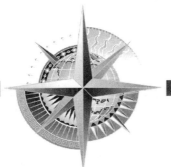

Chapter 17

Information Competence

Kayla read the instructions for the assignment. "Find a research article that addresses the effectiveness of one of the treatment techniques covered in the following list. Write an abstract outlining the study and then a two-paragraph critique of the study. Address any sampling, methods, measurement, and data analysis issues that affect the application of the results of the study." She turned on her computer and signed onto PubMed through her university library. She thought to herself, "I am so much better at this than I was when I started a year ago. I don't know what I would have done without the help of these great librarians."

What Is Information Competence?

Information competence is the process of finding, evaluating, using, and communicating information.[1] Our world has mushroomed with respect to available information. We are bombarded daily with television advertisements, telemarketing opportunities, e-mail, new websites, in addition to traditional print resources such as newspapers, magazines, and books.

Information competence is a critical process to master because our abilities to find, process, and use information are critically linked to our being able to undertake and integrate the following key processes:

- Recognize the need for information.
- State a research question, problem, or issue.
- Determine information requirements in various disciplines for the research questions, problems, or issues.
- Use information technology tools to locate and retrieve relevant information.
- Organize information.
- Analyze and evaluate information.
- Communicate using a variety of information resources and technologies.
- Understand the ethical and legal issues surrounding information and information technology.
- Apply the skills gained in information competence to enable lifelong learning.[1,2]

Researching the Topic

The first step in finding information is knowing what you need to know and where to look. Both of these processes may depend on your ability to conceptualize your needs in *language* that is consistent with the ways in which this information is stored.

Key words become critical in searching for information. Key words follow established conventions for searching that are universally accepted by librarians and others who establish and maintain databases.

Medical Subject Headings

Medical subject headings (MeSH) are the controlled vocabulary used by the National Library of Medicine for indexing articles, for cataloging books and other holdings, and for searching MeSH-indexed databases, including MEDLINE. MeSH terminology provides a consistent way to retrieve information that may use different terminology for the same concepts.[3]

The National Library of Medicine offers an online browser that provides a guide to terminology. This tool is designed to help quickly locate descriptors of possible interest and to show the hierarchy in which these descriptors appear. The browser shows MeSH records and also provides qualifiers that will narrow a search. The URL for the browser is: http://www.nlm.nih.gov/mesh/MBrowser.html

Databases

Databases are indexed lists of resources, journal articles, conference proceedings, and other materials that are often discipline-specific. Some of the most useful databases for the health-related fields are MEDLINE, CINAHL, and Psycinfo.

MEDLINE: 1966 to Present

Provided by the National Library of Medicine, this database indexes thousands of medical journals published throughout the world. Primarily for health professionals, this is the most comprehensive database of medical literature available. Not all journals are indexed in MEDLINE. For example, although the journals *Physical Therapy* and the *Journal of Orthopaedic and Sports Physical Therapy* are indexed in this database, *PT-The Magazine of Physical Therapy* is not.

CINAHL: 1982 to Present

CINAHL (Cumulative Index of Nursing and Allied Health Literature) contains more than 250,000 references to journal articles, meeting abstracts, audiovisuals, and dissertations in nursing and allied health sciences. This index covers more than 1000 nursing, allied health, biomedical, and consumer health journals. CINAHL also provides access to health care books, nursing dissertations, selected conference proceedings, standards of professional practice, and educational software in nursing. Additional physical therapy-related resources are indexed in CINAHL.

Psycinfo: 1967 to Present

The American Psychological Association's index to 1300 journals covers all aspects of psychology. Psycinfo also indexes books, chapters in books, technical reports, and dissertations. This is the first place to look for published research in psychology.

Most databases today exist online or on CD-ROM and are accessible in university libraries. Your access to a database, however, may be limited. There may be a fee or you may have to register as a student to gain access to a library's databases.

Table 17-1 provides examples of online databases that provide access to health-related literature. In addition, your university library probably provides access to many additional resources. Consult with the reference librarian in your library to guide you to these resources.

Conducting a MEDLINE Search

> *MaryAnne was preparing a case study on a 12-year-old girl with whom she worked during her last clinical experience. The patient had a diagnosis of osteogenic sarcoma, a malignant bone tumor. She wanted to research the functional outcomes of limb-sparing surgical procedures on MEDLINE. On entering the term "osteogenic sarcoma," she initially finds 12,459 articles!*

Narrowing the Search

When there are too many references, we can have a database do the work for us. By using the MeSH browser, we can find the terms under which the best articles should be indexed.

For example, on entering the search term "osteogenic sarcoma," the MeSH browser tells us that the correct terminology for searching MEDLINE is "osteosarcoma." It also gives us a possible qualifier RH, which stands for rehabilitation. We can use this qualifier to narrow the search by placing the letters /RH after our search term, osteosarcoma. Table 17-2 provides a sample of MeSH browser output.

> *MaryAnne runs a MEDLINE search using the term "osteosarcoma/RH" and finds 24 articles. She selects three that seem most applicable. She searches through the key words (MH) in the output for other possible search terms.*

The MEDLINE output of one of these articles is listed in Table 17-3. We can widen or further our search by using terms listed under MH. This is often helpful, as there may be terms that we have not used in initiating this type of search.

Table 17-1
HEALTH-RELATED ONLINE RESOURCES

HealthGate Data Corp—http://www.healthgate.com
(USA) Medical site, includes MEDLINE, Ageline, Psycinfo, EMBASE, drug information, and other databases.

Internet Grateful Med V2.6.2—http://igm.nlm.nih.gov/
Free and flexible MEDLINE gateway.

MEDLINE—http://www.nlm.nih.gov/databases/freemedl.html
Free MEDLINE from the National Library of Medicine. Access to 11 million references and abstracts.

Medscape—http://www.medscape.com
(USA) Award-winning free MEDLINE access back to 1966.

PubMed Central Home—http://www.pubmedcentral.nih.gov/
National Institutes of Health repository for peer-reviewed primary research reports in the life sciences. View full-text articles online.

PubMed Medline—http://www.ncbi.nlm.nih.gov/PubMed/
(USA) The National Library of Medicine's MEDLINE and pre-MEDLINE database (WWW access). This is the gold standard for MEDLINE searches.

The Medline Fool—http://www.medportal.com
(Canada) Search PubMed, MEDLINE, and pre-MEDLINE from the National Library of Medicine. Includes an award-winning interface and links to MEDLINE, Canadian and international medical sites, as well as health news feeds.

Internet Directories and Search Engines

To search the Internet, it may be helpful to use either a search engine and/or a directory. Not everybody understands the difference and when it is best to use one or the other.

Directories

Directories provide lists of websites, categorized by topic area with brief descriptions. The categories and descriptions are based on submissions by website masters, reviewed and edited by professional or volunteer editors. The following are examples of directories:

- Yahoo
- Librarian's Index to the Internet
- The Argus Clearinghouse
- Infoseek: Ultrasmart
- Magellan: McKinley's Internet Directory

Search Engines

In contrast to a directory, which categorizes websites and contains very little information about them (just the description), a search engine indexes all the information on all the web pages it finds.

A website might have a few, hundreds, or thousands of pages. The search engine sends out robot programs (called "crawlers") that bring back the full text of the pages they find.

The search engine indexes every word of every page found by its numerous crawlers. It organizes this information not just by the words, but by the order of the words, so you can search for phrases or entire sentences. The following are examples of search engines:

Table 17-2
MeSH Browser Output

MeSH Heading:	Osteosarcoma
Tree Number:	C04.557.450.565.575.650
Tree Number:	C04.557.450.795.620
Annotation:	blood supply / chem / second / secret / ultrastruct permitted; coord IM with BONE:NEOPLASMS (IM) or specific precoord bone/neopl term (IM) or specific bone (IM) + BONE:NEOPLASMS (IM)
Scope Note:	A sarcoma originating in bone-forming cells, affecting the ends of long bones. It is the most common and most malignant of sarcomas of the bones and occurs chiefly among 10- to 25-year-old youths. (From Stedman, 25th ed)
Entry Term:	Sarcoma, Osteogenic
Allowable Qualifiers:	BL BS CF CH CI CL CN CO DH DI DT EC EH EM EN EP ET GE HI IM ME MI MO NU PA:PC PP PS PX RA RH RI RT SC SE SU TH UL UR US VE VI
Online Note:	use OSTEOSARCOMA to search SARCOMA, OSTEOGENIC 1966-88
History Note:	89; was SARCOMA, OSTEOGENIC 1963-88
Unique ID:	D012516

Table 17-3
Sample MEDLINE Output

One result of the search using osteosarcoma/RH:
UI - 93129098
AU - Frieden RA
AU - Ryniker D
AU - Kenan S
AU - Lewis MM
TI - Assessment of patient function after limb-sparing surgery
LA - Eng
MH - Adolescence
MH - Bone neoplasms/rehabilitation/*surgery
MH - Child
MH - Early ambulation
MH - Female
MH - Femoral neoplasms/rehabilitation/*surgery
MH - Gait
MH - Human
MH - Joint prosthesis/*rehabilitation
MH - Male
MH - Osteosarcoma/*rehabilitation/*surgery
MH - Outcome assessment (health care)
MH - Physical therapy/methods
MH - Range of motion, articular
MH - Sarcoma, Ewing's/rehabilitation/surgery
PT - JOURNAL ARTICLE

Table 17-3, continued

DA - 19930211
DP - 1993 Jan
IS - 0003-9993
TA - Arch Phys Med Rehabil
PG - 38-43
SB - A
SB - M
CY - UNITED STATES
IP - 1
VI - 74
JC - 8BK
AA - Author
EM - 199304
AB - Cancer rehabilitation is becoming more of a focus for the field of physiatry due to increased longevity and the side effects of treatment. In order to investigate the rehabilitation needs of patients undergoing limb-sparing procedures, chart analysis was conducted on 17 children treated for primary bone tumors by resection and an expandable endoprosthetic replacement. Each patient underwent a course of postoperative inpatient and outpatient physical therapy and was followed over an average of 2.5 years. Gait training was relatively straightforward and in seven patients required neither orthosis nor ambulatory aid. The other 10 patients walked with a knee orthosis, axillary crutches, or both. Until the time came for reoperation to lengthen the implant, a shoe lift of 1-inch maximum was added to compensate for the limb length discrepancy. These findings compare favorably with the more complex requirements of high proximal amputees with external prostheses, including more difficult gait training and the need for frequent adjustments, as well as prosthetic replacement as the children grow. It is clear that children undergoing limb-sparing surgery have special needs that should be addressed, including early mobilization, gait training, adjustment to repeated brief hospitalizations for lengthening, and continued follow-up to monitor their activity restriction.
AD - Department of Rehabilitation Medicine, Mount Sinai Medical Center, Mount Sinai School of Medicine, New York, NY 10029
PMID- 0008420518
EDAT- 1993/01/01 00:00
MHDA- 1993/01/01 00:00
SO - Arch Phys Med Rehabil 1993 Jan;74(1):38-43

- Google
- AltaVista
- HotBot
- Infoseek
- Ultraseek
- Lycos

There are even search engines that search in multiple search engines simultaneously:

- *DogPile*: Searches 13 web search engines, six Usenet sources, and two FTP archives.
- *All-in-One Search Page*: Compiles form-based Internet search tools divided into the subject areas of general and specialized interest, software, people, news/weather, literature, technical reports, documentation, and desk reference.

- *Ask Jeeves*: User can enter his or her own language to search the Ask Jeeves database as well as other search engines.
- *Hotsheet*: Provides access to both search and multisearch engines as well as links to wire services, investing services, and much more.
- *MetaCrawler*: Searches six search engines and produces a ranked, annotated list of sites.
- *Savvy Search*: Searches 20 search engines at once.
- *Profusion*: Allows the choice of search engines or chooses what it believes are the best three. Also offers an alert feature that notifies you of new websites in your area of interest.

Table 17-4

EVALUATING ARTICLES[4]

Criteria for Evaluation of Articles

1. How recent is this source? Is it written in the last 2 to 5 years? Are there more recent sources?

2. Is it a primary or secondary source? Is it a review article, a position paper, or a research report?

3. Is there a single author or multiple contributors? With what institution(s), universities, or medical centers are the authors affiliated?

4. Who is the intended audience? Is it a scientific or scholarly journal, a popular magazine, or newspaper article?

5. What theoretical approaches or methodologies are used?

6. What findings, facts, or statistics are useful to you? What new information does this source provide?

Evaluating the Quality of the Information You Find

The various searches may turn up journal articles, internet-based bibliographies, testimonials, and commercial sources selling medical products. The next step is to evaluate the credibility of the source. Tables 17-4 and 17-5 give some useful tips for evaluating articles and Internet resources.

Organizing Information

Once the search is done, the next step is to organize the information. It may be helpful to use outlines, two-dimensional grids, or more flexible mapping techniques.[5] Examples are given below.

Outline

An outline is useful to list and categorize information. This is always a good start to classify and list information.

Osteosarcoma
I.   Prevalence and incidence
II.   Pathology
III. Nonsurgical treatment
    A. Radiation
    B. Adjuvant chemotherapy
IV.   Surgical treatment
    A. Amputation
    B. Limb-saving approaches

V.   Rehabilitation issues
    A. Timing
    B. Gait training
    C. Complications
VI.   Case study

Two-Dimensional Grid

This method is often useful to compare and contrast approaches, techniques, or sources of information by pre-determined categories.

It might be useful in this case to contrast the outcomes of amputation and limb-saving procedures by some predetermined categories. Under each category, one could list articles that address the relevant categories (Table 17-6).

The Concept Map

The "mind-map" provides a flexible means to portray and relate information. The "mapper" sketches concepts and draws relationships between them. See the mind map in Figure 17-1. The value of this approach to organizing information is the ability to include relationships, contingencies, and feedback systems.

Summary

The acquisition, evaluation, and use of information may be technically complex and overwhelming. Information competence involves using effective strategies for searching, organizing, and presenting

Table 17-5

CRITERIA FOR EVALUATING INTERNET RESOURCES[4]

1. Who is the intended audience of the page based on its content, tone, and style? Does this meet your needs?
2. What is the source of this information? Web search engines often amass vast results, from memos to scholarly documents. Many of the resulting items will be peripheral or useless for your research.
3. Is there an identifiable author/producer? Does this author have expertise on the subject or published credentials? You may need to trace back in the URL to view a page in a higher directory with background information.
4. What is the location of the site? Is it the site of a larger institution? Sponsor/location of the site is appropriate to the material as shown in the URL.
   Examples:
   - .edu for educational or research material
   - .gov for government resources
   - .com for commercial products or commercially sponsored sites
   - A name (~NAME) in the URL may mean a personal home page with no official sanction.
5. Is there a mail link that is offered for submission of questions or comments?
6. Is the information referenced? Just because it is written, it is not necessarily true. Websites are rarely refereed or reviewed, in contrast to scholarly journals and books. The source of the information should be clearly stated, whether original or summarized from elsewhere.
7. Is the information comprehensive, or does it cover a specific time period or aspect of the topic?
8. Is the information current? Has the site been updated recently?
9. Are links relevant and appropriate? Do they work? Is there a search function on the site?

Table 17-6

TWO-DIMENSIONAL GRID

Surgical Treatment	Author, Year	Long-Term Survival	Sensory and Motor Function	Gait
Amputation	Greenberg, 1994	Quality of life good in long-term survivors	Phantom pain common	
Amputation	Renard, 2000			Function improved after limb salvage surgery
Limb-Saving Procedure	Frieden, 1993			Require gait training and assistive devices
Limb-Saving Procedure	deVisser, 2001		Balance worse with eyes closed	Documented balance difficulty
Limb-Saving Procedure	deVisser, 1998			Slower walking speed and stride duration

Figure 17-1. Mind map.

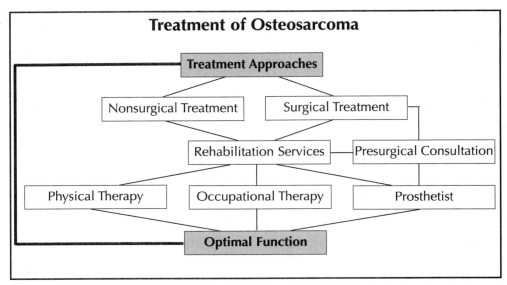

information. Attention to the technical aspects of searching literature and databases will accelerate the acquisition of relevant information. Developing skills in information competence will assist the student to effectively search the literature and appropriately use the information found.

References

1. Gavilan Community College Library. *Information Competence Plan for the California Community Colleges Webpage.* Available at: http://www.gavilan.cc.ca.us/library/infocomp/intro.html#what. Accessed July 6, 2000.

2. California State University, Northridge Library. *Information Competence. A Set of Core Competencies web page.* Available at: http://library.csun.edu/susan.curzon/corecomp.html. Accessed September 3, 2000.

3. Searching PubMed. *Gratefully Yours.* Bethesda, Md: US Department of Health and Human Services, Public Health Service, National Institutes of Health, National Library of Medicine. Webpage available at: http://www.nlm.nih.gov/pubs/gyours/janfeb98.html. Accessed August 3, 2001.

4. Curtis KA. *Library assignment. UNIV 001. University Orientation.* Fresno, Calif: California State University; 1998.

5. Carter C, Bishop J, Kravits SL. *Keys to Effective Learning.* Upper Saddle River, NJ: Prentice-Hall Inc; 1998.

PUTTING IT INTO PRACTICE

1. Go the PubMed Internet site: http://www.ncbi.nlm.nih.gov/PubMed/

2. Enter a topic (word or phrase) for a search:

3. Enter the number of articles you found:

4. Narrow the search using the MeSH browser, located at: http://www.ncbi.nlm.nih.gov:80/entrez/
    meshbrowser.cgi

5. What MeSH terms are applicable for your topic?

6. Enter the number of articles you found using this term:

7. Narrow the search using a qualifier by following the MeSH term with /[qualifier].
    List of possible qualifiers: BL BS CF CH CI CL CN CO DH DI DT EC EH EM EN EP ET GE HI IM
                                 ME MI MO NU PA PC PP PS PX RA RH RI RT SC SE SU TH UL UR US
                                 VE VI

8. Now, how many articles did you find?

9. Select and print one or two of the abstracts that look most applicable to your interests.

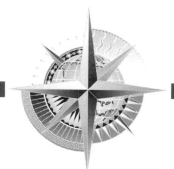

Chapter 18

Diversity And Cultural Competence in Physical Therapy

Mike opened his mailbox and saw the letter from the physical therapy program where he hoped to be admitted. He opened the letter quickly and scanned the text. "You have been admitted to the Class of 2006, pending successful completion of all prerequisite courses prior to beginning the program." He ran into his apartment to tell his roommates. Only Darryl was home. He congratulated Mike and asked if he would be the only African-American male in the program.

Diversity in the Physical Therapy Profession

Who works in the physical therapy profession? Take a look at the demographics of the physical therapist membership of the American Physical Therapy Association in Figures 18-1 to 18-4.[1] As you can see, the profession of physical therapy includes members of all age and ethnic groups. By these comparisons, we can see that the majority of physical therapists are under age 45, female, caucasian, and educated at the baccalaureate degree level.

Most practicing physical therapists fall between the ages of 25 and 44. In contrast, physical therapists are most likely to provide care to the elderly, 35 million strong and growing in numbers daily.

Estimates indicate that there are approximately 100,000 physical therapists in practice in the United States. Even though that seems like a large number, that amounts to less than one physical therapist for every 2800 people who live in the United States.

Even though women outnumber men in the physical therapy profession, recent surveys indicate that there are widespread inequities in salary and positions by gender.[2]

Comparing the Physical Therapy Profession to the Population

The US population estimates have quite different demographics than the members of the physical therapy profession.[1,3] There are large differences between the distribution of physical therapists and the general population by age, gender, and ethnicity. Therefore, it is likely that a physical therapist will provide services to persons unlike themselves in age group, gender, or ethnic origins. It is therefore critical that physical therapists learn skills that will help them to deliver services across this diverse population.

The population of the United States is becoming more culturally diverse. Almost 30% is from African-American, Hispanic/Latino, Asian-American,

Figure 18-1. Comparison of physical therapists and US population by age group (adapted from APTA. *February 2000 and Resident Population Estimates of the United States by Age and Sex, US Census.* Webpage available at: http://www.apta.org/ Research/survey_stat/pt_demo/ pt_age, with permission from the American Physical Therapy Association).

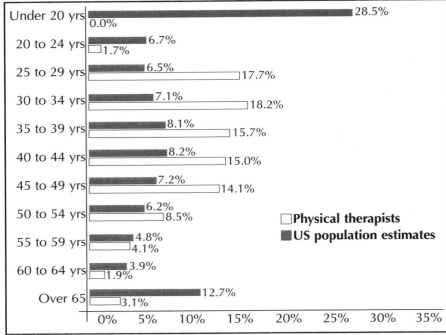

Figure 18-2. Comparison of APTA members and US population by gender (physical therapists) (adapted from APTA. Webpage available at: http://www.apta.org/Research/ survey_stat/pt_demo/pt_sex with permission from the American Physical Therapy Association).

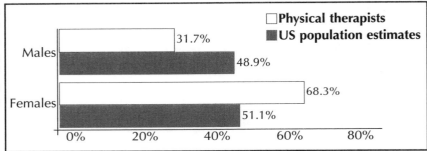

Figure 18-3. Comparison of physical therapists and US population by ethnic group/race (adapted from APTA. *Resident Population Estimates of the United States Ethnic Group/ Race, US Census.* Webpage available at: http://www.apta. org/Research/survey_stat/pt_de mo/pt_race with permission from the American Physical Therapy Association).

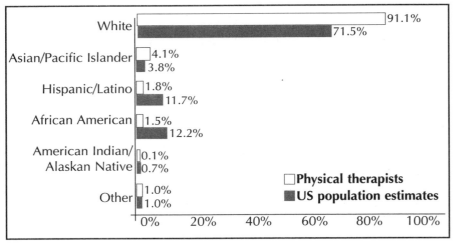

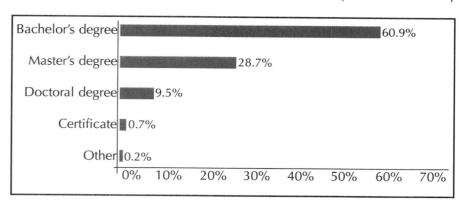

Figure 18-4. Professional education program completed by APTA members (physical therapists) (n=38,355) (adapted from APTA. Webpage available at: http://www. apta.org/Research/ survey_stat/pt_demo/pt_prof_e duc with permission from the American Physical Therapy Association).

Native Hawaiian/Pacific Islander, and American Indian/Alaska Native backgrounds. In contrast to the US population, *fewer than 10% of APTA members* (either physical therapists or physical therapist assistants) are from these backgrounds. What can we do about this?

The APTA is committed to enhancing cultural diversity and awareness of differences in the profession of physical therapy. The association's activities are directed toward promoting minority representation among the APTA membership and leadership; recruiting minority physical therapy students, educators, and researchers; inclusion of issues of cultural diversity in physical therapy educational programs; and promoting physical therapy service delivery to minority group members. There are scholarships, educational materials, workshops, fund-raising events, and public relations efforts that are committed to realizing this agenda.

Increased Minority Representation Among Students

The news is improving as we look at who is entering the physical therapy profession. Recent student data indicates 1853 of the current 11,664 physical therapy students are members of minority groups, increasing minority representation to almost 16%. Among physical therapist assistant students, 213 of 1017 students (21%) are members of minority groups.[4] However, this encouraging data is only the beginning. Profession-wide initiatives will continue to foster increased minority participation in physical therapy education and practice.[5]

Culture

Culture provides a lens through which people see their world and largely determines the characteris-

> *Linda was assigned for a 3-week practicum to a clinic that provides health care services to migrant farm workers. Although many of the clinic staff members were bilingual, Linda struggled to communicate in Spanish. Her patients seemed to appreciate her efforts, and she was surprised on her last day when a patient and his wife brought her a large plate of tamales.*

tics of their community and family life.[6,7] A *cultural group* shares values, norms, symbols, language, and living practices that are repeated and transmitted from one generation to another.[7] Culture goes far beyond race and ethnicity. Where you live, your lifestyle, and your age often form values that cross ethnic and racial lines.

We traditionally associate the term *culture* with the food, music, dance, and clothing that are unique to groups of people. Although cultures differ from one another, there are also *subgroups*, or subcultures, within cultures. We do not always associate the concept of culture or *subculture* with the values of a professional group or roles within organizations. Yet, we experience the effects of these cultures daily.

Cross-cultural experiences involve our moving into a different culture.[6,7] Although we often associate this term with experiencing the customs of a different ethnic group, we can use this term in many contexts. For example, university students live within a very specific subculture of the university; they often find it difficult to make the transition to the subculture of work upon graduation.

Cultural competence is a term that describes a set of skills that grow from the foundation that culture is the key force in shaping behaviors, values, and institutions, including some concepts like family and community.[6-8] Providers, clients, and patients have unique culture-specific needs that influence service delivery. This perspective encompasses the view that people from different racial and ethnic groups can be best served by persons who are part of or sensitive to their culture.

A Culture of One

Despite your ethnicity, geographical area of origin, occupation, gender, or age, you may be quite different from others in groups with whom you might be associated. Appreciating the *culture of one* requires an appreciation of the unique characteristics of every person. There is wide variation within every culture; therefore, a care provider must be sensitive not only to the cultural context in which a person lives but also sensitive to the individual's needs.

See how aware you are of the language of cultural competence. Which of the terms in Table 18-1 are familiar to you? Let's look more closely at your culture and how it may affect the expectations you have of others.

Assess your cultural competence. The questions in Table 18-2 may stimulate you to critically assess your beliefs and practices with persons from cultures other than yours.

If some of the situations in Table 18-2 made you feel uncomfortable or question your tolerance, be assured that you are normal. Cultural competence involves gaining an awareness of your values and the common experiences around differences so that you can develop the skills to provide culturally appropriate services.[7]

Implications of Culture on Physical Therapy Practice

The following are just a few areas in which culture may have a profound influence on what physical therapists and their patients/clients experience.[9,10]

Health Beliefs

> Francine felt the lump in her breast for months before she mentioned it to anyone. By the time she visited the clinic, the lump had doubled in size. A biopsy showed an infiltrating ductal carcinoma, almost 2 cm in diameter. The oncology nurse encouraged the physical therapy students to explore Francine's beliefs to understand why she waited to seek attention.

Health beliefs are related to our perceptions of our vulnerability and the seriousness of an illness or injury. We also hold beliefs about our likelihood of recovery and the seriousness of the problem. Health beliefs and related fears may keep a person from taking action or may cause a patient to seek assistance for an alternative healer.

Cultural Beliefs

> Fatima waited nervously in the chairs outside the clinic doors. Eric, the student physical therapist, called her name. She asked, "Excuse me, I'd prefer to be seen by a female therapist. Is that possible?" Eric asked Carla, his supervisor, to work with Fatima. Carla, afterward, complimented Eric on his cultural sensitivity and told him that the patient's religious beliefs did not permit her to disrobe in front of a man.

Cultural beliefs may dictate assignment of a physical therapist of the same gender. It may not be acceptable for male therapists to provide care to female patients or for female therapists to care for male patients. Beliefs may also preclude some forms of treatment.

Concepts of Time

Time is a culturally defined phenomenon. "Early" and "late" are cultural concepts. Therapists may be quite surprised or frustrated by the unexpected or delayed arrival of a patient.

Food and Lifestyle Habits

Diet, exercise, "type A" behavior, stress, and expectations of ourselves are all influenced by culture. It may be very difficult to change behavior, even when unhealthy, due to the strong influence of the family, environment, social customs, and habits. Consider how difficult it would be to change foods when a certain dish symbolizes prosperity, love, or hope.

Meaning of Illness, Aging, Death in Patient Culture

The meaning of an illness or death within a culture largely determines actions around these events. You can imagine that advice regarding prevention or healing might be taken quite differently by people who see illness as the effect of an external force out of one's control and people who believe that illness has internal causes that can be controlled.

> Mrs. Chen fractured her hip in a fall in her bedroom. This was the third hospital admission in the past 6 months. Although the orthopedic team recommended placement in a subacute facility, her son and daughter-in-law insisted on home-based rehabilitation services. She was discharged 2 days later.

Table 18-1
CULTURAL VOCABULARY[7]

Beliefs	Acceptance of something as true.
Culture	The learned and shared knowledge, beliefs, and rules that people use to interpret experiences and generate social behavior. The guiding force behind the behaviors and material products associated with a group of people.
Cultural competence	A set of practice skills, knowledge, and attitudes that encompasses: (1) awareness and acceptance of difference; (2) awareness of one's own cultural values; (3) understanding of the dynamics of difference; (4) development of cultural knowledge; (5) ability to adapt practice skills to fit the cultural context of the client or patient.
Cultural group	A group of people who consciously or unconsciously share identifiable values, norms, symbols, and some ways of living that are repeated and transmitted from one generation to another.
Culture shock	A form of anxiety that results from an inability to predict the behavior of others or act appropriately in a cross-cultural situation.
Ethnicity	A group identity based on culture, language, religion, a common attachment to a place, or kin ties.
Ethnocentrism	The interpretation of the beliefs and behavior of others in terms of one's own cultural values and traditions with the assumption that one's own culture is superior.
Language	The form or pattern of speech (spoken or written) used by residents or descendants of a particular nation or geographic area or by any large body of people. Language can be formal or informal and includes dialect, idiomatic speech, and slang.
Norms	A standard, model, or pattern for a group.
Social customs	A usual practice carried on by tradition by a group.
Values	Acts, customs, and institutions regarded as especially favorable by a group.

Are the elderly valued and revered or discounted as a burden? Cultural beliefs may determine the structure of the health care system as well. In some cultures, placing a loved one in a long-term care facility is an unthinkable option.

Developing Cultural Competence

Students will have many opportunities to develop cultural competence. Take this responsibility seriously. Culturally sensitive care is your responsibility as a health care provider. There are many aspects to consider.[8-16]

Show Respect

Demonstrate respect for the diverse cultures, heritages, and experiences of the patients you encounter. Gain experience in working with racially, ethnically, and culturally diverse populations. Seek experiences that challenge you to work with individuals who are unlike yourself.

Develop Self-Awareness

Rita, a student physical therapist, was assigned to the spinal cord injury unit. Her patient had sustained a spinal cord injury just 2 weeks earlier. She was not hopeful that he would regain muscle function because his injury was complete and he had no signs of neurological function below the level of the spinal cord lesion. She approached his room for his initial visit on Tuesday afternoon and was told that a healing session was in progress and that he would not be finished for at least another hour. Rita felt inconvenienced and wondered later why the hospital would allow such practices.

Examine the influence of the similarities and differences of your own culture, ethnicity, language,

Table 18-2
CULTURAL AWARENESS EXERCISE

Answer the following questions to test your cultural competence:

1. Someone in your workplace has practices different from your own. This might involve a religious practice, a style of dress, or a lifestyle. How do you react? Are you judgmental or critical of this person either openly or silently?
2. What diverse groups of individuals live in your neighborhood, attend school, or work with you? How are different cultural practices honored? How do you feel about a colleague requesting a delay of an examination or asking for a day off from work for celebration of ethnic or religious holidays?
3. How were you raised as a child? What are your cultural origins? What beliefs, stories, and values did your family share with you? How did your upbringing differ from those of your friends and neighbors? What did you learn about alternate lifestyles or belief systems? If you have children, what beliefs, stories, and values do you share with them? How would you feel about your children, nephews, or nieces learning about alternate lifestyles or belief systems? What might you teach them?
4. What health behaviors do you practice that are related to culture? How much are the foods you eat, your attitudes about sickness and health, and the care you seek when you are ill influenced by your cultural beliefs? How tolerant would you be of a patient or client who failed to change the behavior (such as a dietary habit) that resulted in a serious and preventable health problem?
5. What are your expectations in receiving health care? How do you feel about receiving expert care that is insensitive to your experience, beliefs, or family situation? What assumptions does your health care provider make about you or a family member? What recommendations of a health care provider have you or a family member ignored because they did not fit with your lifestyle, your traditional diet, or social customs?

and/or race on your interactions with others. Identify how your own biases might influence service delivery. Examine how your professional values may conflict with the needs of the individual. Recognize the need to address these differences and possibly refer the patient to another provider to receive the most beneficial treatment.

Learn as Much as You Can

Read about the differences in cultures related to history, traditions, values, belief systems, acculturation and migration patterns, reasons for immigration/migration, and dialect and language fluency. Examine particular stressors and traumas that a group of people may have experienced related to war, trauma or violence, political unrest, racism, or discrimination. Identify unique aspects of cultural survival and maintenance, socioeconomic status, and culturally based belief systems.

Communicate in Many Ways

Develop sensitivity to verbal and nonverbal lan-

guage, speech patterns, and communication styles. Conduct interviews that incorporate sensitivity to the potential influence of psychological, social, biological, physiological, cultural, political, spiritual, and environmental aspects of the patient or client's experience.

Services for non-English-speaking patients should include informing them that they have the right to receive no-cost interpreter services. Signs and commonly used written patient education materials should be translated for the predominant language groups in a service area.

Try to use the patient/client's preferred language whenever possible. Use interpreters as needed when bilingual clinicians are not available. Interpreters and bilingual staff should have bilingual proficiency, be trained in the skills and ethics of interpreting, and have knowledge in both languages of the terms and concepts needed in the clinical encounter. Family members are not considered suitable substitutes for trained interpreters because they usually lack these skills and knowledge. Avoid using a patient's children or grandchildren as interpreters.

Be Flexible Regarding Treatment

> *Rita reflected further on her patient's needs. She thought about her own beliefs and how she might react to a catastrophic injury. Would she cling to hope from anyone who offered it?*

Acknowledge differences in the acceptability and effectiveness of various treatment modalities for individuals from different groups. Consider social, political, and economic conditions that may influence the nature of the intervention that you can provide. Incorporate indigenous healing practices and the role of belief systems (religion and spirituality) in the intervention whenever possible.

See Through Cultural Lenses

Develop an intervention that fits the patient/client and family's concept of illness or injury. Create collaborative plans for service delivery that incorporate the culture, family, and community. Use resources that are culturally appropriate, such as the family, clan, church, community members, and other groups.

Take Cultural Competence as Seriously as Other Clinical Skills

See the Seven Domains of Cultural Competence in Table 18-3. Incorporate these elements into your practice as diligently as you would a patient assessment or treatment technique. It will make a big difference to all whose lives you touch.

Summary

With increasing diversity in our population, it is likely that the physical therapist will frequently work with patients and clients of a different ethnicity, age, or gender group. Cultural competence involves the acquisition of skills that enable the therapist to provide culturally and linguistically sensitive services to all persons.

References

1. APTA. *PT Membership Demographics Webpage.* Available at: http://www.apta.org/Research/survey_stat/pt_demo. Accessed June 21, 2000.

2. US Census. *Resident Population Estimates of the United States by Age and Sex.* Available at: http:// www.census.gov/population/estimates/nation/intfile2-1.txt. Accessed June 21, 2000.

3. Rozier CK, Raymond MJ, Goldstein MS, et al. Gender and physical therapy career success factors. *Phys Ther.* 1998;78(7):690-704.

4. APTA. *Minority Membership Statistics.* Available at: http://www.apta.org/About/special_interests/minorityaffairs/minoritymembershipstats. Accessed June 21, 2000.

5. Monahan B. The quest for diversity in the classroom. *PT-Magazine of Physical Therapy.* 1997;5(1):72-77.

6. Shaw-Taylor Y, Benesch B. Workforce diversity and cultural competence in healthcare. *J Cult Divers.* 1998;5(4):138-148..

7. Bureau of Primary Health Care. Office of Minority and Women's Health. *Guidelines To Help Assess Cultural Competence in Program Design, Application, and Management.* Available at: http://158.72.105.163/cc/guidelines.htm. Accessed July 16, 2000.

8. Bureau of Primary Health Care. Office of Minority and Women's Health. *What is Cultural Competence?* Available at: http://158.72.105.163/cc/7domains. Accessed July 16, 2000.

9. Noorderhaven NG. Intercultural differences: consequences for the physical therapy profession. *Physiotherapy.* 1999;85(9):504-510.

10. Padilla R, Brown K. Culture and patient education: challenges and opportunities. *Journal of Physical Therapy Education.*1999;13(3):23-30.

11. Jecker N, Carrese J, Pearlman R. Caring for patients in cross-cultural settings. *Hastings Center Report.* 1995;25(1):6-14.

12. Lajkowicz C. Teaching cultural diversity for the workplace. *J Nurs Educ.* 1993;32(5):235-236.

13. Like R, Prasaad S, Rubel A. Recommended core curriculum Guidelines on culturally sensitive and competent health care. *Fam Med.* 1996;27:291-297.

14. Millon-Underwood S. Educating for sensitivity to cultural diversity. *Nurse Educator.* 1992;17(3):7.

15. Rankin S, Kappy M. Developing therapeutic relationships in multicultural settings. *Academic Medicine.* 1993;68(11):826-827.

16. Rubenstein H, O'Connor BB, Nieman LZ, et al. Introducing students to the role of folk and popular belief-systems in patient care. *Academic Medicine.* 1992;67(9):566-568.

Table 18-3
THE SEVEN DOMAINS OF CULTURAL COMPETENCE[8]

Cultural competence involves a dynamic interplay between the seven following interdependent factors or domains. These domains, while separate and discrete, are in constant motion and interact with each other. These domains include:

1. Values and attitudes. These include practices that promote mutual respect between provider and patient. For example, screening materials for offensive cultural, ethnic, or racial stereotypes; being aware and intervening where appropriate on behalf of clients when organizations display culturally insensitive behaviors; being aware of the varying degrees of acculturation by persons into the dominant culture and intervening where appropriate; respecting the varying gender roles in cultures; having a client-centered perspective; accepting that religion and other beliefs may influence patients' responses to health, illness, disease, and death.
2. Communication styles. These include provider attitudes and behaviors toward individuals of differing languages and cultures and the sensitivity to use alternatives to written communication for some clients.
3. Community/consumer participation. This includes the active and continuous involvement of community leaders and members in the development, implementation, and evaluation of policy, practices, and program interventions. Involved program participants are more invested in the success of the program; hence, health status outcomes are improved.
4. The physical environment, materials, and resources available to health care. Use culturally and linguistically responsive interior design, pictures, posters, and artwork, as well as magazines, brochures, audios, videos, films, and literacy-sensitive print information that is congruent with the cultures and languages of the populations served.
5. Policies and procedures. These include written policies, procedures, mission statements, goals, and objectives that incorporate cultural and linguistic principles and practices, including hiring multicultural and multilingual staff reflective of the community, clinical protocols, orientation, community involvement, outreach, etc.
6. Population-based clinical practice. Clinical practice that avoids the misapplication of scientific knowledge and the stereotyping of group members while still appreciating the importance of culture. Culturally skilled clinicians have good knowledge and understanding of their own world views, have specific knowledge of the particular groups with which they work, understand sociopolitical influences, and possess distinct skills (intervention techniques and strategies) needed in working with culturally diverse groups.
7. Training and professional development. These include requirements for cultural competence training opportunities, nature of the cultural competence training provided to staff in quality, duration, and frequency of professional development opportunities.

PUTTING IT INTO PRACTICE

1. How would you define your culture? Consider shared values, norms, symbols, language, and living practices that are repeated and transmitted from one generation to the next.

2. In what ways do the similarities and differences of your own culture, ethnicity, language, and/or race influence your interactions with others?

3. Take the Cultural Diversity and Competence Exam at http://www.quia.com/jq/17648.html.

4. Plan a visit to a local physical therapy clinic. What evidence would you look for as indicators of culturally sensitive care? After the visit, summarize your observations.

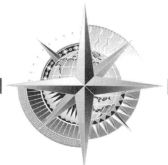

Chapter 19

Collaboration: You're on the Team!

Sam noticed a familiar pattern of bruises on the child's arm, as if someone had grabbed his arm and held too tightly. Although he suspected possible child abuse, he wasn't sure what to do. He excused himself from the treatment room and called the hospital social worker, who referred him to the Child Protective Services hotline. He called and reported his concern. He thought to himself, "I never thought I would be doing this as a physical therapist." It felt good to know that someone would follow up on his observations.

Interprofessional Collaboration

The practice of interprofessional collaboration has been identified as a critical skill for educators, health professionals, and social service providers, especially with the increasing complexity of our educational, health, and social service networks. Collaboration involves team building and building integrated service delivery mechanisms to improve outcomes for recipients of health, education, and social services.[1-5]

The complex health and social issues facing health care providers can only be addressed within the context of culture, language, socioeconomic status, and education. The needs of victims of domestic abuse, rural or inner city children and families who live in poverty, the elderly who are isolated and dependent on a fixed income, people with no insurance, and those with lifelong disabilities are so vast that one health care professional cannot begin to address them.

In addition, our health care and social service systems are tricky to navigate for even those who know the way. It is very easy for critical information and pressing needs to fall through the cracks. Clearly, discipline-specific practice does not work. The needs of a client do not stop at the role boundaries of an individual health care provider.

Consider the following example:

Mr. Feldman was discharged to his home following an open reduction of a hip fracture. The ambulance drivers brought him into his apartment and put him into his bed. He looked at the floor on which he had spent the night after falling on his way to the bathroom. The door shut and he wondered, "Wasn't someone supposed to bring me a hospital bed? How do I shop for groceries? What am I going to do?" He had forgotten what the social worker at the hospital had told him, and his papers were left on the countertop in the other room. Even the telephone was in the other room. He felt scared and alone.

Interprofessional collaboration involves professionals from different disciplines creating systems that help to meet the complex needs of a patient such

Table 19-1
TERMINOLOGY[1,2,3]

Term	Definition
Discipline	A specific body of teachable knowledge with its own background of education and training, procedures, methods, and content.
Interdisciplinary	The use of methods and language from more than one discipline to address common interests or problems.
Multidisciplinary	The juxtaposition of several disciplines side by side, focused on one problem where each discipline works alone.
Cross-disciplinary	The view of one discipline from the viewpoint of another (eg, the biomechanics of performing arts).
Transdisciplinary	A process creating new solutions beyond the scope of the individual disciplines.
Interprofessional	A shared experience that aims to help professionals work together more effectively in the interests of their clients and patients.
Intraprofessional	A specialized approach within a professional group using a common perspective.

as Mr. Feldman. It involves the following elements:[1]

- Comprehensive client-centered interventions and case management systems.
- Referral systems to link patients and clients to a network of other professionals, agencies, and services.
- Clear and effective communication with other service providers.
- Organizational structures to foster integrated service delivery using a collaborative model.
- Decentralized organizations to provide more access to services for clients.
- Mechanisms for linking/collaborating with other service providers.
- Outcome-oriented evaluation systems.

The Disciplinary Alphabet Soup

Interdisciplinary, multidisciplinary, transdisciplinary, cross-disciplinary, cooperation, collaboration. The terminology in this growing educational and practice movement is enough to make you dizzy. These words underlie the issues at the heart of the collaborative process. It is important that we understand their meanings. Take a look at how some authors have defined these terms in Table 19-1.

Teams, Groups, Committees, Task Forces, and Professional Relationships

You're on the Team!

Recognize now and forever more that your effectiveness in your work as a health care professional will be made possible by the efforts, cooperation, and collaboration of others. The outcomes that you hope to accomplish must involve others. The system you live and work in is far too complex (not to mention time-consuming) for a single provider to successfully navigate and reach a conclusion.

At a minimum, you will work with support personnel in the physical therapy profession. More likely, however, you will frequently interface with administrators, managers and clerical staff, physicians, social workers, nurses, occupational therapists, case managers, and counselors who will also provide services to your clients and patients.

Working well with others requires several key behaviors. Review Table 19-2 and see how you rate your collaboration quotient.

Table 19-2

COLLABORATION QUOTIENT

Collaboration Quotient

Consider your experiences when working on a team or on a group project in responding to the following questions.

Score

Always = 0
Frequently = 1
Sometimes = 2
Never = 3

_____ 1. Have you experienced communication problems with one or more members of the group?

_____ 2. Have you taken action before consulting others, just to "get it done"?

_____ 3. Have you expected others to recognize the value of your contributions?

_____ 4. Have you missed scheduled group or team meetings for any reason even if it's a "good" reason?

_____ 5. Have you resented the limited cooperation or lack of productivity of some group members?

_____ **Total**

If you score 13 to 15, congratulations! You are a master collaborator. Your communication skills, patience, commitment, and nonjudgmental attitudes are key to successful collaboration.

If you score 8 to 12, you need to be aware that communication is the key to successful collaboration. Put your efforts into an outcome, not your personal needs. Hold others accountable for their commitments instead of passing them off as unreliable or disinterested.

If you score below 8, your focus is on yourself and your experience, not the group outcome. Although your contributions may be valuable, you cannot do this alone. You need help in changing your perspectives. Enroll in a course on group dynamics and examine how your behavior contributes to the outcomes of the group.

Keys to Success in Collaboration

Communicate, Communicate, Communicate!

There is no substitute for communication. Include all group members in written communications. Make sure that all group members are heard. Make a special effort to reach out to those who seem to be less vocal or less involved.

Perspective-Taking

Our perceptions of our professional roles and perspectives on any problem are the product of a long series of events that we have experienced both before and during professional education. Others with whom you work have their own unique perspectives and experiences.

Take another's perspective. What does the client experience when telephoning into the office to change an appointment? What does the clerk who works for an insurance company experience when patient-related documentation is incorrect or incomplete? Looking at the situations you experience from another perspective increases your empathy.

"It must have been [exciting, difficult, frustrating, upsetting] for you when..." is a good starter to indicate your awareness of another's perspective.

Acknowledge the Contributions of Others

Although you might disagree with a particular suggestion or approach, make sure that other group members know that you heard them. A statement such as "What I like about what you said..." is an effective opener for then proposing a different perspective.

Meetings, Schedules, and Systems

Schedule meetings and create communication systems that will ensure success. Get group member commitments to attend meetings as they are scheduled. Create e-mail or distribution lists, which will simplify communication. Write minutes of meetings and record action plans for distribution to all group members.

Identify and Challenge Your Assumptions

Your assumptions about other group members will interfere with group activity. We all have stereotypes, biases, and our own ideas about others. Others have their own stereotypes, biases, and ideas about you. Spend time up front to get to know other group members and listen.

Identify for yourself what stereotypes you hold about members of other professional groups; clients; patients; ethnic, gender, or age groups. There are many interesting group exercises that can assist you to examine your biases. Acknowledging that you hold biases is the first step to limiting their power over your thoughts and actions.

Break Down Role Boundaries

Our beliefs about our roles determine the ways in which we act and what we expect of others. Role conflicts occur when we perceive that we are not able, in some way, to perform our roles. Learning more about the way that other professionals view a problem is a key step to successful collaboration. Help others to see and hear you in the way that you would like to be seen and heard.

What Is Your Professional Identity?

Examine your ideas about what physical therapists do. Did those ideas evolve as you gained more exposure to the field? Have those ideas changed after reading the first few chapters of this book? What do *others* think that physical therapists do? You will not find out unless you ask. Then, educate others as to your skills, capabilities, experience, and the scope of your professional role.

Focus on the Outcome

What outcome are you trying to achieve? Be very clear and get the commitment of all group members to this outcome. Acknowledge steps that will help you to achieve the outcome. Use the outcome to keep your focus and direction. Constantly evaluate, "Is this (meeting, activity, discussion, communication) going to help us achieve this outcome?" Use your time wisely!

The Role of Physical Therapy Education in Promoting Collaboration

Consider the educational experiences that can help you to acquire these skills and perspectives. Not all universities and professional training programs incorporate specific training in these skills. Increasingly, physical therapy educators are becoming aware of these needs and instituting university-based programs that support these skills (Table 19-3).

Recent authors in health care summarized the situation well:[5]

> Changes in the nation's health and education systems have mandated that professionals work together in a more cost-effective, collaborative manner. Academic institutions need to provide training to enable graduates to work in interdisciplinary settings, such as school-based health centers, so they can learn the skills needed to work in a truly collaborative manner. Basic knowledge about team building, communication skills, negotiation, conflict resolution, and family-based models of practice needs to be combined with opportunities for group work and decision making. This approach fosters the transformation of a group of individuals from different disciplines to a truly collaborative functioning team.

Training in Interprofessional Collaboration

Sonya, a physical therapy student, wrote in her class journal, "I never considered what others thought that we did. I was really shocked to hear that they thought we just did massages for people. Why would I need to get a graduate education to do that? The exercise in our last class helped so much to open my eyes to what others thought about me, in addition to helping me understand my thoughts about others."

Some institutions (see Table 19-3) offer specific training in interprofessional collaboration. These courses involve graduate students and practicing

Table 19-3

UNIVERSITY-BASED TRAINING IN INTERPROFESSIONAL COLLABORATION

Certificate for Advanced Study in Interprofessional Collaboration

Program Objectives

On completion of the program, students will be able to:

1. Explain the purpose, function, and structure of interprofessional practice.

2. Distinguish the roles of various professionals in meeting the needs of clients receiving services.

3. Describe theoretical framework and communication skills involved in interprofessional collaboration.

4. Discuss organizational structures for integrated service delivery using a collaborative model.

5. Use collaborative skills to provide more effective services to clients.

6. Demonstrate skills for linking/collaboration with other service providers.

7. Increase involvement with other service agencies.

8. Participate in team interaction in integrated service delivery settings.

9. Assess, develop, and implement methods for interprofessional collaboration with other service providers.

Course Descriptions

IPC 201: Interprofessional Collaboration Foundations (3 units)
Course description: Examination of beliefs and biases affecting professionalization and discipline-specific culture. Group process and team-building skills, including active listening, conflict mediation, and cultural competence. Principles of integrated service delivery models of team practice in a multicultural and interdisciplinary context.

IPC 202: Integrated Service Delivery Models (3 units)
Course description: Analysis of local community health, education, and economic challenges. Issues in working with families, agencies, and community, including access and equality. Organizational development and systems to build interagency partnerships for collaborative practice. Measuring outcomes of integrated service delivery programs.

IPC 203: Practicum in Interprofessional Collaboration (3 units)
Course description: 30 hours of supervised practice in an agency using an integrated service delivery model. This will be supplemented by a weekly 2-hour seminar on campus, which provides a forum for reflection, analysis, and synthesis of experiences and observations.

Reprinted with permission from Interprofessional Collaboration Program, California State University, Fresno (http://www.csufresno.edu/interprof).

professionals from many disciplines to participate in learning experiences that address the key beliefs and skills for successful collaboration.

Summary

Successful collaboration depends on our perspectives and actions toward others. Spending time to work on the collaborative process is an investment with tremendous returns. Education and experience in collaborative processes can change the way we think and the ways in which we deliver services to our patients and clients. The diversity of our population and complexity of our social service and health care systems requires interprofessional collaboration to ensure that our clients and patients have access to and receive appropriate services.

References

1. California State University, Fresno. *Interprofessional Collaboration Program webpage*. Available at: http://www.csufresno.edu/interprof. Accessed July 16, 2000.

2. Jacobs HH. *Interdisciplinary Curriculum: Design and Implementation*. Alexandria, Va: Association for Supervision and Curriculum Development; 1989.

3. Soothill K, Mackay L, Webb C. *Interprofessional Relations in Health Care*. London: Edward Arnold; 1995.

4. Hooper-Briar K, Lawson H. *Serving Children, Youth and Families Through Interprofessional Collaboration and Service Integration. A Framework for Action*. Oxford, Ohio: The Danforth Foundation; 1994.

5. Papa PA, Rector C, Stone C. Interdisciplinary collaborative training for school-based health professionals. *J Sch Health*. 1998;68(10):415-419.

PUTTING IT INTO PRACTICE

1. Review your university catalog or website. What other professional education programs exist at your university? What is the degree awarded, the length of the program, and the required semester hours of study? How are these programs similar to the physical therapy professional education program? How do they differ?

    What classes or educational opportunities will you share with students entering other health and human services professions?

2. Visit the University of Missouri-Columbia Virtual Health Care Team at http://www.hsc.missouri.edu/~shrp/vhctwww/

    Complete one or more of the case studies. Write your comments and reactions below:

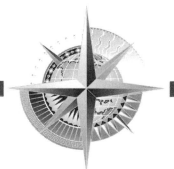

Student Involvement in the American Physical Therapy Association

American Physical Therapy Association

The American Physical Therapy Association (APTA) is an organization of more than 65,000 physical therapists, physical therapist assistants, and students. The APTA offers several categories of membership for students in physical therapist or physical therapist assistant educational programs.[1] Student membership is offered at a fraction of the active membership costs, making it one of the best deals in your career.

Students in Physical Therapist and Physical Therapist Assistant Programs

Student membership requires enrollment in a physical therapy education program that is accredited or is seeking or granted candidacy status by the Commission on Accreditation in Physical Therapy Education. *Student affiliate membership* requires enrollment in a physical therapist assistant education program that is accredited or is seeking or granted candidacy status.

Physical Therapists in Graduate School

There is a special membership category, called *active graduate student status*, for licensed graduate physical therapists who return to graduate school. This membership is also offered at a reduced fee.

Members in this category must be a graduate physical therapist enrolled full-time in a graduate program in any field. This membership status is limited to 2 years in a master's degree program and 4 years in a doctoral degree program.

Physical Therapists

Active membership is offered to physical therapists who have graduated from US physical therapy education programs that have met approval standards defined by the APTA. Membership is also open to physical therapists from other countries who have an equivalent education, as certified by an authorized agency, state board or institution, and have citizenship, legal residence, or a legal permit to work in the United States.

Physical Therapist Assistants

Affiliate membership is offered to physical therapist assistants who have graduated from US physical therapist assistant education programs that have met approval standards defined by the APTA. Membership is also open to physical therapist assistants from other countries who have an equivalent education, as certified by an authorized agency, state board or institution, and have citizenship, legal residence, or a legal permit to work in the United States.

All membership categories require members to sign a pledge to be guided by the *Code of Ethics* of the APTA.

APTA Career Starter Dues Program

There is a helpful plan to assist students with the financial burden of membership in the first few years of their careers in the physical therapy profession. New graduates who renew their memberships within 90 days following graduation pay only one-third of the active membership costs for the first year and two-thirds of these costs for the second year out of school. Graduates do not pay the full costs of active membership until the third year out of school. This ensures that new graduate therapists will have the continued support of the APTA and access to valuable news and information while establishing themselves in their careers.

Benefits of APTA Membership

APTA membership is one of the best investments that students can make in their future. Through APTA publications and student programs, they will have access to the latest developments in the profession, sources of financial aid, and building networks for future employment and professional activities.[1,2]

Information on New Developments and Research

- APTA monthly publications include *Physical Therapy* and *PT—Magazine of Physical Therapy.* These two publications include articles and information on the latest events in the profession, conference announcements, latest research, and current professional issues.

- The APTA website (http://www.apta.org) and the student assembly webpage (http://www. aptastudent.org) are valuable sources for information that students can use for everything from class projects to future job searches.

- *PT Bulletin Online* (http://www.apta.org/ Bulletin), a weekly newsletter, features current news and classified employment listings.

- *The Flash,* a biannual publication, is a news bulletin for liaisons and contains articles and information written by students from across the country. Twice a year, in the fall and spring, *The Flash* is distributed to APTA student liaisons. There are also monthly e-mail newsletters that are distributed to APTA student liaisons in each educational program.

Financial Aid for Students

There are several scholarship and loan programs, and competitive financial awards available for students in physical therapist and physical therapist assistant programs, as well as physical therapists who are enrolled in graduate programs. Specific research-related funding is available through the Foundation for Physical Therapy.[3] More information is available on the APTA website at http:// www.apta.org. Also look through the Foundation for Physical Therapy website at http://www.apta.org/ Research/foundationforpt.

Professional Networks

The APTA is the gateway for developing a professional network through chapter and district meetings, national conferences, and the National Student Conclave, an annual meeting for students of physical therapy. Membership gives students access to policymakers, researchers, expert clinicians, and leaders in the field.

Specialization

Within the APTA structure, there are 19 specialty sections that focus on particular areas of physical therapy practice, such as pediatrics, sports physical therapy, or geriatrics. Involvement in a section gives you access to specialized publications, directories of other members with similar interests, and opportunities to learn about state-of-the-art clinical techniques and residency programs available after graduation.

Professional Books and Conference Discounts

APTA membership also entitles members to discounted rates on all APTA publications and conferences. Special "member" prices also apply to t-shirts, promotional items, and public relations materials about the physical therapy profession. Further, students who volunteer for a few hours to help at state and national conferences can often attend at a markedly reduced rate.

Insurance Plans

Most clinical facilities and academic programs require that students enroll in a malpractice insurance program prior to beginning the clinical education portion of the curriculum. APTA-affiliated malpractice plans offer professional liability insurance to students at a low cost. In addition, the APTA has negotiated reasonable rates on many other forms of auto, home, and life insurance.

Leadership Skills

Students can actively participate in local district, state chapter, and national activities through student special interest groups (SSIG), the Student Assembly (SA), and the National Student Conclave. These valuable learning opportunities offer critical insights into professional organizational and governance processes. There are scholarship programs available for internships in government affairs as well. These experiences develop leadership skills for future career opportunities.

Land that Position

The APTA sponsors a Career Center at the Annual Conference and the Combined Sections Meeting, which offers guidance on resumé writing and interviewing skills. Employers and recruiters often exhibit at these meetings and at the National Student Conclave.

APTA membership should be listed on *your resumé*. APTA membership and voluntary student activity in the profession reflects a commitment that is recognized by employers and professionals across the country. It indicates that you are current and in touch with the latest educational and research information.

Student Leadership and Involvement

Here are some of the many ways that students can get involved in activities that promote the profession of physical therapy.

On-Campus Organizations

Serve in the leadership of an on-campus organization that promotes physical therapy education or awareness. Established physical therapy student organizations can usually receive financial support from university student organization funds. Such groups sponsor physical therapy awareness and disability awareness events, fundraising, lecture series, and serve as a valuable resource for the campus community.

Fundraising Activities

Work on a fundraising event. There are many potential fundraising projects that directly support student interests in the physical therapy profession. Campus organizations that support physical therapy students, political action committees, and foundations for research are all in need of support.

Campus and District/State APTA Activities

Every campus has funds and mechanisms for donations for student scholarships or resources to support student attendance at professional conferences and other activities. Students can become actively involved in raising funds to support their activities as students. Students may also become involved in district and statewide APTA fundraising efforts for particular initiatives and organizations.

Political Action

Public policy, state and federal legislation plays a major role in the future of the physical therapy profession. Political action committees are critical to ensure that legislators are well-informed about the physical therapy profession. Support of political action groups ensures that the physical therapy profession will also have a strong voice in the state and federal legislative processes.

Physical Therapy Research

The Miami Marquette Challenge is an annual fundraising competition between academic programs that donates funds to the Foundation for Physical Therapy. These funds are used to support physical therapy research. There may be similar organizations in your state or local community as well.

Observe the APTA House of Delegates

Students may observe the annual APTA House of Delegates. This session is held in conjunction with the Annual Conference in June each year. Students can see organizational governance in action on the floor of the House of Delegates. The APTA Student Assembly also sends two delegates to the House of Delegates.

Volunteer at State and National Conferences

Attending a conference is one of the best ways to see and hear the latest information, meet other students and potential employers, and develop a professional network. Students who volunteer receive discounted registration rates. Call well in advance to offer your services.

Join the APTA Student Assembly

The APTA Student Assembly (APTA-SA) was formed in 1991 to address the needs of student and student affiliate members.[2] Students share similar needs and interests in answering the challenges, issues, and pressures placed on them by their learning environment. Students share challenges such as financial and time constraints, school pressures, and concerns about future employment. The APTA-SA includes both student and student affiliate members and provides a strong base of support for future professional development.

The APTA-SA serves several functions in providing information for assembly members, promoting the role of students in the physical therapy profession, encouraging student membership, and representing the interests of APTA-SA members to APTA leadership and components. The APTA-SA sends both a PT student delegate and PTA student delegate to the House of Delegates. Although they cannot vote, they represent the APTA-SA on important issues.

There are many leadership opportunities for APTA student members on the SA Board of Directors. A new slate of candidates is nominated annually, and the election of a new board is held each June. Interested candidates can contact the nominating committee.

The APTA-SA has a webpage at http://www. aptastudent.org. A popular feature is an Assembly Bulletin Board that enables students to post messages concerning everything from good sites to clinical affiliations to requesting to find roommates for conferences. This site includes information on the latest developments, students, student issues, awards, and contact information for the APTA-SA Board members and Nominating Committee.

Serve as the APTA Student Liaison on Your Campus

Student liaisons link the APTA-SA with physical therapy and physical therapist assistant students around the country. Student liaisons disseminate information received from the Board of Directors of the APTA-SA to their classmates via public announcements, a centrally located bulletin board, and monthly e-mail letters. This information includes developments in the world of physical therapy as it relates to students. It provides a vehicle for students to communicate with each other as well. *The Flash*, the biannual publication for students, is distributed through student liaisons.

Student liaisons must currently be enrolled in either an accredited or developing PT/PTA program and be a member of the APTA. Information about becoming a student liaison and an application form can be downloaded from http://www.aptastudent.org.

Join or Start a Student Special Interest Group

Student Special Interest Groups (SSIGs) are groups of student and student affiliate members who are organized on a statewide basis in conjunction with APTA state chapters. SSIGs promote membership in the APTA and represent the interests of SSIG members to the APTA state chapter leadership. SSIGs frequently communicate by newsletters and organize meetings, educational sessions, and social events in conjunction with chapter conferences. Take a look at the sample California SSIG newsletter (Figure 20-1).

There are leadership opportunities to serve as officers of SSIGs as well.

At the time of publication, only the following 10 APTA state chapters had SSIGs: Alabama, California, Florida, Georgia, Louisiana, Massachusetts, Ohio, Pennsylvania, Tennessee, and Texas. The steps to form a SSIG are outlined on the APTA Student Assembly webpage: http://www.aptastudent.org.

APTA National Student Conclave

The National Student Conclave is an annual weekend conference sponsored by the APTA, designed to support students, expose them to advances in the field, and introduce them to the APTA governance process. It is a tremendous networking and educational opportunity that should not be missed.

Students attend educational sessions regarding career strategies, interviewing skills, legislative initiatives, and clinical sessions in areas such as orthopedics, home health, and sports physical therapy. There is an exhibition area, and many employers recruit students at this event. A popular event is the Mock House of Delegates in which students learn about the APTA governance process and parliamentary procedure. In addition, social events top off the conference activities with talent shows and receptions. Take a look at the letter (Figure 20-2) from an enthusiastic student who attended a recent student conclave.

This annual meeting occurs in the fall (usually

California Student Special Interest Group Newsletter
Pre-millennium Edition, October

The CSSIG is a peer support group in which students will have a chance to be heard and build confidence for a successful transition from school to the workforce.

Why Get Involved?

The coming of the 21st century brings many challenges for physical therapists, as managed care and capitation literally dictate our profits and survival. As young physical therapists, we need to diversify and maximize our potential. We must become educated in areas not taught in most schools, such as third-party payer interface, direct access, legislative issues, and the political base.

What Does the CSSIG Have to Offer?

- Learn about alternative practice sites and how to get the most out of the external market, such as community centers, schools, health clubs, assisted living facilities, corporations, and municipalities.
- Receive education on self-promotion and marketing, reimbursement, entrepreneurship, and alternative practice sites.
- By joining the CSSIG, you will receive monthly newsletters from a student point of view. The text will be derived from student questions and concerns as well as information confronting the chapter board.
- You will be afforded the opportunity to be involved in legislative issues and receive information on pending bills.
- You will be able to network and interact with your future colleagues and current mentors.

Some Current Issues Confronting the California Chapter Board:

- The Diagnosis PR Fund: This is an attempt to raise monies in order to support the efforts of our legislators. By supporting this fund, we can play an integral part in becoming a direct access profession.
- The Occupational Therapy Licensing Bill: As this bill sits on the governor's desk, we await the outcome and effect it will have on our profession. The bill is to be signed or vetoed by Monday, October 11.
- The job market: What means are available to make it easier?
- The status of student treatments and documentation in regard to Medicare.
- The role of the DPT and residency programs.
- Ways to increase continuing education.
- Preventative medicine and wellness programs.
- Student leadership opportunities.

California Chapter APTA SSIG Newsletter, October 1999.

Figure 20-1. Sample Student Special Interest Group newsletter (reprinted with permission from California Physical Therapy Association, Sacramento, Calif).

Greetings!

For those that did not attend, I would like to take a moment to describe my recent experience at Student Conclave in Dallas this past October. Those that did attend know how much fun it was and, like me, are probably eager to attend again next year.

Despite a 45 minute, $36 dollar cab ride to the city from the airport, everything about Conclave was fun. When we did decide to take the trip, we had some interesting experiences at downtown clubs in Dallas, and we saw where President Kennedy was shot.

Practically a small city itself, we did not have to leave the Dallas/Fort Worth airport to have fun. The first night featured a talent show put on by the student assembly. I expected to see at least enthusiastic, if not world class, offerings of singing, dancing, and other performances. I was pleasantly surprised to see the level of talent on display that night! Examples included third place Howard University's dazzling Dance Therapy for Ataxia; second place Texas Tech's PT version of "Stomp" with walkers, canes, and gym balls and a gentleman who took first place by putting on a magic show that I would probably have paid $20 to see back home in California. There were other great acts in the tough field as well, including the crowd favorite from Puerto Rico (with the guys at least). There was a Ricky Martin character singing "La Vida Loca," accompanied by some talented young female PT students with some... amazing dance moves. I met the Puerto Rico contingent as I was checking in, and I was excited to see the level of commitment it took to get 17 students to Dallas from so far away.

Along with student-oriented seminars on mentoring, how to use the *Guide to PT*, the licensing exam, networking, funding tips, and two hands-on workshops, my favorite activity was the Mock House of Delegates. APTA Speaker of the House Pam Duffy was kind enough to share her experience by presiding over the Mock House, assisted by Student PT Delegate and natural people-person Troy Bourgeois. I got a chance to see how APTA policy is determined and how different RCs are created, deleted, or amended. Of course, being in Texas, the large home state vote was important to any changes that were proposed. I know I feel much more prepared to participate in the voting proceedings on Student Assembly policy when I return to the National Conference this year in June.

Along with the fun activities, new friends and contacts, informative speakers, and fine surroundings, we were lucky enough to have APTA Vice President Jane Snyder describe to us how the political process works concerning physical therapy. She was in Washington, D.C. on Thursday, and telling us about it in Dallas on Friday. She informed us of the proposed bills in the House and Senate that came up the day before concerning the Medicare caps on reimbursement. We took the news home on Monday and spread the word to the rest of the grass roots constituents. The wave of letters from our letter writing campaign helped achieve a huge victory within just a few weeks. The Senate bill proposing a moratorium on all caps for 2 years has been agreed to. Not to be redundant, but this is huge!! Some of you graduating will have jobs because of this!

All in all, I give the conference an A+, but I am getting long-winded so I'll wrap it up. See you in New Orleans in February for Combined Sections Meetings!

P.S. Stop by the Student Assembly Booth and say hi to the officers, they will appreciate it. I had the opportunity to spend some time with them, and I found them to be bright, friendly, enthusiastic, generous with their knowledge, and eager to share.

Figure 20-2. Sample of student impressions of the APTA National Student Conclave (reprinted with permission from James Moore[4]).

October), and all student and student affiliate members are invited to attend.

Student Awards

There are several awards that recognize outstanding students in the physical therapy profession. Information about these awards and nomination forms are available through the APTA webpage (http://www.apta.org) or the Student Assembly webpage (http://www.aptastudent.org). Is there someone deserving of recognition in your educational program?

- Outstanding PT Student Award
- Outstanding PTA Student Award
- Outstanding Student Liaison Award
- Outreach for Cultural Diversity Award
- Miami-Marquette Challenge

- Dorothy Briggs Scientific Inquiry Award
- Mary McMillan Scholarship Awards
- Minority Scholarship Awards for Academic Excellence
- APTA Section Student Awards (eg, Oncology Section Student Research Award)

Internships

The R. Charles Harker Internship is a tremendous opportunity for students with an interest in legislative and public policy issues to gain valuable experience at APTA headquarters in Alexandria, Va in the Government Affairs Department. The intern is involved in hearings, fundraisers, and other events on Capitol Hill, in addition to special projects and administrative duties at APTA headquarters.

The intern must be an APTA member and enrolled in a postbaccalaureate program in physical therapy. A stipend is provided for the intern. Obtain application details through R. Charles Harker Internship, Human Resources Department, 1111 N. Fairfax Street, Alexandria, VA 22314-1488.

Summary

Student membership in the APTA offers many benefits, including access to the latest research and health policy developments in the field, connections to professional networks, opportunities for specialization, discounts on conference registration, APTA publications, and group insurance programs. Numerous opportunities exist for students to organize on-campus activities and take leadership roles in the APTA through the SA and SSIGs.

References

1. APTA. *Step Into Your Future with APTA: The Benefits of Belonging to the American Physical Therapy Association*. Available at: http://www.apta.org/About/apta_membershipinfo/informationstu. Accessed July 22, 2000.

2. APTA. *Student Assembly Home Page*. Available at: http://www.studentapta.org. Accessed July 22, 2000.

3. APTA. *Foundation for Physical Therapy*. Available at: http://www.apta.org/Research/foundationforpt. Accessed July 22, 2000.

4. Moore JH. *Student Conclave*. Report to Student Assembly. January 10, 2000.

PUTTING IT INTO PRACTICE

1.   Who is the APTA student liaison for your program?

2.   When and where is the next National Student Conclave? How many students from your program will attend this conference?

3.   Access the Student Assembly webpage at http://www.studentapta.org.
      Is there a student special interest group in your state? List the contact person below:

4.   Does your program participate in fundraising for the Miami-Marquette Challenge? Generate several fundraising ideas and write them here. How can you initiate and/or add to the efforts of fundraising for the Foundation for Physical Therapy?

5.   Check the Student Assembly webpage at http://www.aptastudent.org. Is there a student in your program who would qualify for a student award?

      List the requirements and application/nomination deadline.

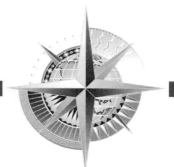

Chapter 21

Attending Professional Conferences

Kelly saw the announcement for the state APTA conference and heard other students talking about attending. It was a 3-hour drive, and then she would have to stay in a hotel. She worried, "I've never been to a conference before. I have no idea what to do there."

Why Attend Professional Conferences?

Conferences provide multiple opportunities for students to hear about new developments in the field, network with colleagues, try out new equipment, and make essential contacts for a first position.

Access to Information and Research

The latest information, trends, and developments are communicated at professional conferences long before they are in textbooks and often even before they are in journal articles. Although access to information is almost instantaneous in the electronic age of Internet and e-mail, conferences provide an opportunity to hear about and discuss these types of findings. Many conferences also feature equipment vendors and publishers. You may have an opportunity to try out a new piece of equipment, peruse the latest publications, and make purchase decisions at a discount, just because of have made the contact at the conference.

Sharing Experiences and Ideas

The greatest advantage of attending a professional conference is the opportunity to share your experience and interact with others. Your experiences in your academic program, questions about job searching, your career goals, and contributions to professional organizations are all better shared in a large setting. You may have a chance to meet the authors of your textbooks and reading materials, talk with leading researchers in the field, and explore new areas that have not been covered in school.

Networking with Other Students and PTs

There is really no better place to meet potential employers, future colleagues with similar interests, or students and faculty from other universities. In addition, your chances of finding someone who knows someone that can help you are far greater than when you circulate solely among your own contacts. Become a master networker and use conferences to both develop and strengthen your professional network.

Bigger Picture of the Profession and Opportunities

Job-hunting is always a concern for students. Student physical therapists, however, are often confined by the images of the profession that they have personally seen and experienced. Professional conferences open up a much wider view, including dif-

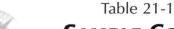

Table 21-1

SAMPLE CONTINUING EDUCATION COURSE LISTING

Title: One Step Ahead: Prosthetics and Amputee Rehab
Description: A dynamic 3-day presentation featuring acute care of the amputee, prosthetic componentry, biomechanics of gait, beginning to advanced prosthetic gait training, functional skills, and running gait. 2.1 CEUs for PTs, PTAs, and ATCs. Cost is $425.00.
When?   From: 27-Apr-01 To: 29-Apr-01
Where?   Raleigh, NC
Sponsor: Advanced Rehabilitation Therapy, Inc
Instructor: Robert Gailey, PT, PhD
Topic Area: Other

Contact Information
Name: Ann Gailey
E-mail: rgailey@bellsouth.net
Phone: 305-378-0855
Fax: 305-378-4107
Address:
7641 SW 126 Street
Miami, FL 33156

Reprinted with permission from the American Physical Therapy Association and Advanced Rehabilitation Therapy, Inc.

ferent geographical areas, treatment techniques, and practice opportunities, as well as provide a means for comparing and seeking future opportunities.

Types of Conferences

There are many types of conferences, seminars, and workshops available for professionals. Often, student physical therapists are offered a discounted registration, especially if they offer to assist with some aspect of the conference administration.

Continuing Education Courses

Continuing education courses are frequently held all over the country. There are many continuing education companies that sponsor multiple speakers. Most speakers are specialized, and many courses are held in a series. Take a look at the following website for a sample of the courses offered in your area. Site visitors can sort listings by area, subject, dates, or instructor: http://www.apta.org/Bulletin/Course_ Listings. Table 21-1 illustrates a sample course listing from this site.

Continuing education courses frequently offer continuing education units (CEUs). Some states require licensed physical therapists to attend continuing education courses that offer CEUs to meet state license renewal requirements. Check on the requirements in your state.

It is important to differentiate between *contact hours* and *CEUs*. A contact hour is defined as a 50-minute period of organized learning activity.[1] One CEU is equivalent to 10 contact hours.[1]

Some states require continuing education for license renewal. Consider the continuing education needs of therapists who live in a state that requires 2.4 CEUs per 24-month period. For example, a day-long continuing education course that runs from 9 am to 12 noon and 1 to 4 pm would award 0.6 CEUs for attendees. Physical therapists would need to attend four such courses over the 2-year period to meet their state requirements for license renewal.

Some conferences are focused on particular problems as a way of bringing together many experts to contribute to the resolution of an important issue. It might be a clinical issue such as lymphedema management or an administrative issue such as government affairs.

Frequently, the proceedings of such a conference are a valuable reference for future direction.

Look at the example in Figure 21-1 of an annual

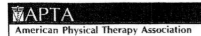

American Physical Therapy Association

Coding 2002 and Beyond

Have changes in coding and reimbursement affected you? APTA can help.

Whether you're an experienced user of coding or just starting out, here is an opportunity to explore in-depth coding techniques and get up-to-date information on the latest changes.

APTA's *Coding 2002 and Beyond* seminar is designed to educate the physical therapy professional about the best possible methods to deal with changing regulations in today's environment.

Why Should You Attend *Coding 2002 and Beyond*?

This seminar was designed to educate the physical therapy community on the changes in today's coding practices. By attending the one-day seminar you will receive the latest, most up-to-date information in the field.

- **Calculate** relative values for any CPT code.
- **Describe** the American Medical Association's CPT/ Resource-Based Relative Value System methodology that includes code and related relative value development and implementation.
- **Discuss** how coding can affect reimbursement levels and speed of payment.
- **Use** the proper nomenclature for and application of the 2000 CPT reimbursement codes.

Who Should Attend *Coding 2002 and Beyond*?

PTs in all of the following settings can benefit from APTA's *Coding 2002 and Beyond* seminar!

- Physical Therapists in Outpatient Hospitals, Rehab Agencies, CORFs, SNFs, Private Practice
- Office Managers
- Administrators and Program Directors
- Anyone who uses procedure codes to describe their services
- Anyone who is interested in improving their reimbursement levels, reducing denied claims, and successfully appealing problem claims

Seminar Schedule

8:00-8:30 am	Registration/Continental Breakfast
8:30-10:30 am	Welcome/Overview of CPT/RBRVS System
10:30-10:45 am	Break
10:45 am-12:15 pm	Current Codes and Coding Challenges
12:15-1:30 pm	Lunch (on your own)
1:30-3:00 pm	Payment Policy Challenges
3:00-3:15 pm	Break
3:15-5:00 pm	Coding Situations, Questions, and Wrap-up

Continuing Education

Equivalent to .65 CEU or 6.5 Contact Hours

Registration Fees

Advance Registration Fees:
APTA members and Life members: $195
APTA member's Office Manager (must be registered by the APTA member): $195
Nonmembers: $350

Onsite Registration Fees:
APTA members and Life members: $250
APTA member's Office Manager (must be registered by the APTA member): $250
Nonmembers: $450

To obtain further information about the seminar or to register, phone the APTA Service Center at 800/999-APTA (2782), ext 3395. Remember to check APTA's online Calendar for seminar updates and schedule information.

APTA members save $150! If you're not already a member, join APTA today!

Cancellation Policy:

Cancellations must be received 72 hours prior to seminar. Requests for refunds must be made to APTA in writing prior to the seminar, and will be subject to a 20% service charge per registration. APTA reserves the right to cancel a seminar up to two weeks prior to the start dates. In the event of cancellation due to circumstances beyond our control, APTA is at no time responsible for expenses incurred by seminar registrants, including but not limited to costs of airline tickets, other travel, food, or room.

Figure 21-1. Sample of a problem-focused conference (adapted with permission from the American Physical Therapy Association).

special interest conference on government affairs sponsored by the APTA.

State or Chapter Conferences

State chapters of the APTA usually sponsor annual or semi-annual conferences that include educational programming, social events, equipment exhibits, and organization business meetings. Such conferences are usually fairly low cost and convenient for students to attend. Many offer special events for students as well. Check your state listings at: http://www. apta.org/Components/comp_mtgs

National Conferences of the American Physical Therapy Association

There are two national conferences of the APTA each year. Student physical therapists are encouraged to attend both conferences. Students who volunteer to provide services at the conference often receive a discounted registration fee. Both of these meetings publish a *Call for Papers* during the preceding summer. More information about the meetings listed below can be found on the APTA website: http://www.apta.org/Meetings

Combined Sections Meeting

This is a 4- to 5-day meeting of all 19 sections of the APTA, which includes special programming specific to each section. Many clinical trends, new developments, and instructional courses are offered at this conference. In addition, each section holds business meetings for its membership. Each section also sponsors an original paper platform and/or poster session. This is an exciting conference because it always features indepth, practice-oriented information. This meeting is held usually in early to mid-February.

Annual Conference and Exposition of the APTA

This is a larger conference that includes the annual House of Delegates meeting, which is followed by a 4- to 5-day meeting of the association membership. There are many social events, educational and special interest sessions, exhibits, research presentations, and career networking opportunities. This meeting is held usually in early to mid-June.

International Physical Therapy Conferences

The World Congress of Physical Therapy (WCPT) meets every 4 years in a different country. This conference includes representatives from many nations who meet each quadrennium to discuss and plan for physical therapy needs on a global basis. There are numerous social events, educational and research sessions, and many opportunities for networking with international colleagues.

Interdisciplinary Conferences

There are many conferences that include professionals from several disciplines. These conferences are usually focused around a particular clinical area or a specialty interest. Physical therapists frequently attend such conferences on issues such as spinal cord injury, pain management, rehabilitation technology advances, and pediatrics. Attending an interdisciplinary conference not only helps physical therapists understand how individuals from other disciplines approach a problem, it enables a dialogue to begin between professionals that ultimately improves service delivery (see Chapter 19 on interprofessional collaboration).

Strategies for First-Time Conference Attendees

Before attending a conference, there are several ways that you can maximize your time and resources:

- *Read abstracts and the conference program; highlight interests.* Conference abstracts for several meetings are published in advance of the conference. If not, a package of conference abstracts is usually available at registration. It is well worth the time to read through the abstracts to see what is involved in each session.

- *Plan attendance at specific sessions.* Highlight and plan to attend those sessions that interest you. Going to the conference with a plan will help you to focus your efforts and maximize your time use. You will know where you want to be, which will make it much easier to ask directions and arrive there! Do not wait until the last minute, because some sessions require preregistration and fill up quickly. Latecomers are often left out.

- Make an overall schedule of events. Outline conference events you intend to attend on an hour by hour basis for the duration of the conference. Conferences usually run 10 to 20 competing events at a time. It is difficult to choose, but committing yourself in writing will minimize your confusion. Go through conference programs and note the room and building in which each session will be held. Conference sessions are sometimes in different hotels blocks away from each other or from your hotel. You'll need to plan to get there.

At the Conference

- *Arrive early at popular sessions.* Arrive early at each session you plan to attend. There are usually limited handouts and seats. Popular sessions fill up quickly, and those who do not fit are usually left out.

- *Sit up front.* Choose your seat to maximize what you can see. There are a lot less distractions toward the front of the room. Another reason to arrive early!

- *Exchange business cards.* You will meet dozens of new colleagues. Ask for the business cards of speakers, researchers, and potential employers with whom you wish to stay in contact. You may want to prepare some business cards with your name, address, phone number, and e-mail address. Office supply stores offer business cards very inexpensively. Do not pass up the opportunity to make and keep a contact.

How to Submit an Abstract

Call for Papers

A *Call for Papers* is published 6 to 9 months prior to the conference. It may be called a *Call for Proposals* or a *Call for Abstracts*. Several categories of submissions may be included, such as research, special interest of theory presentations, video, or multimedia technology programs.

Research reports are presentations of original scientific data collected by the author. *Special interest presentations* cover important issues or new developments in education, administration, or clinical practice. *Theory presentations* address a theory, idea, concept, or model that describes a foundation for administration, education, or clinical practice. *Multimedia presentations* are demonstrations of computer or video-based programs that serve an educational or research purpose.[2]

Participants who submit an abstract generally are given the choice of how to present—by a platform or poster presentation. A *platform presentation* is a delivered address to an audience in a meeting room at a podium. Conference participants attend the platform session, which is usually one of several papers, each lasting 15 minutes.

A *poster presentation* is a display that is mounted on a large bulletin board but not presented orally to an audience. In a poster presentation, the content is summarized using brief written statements and graphic materials such as photographs, charts, graphs, and/or diagrams. The poster is usually displayed for most of the conference. Conference participants may visit posters during designated hours to interact with the authors. A multimedia presentation is generally defined by the format of the presentation, such as video or computer. A presenter is given a time to interact with conference participants similar to the arrangements for a poster session.

Deadlines

A firm deadline for receipt of proposals is established. Look carefully at the instructions and see if the date is for receipt or postmark of the materials. It is a good idea to either send an abstract well in advance or by express mail to ensure delivery by the designated deadline. Do not miss the deadline!

Guidelines for Submission

The conference abstract must be formatted in a prescribed way. Take a look at the guidelines and sample abstract in Figures 21-2 and 21-3. Careful preparation of the abstract is critical, because abstracts will be published as submitted.

A recent *Call for Abstracts* published by the APTA is typical of the specified requirements of an abstract for a research report (Table 21-2).

Preparing a Presentation

After an abstract is accepted for presentation at a conference, presentation planning must begin. The presentation must be carefully crafted with the anticipated audience in mind.

Poster Presentations

Check the Size of the Display Space

A typical display space is 4 x 6 feet. (Title should be about 4 to 5 feet long, and 8 to 12 inches tall). Conferences typically provide a bulletin board type of display on which to mount the presentation. Bring push pins with you.

> Susan received the conference packet late on a Friday afternoon. Her abstract had been accepted. Now what? She excitedly called her co-authors one by one to tell them the good news. She scheduled a planning session during the next week. Although she was excited, she worried, "I hope they don't ask a lot of questions about the statistics!"

Submission Sheet for Abstracts
PHYSICAL THERAPY 2002:
THE ANNUAL CONFERENCE & EXPOSITION OF THE
AMERICAN PHYSICAL THERAPY ASSOCIATION
Cincinnati, Ohio, June 5-8, 2002

Submission Deadline: September 4, 2001

Submitter information *(please type or print):*

_____   _____
Name   **Member #** *(if applicable)*

_____
Address   *(If you are providing a company address, please provide name of company)*

_____   _____   _____
City   **State**   **ZIP Code**

_____   _____
Office Tel   **Home Tel**

_____   _____
Fax   **E-mail**

Only list one name: Please print your name (first name, middle initial, last name), credentials (eg, PT, MS, OCS), and affiliation (eg, St Mary's Hospital, Johnstown, NY) as you would like them to appear in the program. *Example: Adam B Smith, PT, MS, OCS, St Mary's Hospital, Johnstown, NY*

FOR ABSTRACTS ONLY

Category of Submission *(check one):*
- ☐ Research Report/Platform
- ☐ Research Report/Poster
- ☐ Special Interest Report/Platform
- ☐ Special Interest Report/Poster
- ☐ Theory Report/Platform
- ☐ Theory Report/Poster
- ☐ Multimedia Technology

Abstract Title: _____
_____
_____
_____
_____
_____

☐ Previously Published Abstract *(identify title, date of all publications*
in which it appeared): _____
_____
_____
_____
_____

☐ Submitted for presentation at: _____
_____
_____

FOR ABSTRACTS

Specify Topic Descriptors *(please check a Primary and a Secondary category):*

Primary	Secondary		
☐	☐	1.	Acute Care/Hospital Clinical Practice
☐	☐	2.	Administration
☐	☐	3.	Aquatics
☐	☐	4.	Cardiovascular and Pulmonary
☐	☐	5.	Clinical Education
☐	☐	6.	Clinical Electrophysiology
☐	☐	7.	Education
☐	☐	8.	Geriatrics
☐	☐	9.	Hand Rehabilitation
☐	☐	10.	Health Policy, Legislation, and Regulation
☐	☐	11.	Home Health
☐	☐	12.	Neurology
☐	☐	13.	Oncology
☐	☐	14.	Orthopedics
☐	☐	15.	Pediatrics
☐	☐	16.	Performing Arts
☐	☐	17.	Private Practice
☐	☐	18.	Professional Issues
☐	☐	19.	Research
☐	☐	20.	Sports Physical Therapy
☐	☐	21.	Technology
☐	☐	22.	Veterans Affairs
☐	☐	23.	Veterinary Physical Therapy
☐	☐	24.	Women'

Please send your submissions as soon as possible.
Submissions must arrive at APTA Headquarters no later than September 4, 2001.

DO NOT FOLD THIS MATERIAL   DO NOT FOLD THIS MATERIAL

Figure 21-2. Sample abstract submission form (reprinted with permission from the American Physical Therapy Association).

Abstract Form

Submission Deadline:
September 4, 2001

PHYSICAL THERAPY 2002:
THE ANNUAL CONFERENCE & EXPOSITION OF THE AMERICAN PHYSICAL THERAPY ASSOCIATION
Cincinnati, Ohio, June 5-8, 2002

THE EFFECTS OF THE USE OF FRONTAL SHOE ORTHOTICS AND PLYOMETRIC TRAINING ON SELECTED FUNCTIONAL MEASUREMENTS IN JUNIOR HIGH FOOTBALL PLAYERS. Reaper E, Longinotti S, Hattlestad M, Carson A, Culpepper H, Campbell M, Bandy WD; Department of Physical Therapy, University of Central Arkansas, Conway, AR, USA.

PURPOSE: Plyometric training incorporates quick, powerful movements involving a pre-stretching (or eccentric muscle contraction) prior to concentric contraction, thereby, emphasizing an "explosive-reactive power training" program. A plyometric training program is allegedly enhanced (according to manufacturers) by the use of a frontal shoe orthotic which is used in an attempt to increase the difficulty of the training but no study to date has examined this claim. Therefore, the purpose of this study was to determine whether the use of the Jumpsole™, a frontal shoe orthotic, will enhance the effects of plyometric training on vertical jump, 40 yard dash time, and calf circumference. SUBJECTS: Thirty-five healthy eighth and ninth grade male participants on the same junior high school football team volunteered to participate in the study. METHODS AND MATERIALS: Stratified sampling scheme was used to ensure similarity of weight and power analysis between a control group (18 males) and experimental group (17 males). The control group completed the six week training program without the Jumpsole™ shoe orthotic, while the experimental group completed the program with the orthotic. The six week training program consisted of 45 minute to 1 hour sessions performed bi-weekly utilizing acceleration activity, skipping, lateral cone hops, bounding, jump rope, and depth box jumps. Vertical jump, 40 yard dash time, and calf circumference were measured before and after the six weeks of training. ANALYSES AND RESULTS: A two-way multivariate analysis of variance with repeated measures on one factor and appropriate follow-up repeated measures univariate analyses revealed that the only significant difference occurred between the pre-test and post-test (irrespective of the influence of whether the subjects were in the experimental group or the control group) for the dependent variable vertical jump. CONCLUSIONS: These results indicate that, although the plyometric training program was effective for enhancing vertical jump, the training program did not improve speed of running or size of the calf muscle. Additionally, the use of a frontal shoe orthotic in an attempt to enhance the plyometric training program was not effective.

PLEASE RETAIN A COPY OF ALL SUBMITTED MATERIALS FOR YOUR FILES

Remember:

Copies may be made using either a photocopier or printer. Please make certain that all copies are easy to read and free from any extra marks or smudges.

In addition to the submission of one original abstract and the Submission Sheet, please provide the following materials:

Two copies of the abstract, including the name of the author(s) and the name and location of the institution in which the work was done.

Seven copies of the abstract from which you have deleted the author name(s) and the name and location of the institution in which the work was done, as well as words within the text that identify the author(s) or institution.

One computer disk from an IBM or compatible PC, in Microsoft Word or ASCII file format, of the complete formatted abstract to include names of all authors.

DO NOT FOLD THIS FORM. USE CARDBOARD BACKING TO AVOID DAMAGE.

Figure 21-3. Sample abstract (reprinted with permission from the American Physical Therapy Association).

Table 21-2
ABSTRACT COMPONENTS[2]

Purpose: What was the major reason for doing this study or for formulating a hypothesis?

Subjects: Describe the number and relevant characteristics of subjects.

Methods and Materials: What techniques were used to collect the data? What materials were included within this methodology?

Analyses: Describe the type(s) of statistical analyses used to address the purpose or hypotheses. Include descriptions of statistics and/or hypotheses testing.

Results: Briefly summarize the data derived from your analysis.

Conclusions: What can you logically conclude through the analysis of your data?

Adapted from APTA. *PT 2001 Call for Proposals/Abstracts*, with permission from the American Physical Therapy Association.

Map Out Your Plan to Scale Ahead of Time

Set up a mock poster in the allowable space, with each of the elements displayed. It will be much easier to see your plan and make needed adjustments this way.

Make it Visually Interesting!

Use photos, graphs, and other illustrations in your presentation. Be aware that visual interest will draw participants to your poster. Let pictures tell the story as much as possible, with words to explain the pictures.

Use high-contrast materials, either light background with dark letters or dark background with white letters. Use color to create interest, but be sure that your message is readable from 5 feet away. A computer presentation program will be helpful to lay out the text for the presentation.

Use Text Sparingly

Limit your text to a simple description of the problem, purpose, subjects, methods, results, and conclusions. Label and explain photographs, graphs, and tables. Use 24-point font and larger, and limit the content on a page to seven or eight lines. Check Table 21-3 for some design guidelines.

Do *not* display pages or a table from a written paper. In addition to being illegible from a distance, this material is far too complex to understand in just a few minutes.

During the Assigned Poster Session

You will be assigned a time during the conference for the poster session. Stand next to your poster during this time.

Be aware that participants may not have an understanding of your subject matter. Draw participants to your poster with questions like, "Do you have a program for _____ in your practice?" Explain your poster briefly and let participants take a look at your findings. Offer to answer questions. Remember that you know far more about your project than participants who visit your poster.

Be sure to bring a supply of business cards and exchange cards with conference participants. If a participant asks for additional information, be sure to write their request on the back of their card. Do not rely on your memory. You may finish the session with dozens of cards.

Provide Materials

Not all participants can attend a poster session when the authors are present. Therefore, some poster presenters find it helpful to provide a flyer, business cards, or some other means for participants to see and take away a summary of the poster, with contact information for the authors. Simple materials can be made available in an envelope attached to the poster display board.

Table 21-3
DO'S AND DON'TS FOR PRESENTATION DESIGN[3]

Do

- Use a landscape view, rather than portrait view, for best projection.
- Plan for single or dual projection of slides and materials (Note: an LCD projector from a computer is limited to one slide and one screen).
- Keep the presentation moving (plan for 30 seconds to 1 minute maximum per slide).
- Use a sequence of information that is logical and builds on itself.
- Define technical terms before using them.
- Use a title at the top of each slide (eg, Introduction, Methods, Results).
- Keep it simple, clear, and concise.
- Use a maximum of seven lines of text in the space below the title of the slide.
- Use phrases, not sentences.
- Use uppercase and lowercase letters; they are easier to read than all capitalized text.
- Use simple transitions from one slide to another (fade).
- Use dark background with light letters (purple/yellow, blue/white, etc).
- Use photos to show methods and setup.
- Create simple tables with a maximum of three columns and three or four rows.
- Use line diagrams or graphics if feasible.
- Create simple graphs and charts and label them clearly.
- Use pie charts to display demographics or proportions.
- Use bar graphs to display differences between groups over time.
- Use line graphs to display multiple points over time.
- Label the x and y axes on all graphs.

Don't

- Display results of different dependent variables on the same slide unless there is a reason to compare them by your experimental design.
- Use more than two types of fonts, colors, and styles. Keep the font type, color, and style consistent throughout the presentation.
- Use a font smaller than 18 points in a projected slide program.
- Use a light background with colored letters.
- Use ALL CAPITALS. This is more difficult to read.
- Use tables with more than three columns or four rows.
- Try to scan in a complicated graph from a written paper.
- Use multiple types of transitions from one slide to another. It may be entertaining for you as a designer, but it will distract your audience to see your text fly in from the right, bottom, top, or appear in a checkerboard pattern.

Platform Presentations

Platform presentations are typically delivered in conference rooms with a podium and a microphone. The sessions are organized with three or four papers in succession. Time is limited to 15 to 20 minutes with a few minutes for discussion. Session moderators introduce participants and keep time.

Preparation and Presentation Design

Computer-based programs are readily available to help presentation design. Think carefully about the visual impact and sequence of the material you present. Table 21-3 lists a few tips for presentation design.

Presentation Materials

Indicate to conference organizers what equipment

you will need for your presentation. If you are doing a computer-based presentation, it is a good idea to bring your own laptop computer with the presentation preloaded and a set of overhead projector transparencies as a backup. Technology is not fool-proof. A backup plan is better than floundering when equipment fails.

You may distribute written material to accompany your presentation. Many speakers give participants a summary of their slide presentation. You may want to consider this option, depending on the length and complexity of your talk. Make 50 to 100 copies of materials, more if it is a very large conference.

The moderator of your session may contact you in advance for information about your background. Bring a copy of all materials that you have sent and received in relation to the conference presentation, in the event that something is lost or misplaced.

Practice Sessions

Write down what you are going to say and practice it until you do not need to look at it. Practice is critical. Practice, revise, and practice again. Practice speaking slowly and allow the audience to see and read each slide. Practice using a pointer to point out notable features on graphs or tables. Refer to colors of lines or bars on the graph. Time the presentation and allow for questions from the audience. Remember that the audience knows far less about your work than you do.

At the Conference

Check the size and location of the room in which you will present. If possible, attend another presentation in the room so that you can see how speakers get to and from the podium and how the lighting and projection system works. Although someone else will be responsible for controlling this equipment, you may be able to plan for visuals more effectively when you see the conditions under which you will present.

Dress professionally in comfortable clothes and shoes. Conference organizers may request that you meet session moderators in advance of your session, often in a speaker preparation room. These rooms typically have audiovisual equipment available so that you can preview your presentation. Use the few minutes before the session wisely. Be sure that all equipment is functioning in the room. Go to the podium and make sure that you know how to turn on equipment to begin your presentation.

Plan to leave copies of written materials at the back of the room. Inform the conference room assistant that you have written materials to accompany your presentation, and he or she may be able to direct participants to these materials as they enter the room.

While Giving Your Presentation

Thank the moderator for the introduction and greet the audience. Make eye contact with at least one member of the audience. Breathe and be conscious of your speed of presentation. Do not dwell on small mistakes that you may make; the audience understands that you may be nervous. Finish the presentation and say, "Thank you. Are there any questions?"

Always repeat the question. Then answer it simply. If it is too complex for a simple answer, state, "That's an interesting question. I'd like to talk with you a little further about that after the presentation if you're available."

One of the greatest fears that new speakers have is not being able to answer a question. If you do not know the answer to a question, tell the participant that you would like to refer to the written manuscript and you will speak with him or her after the presentation. This is an opportunity to get valuable feedback. Spend the time to understand and discuss a point that a participant is making.

Congratulate yourself and go out for lunch or dinner to celebrate!

What Will it Cost?

Conference expenses are fairly predictable and fall into several categories. Table 21-4 shows a typical budget for attending an out-of-state conference.

How Do I Pay for it?

Conference participation is a valuable part of your professional education. Budget for it and plan to attend. If you have an abstract *accepted* for a conference presentation, there are many potential means of support.

Graduate School and University Support

Ask for support! Most universities have some funds to support student research and related travel to conferences. Ask about available programs, scholarships, and aid that may support such expenses. If not readily available, a motivated student may be able to create such funds by meeting with department and university administrators.

Table 21-4

TYPICAL CONFERENCE EXPENSES

Expenses (4-Day Conference)	Costs	To Cut Costs
Conference registration	$300	Volunteer to assist at the conference and the registration fee will be markedly discounted or provided by the organizers.
Hotel (four nights at $150/night)	$600	Share a room with other students or look on student listservs for students in the area who will offer housing to other students.
Roundtrip airfare	$500	Look for student discounts and lower fares from alternate departure cities.
Meals ($35 per day)	$140	Visit exhibit halls and exhibitor parties. While networking, you can often eat for free!
Ground transportation (shuttle to hotel)	$30	Share a cab with other conference participants to often beat "per person" shuttle rates. Check in advance with taxi driver.
Incidentals	$100	Be prepared to find some great deals on books, equipment, and other musts at the conference. Have some fun, too!
Presentation materials	$100	Ask the university to assist you with the preparation costs of presentation materials.
Total	**$1770**	A motivated student can reduce costs by $600 to $800 by using the above tips.

District and State APTA Funds

Contact your district and chapter offices of the APTA. See if they are able to support your travel and conference expenses in some way.

Loans and Grants

Seek other sources of support to augment your available resources. This is an important investment. The contacts you will make and the addition of a presentation to your resume is worth the expense of attending a conference.

Summary

Professional conferences provide multiple opportunities to learn new information, share ideas and experiences, network with other colleagues, and gain additional perspectives of the profession. Successful conference presentations result from careful planning and attention to detail. Student physical therapists should seek opportunities and support to attend and present at professional conferences.

References

1. Corexcel. *CEUs and Contact Hours*. Available at: http://www.corexcel.com/ceus.contacthours.ceus.htm. Accessed August 3, 2000.

2. APTA. PT 2001 Call for Proposals/Abstracts webpage. Available at http://www.apta.org/Meetings/2001call. Accessed August 3, 2000.

3. Curtis KA. Making poster and platform presentations. *Student Research Manual*. Fresno, Calif: California State University; 2000.

PUTTING IT INTO PRACTICE

1.   Find out the Call for Abstracts deadline and the dates and location of the following:
      a. the next Chapter Conference of the APTA in your state

      b. the next Combined Sections Meeting of the APTA

      c. the next Annual Conference and Exposition of the APTA

	Call for Abstracts Deadline	Conference Dates, Location
Chapter Conference		
Combined Sections Meeting		
Annual Conference and Exposition		

2.   Find out about potential sources of support for conference presentations at your university. If you were to present your research, to whom would you apply for assistance to attend the conference?

      Prepare a budget to estimate your costs of attendance at one of the above conferences.

3.   Explore the availability of continuing education conferences in your area. Go to: http://www.apta.org/Bulletin/Course_Listings

      Look for courses listed in your state. How many did you find?

      How many are within 100 miles of where you live?

      What are the average registration fees per day of instruction? Give a range from the lowest to the highest.

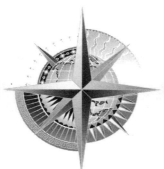

Part Six

First Steps into the Profession of Physical Therapy

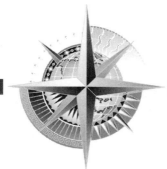

Chapter 22

Preparing for Licensure

Ellen looked at the travel brochures and was anxious to see the world after she completed her professional education. She wondered, "Will it be complicated to get my license in another state?"

State Laws for Licensure and Registration

Each state licensing board has its own criteria that applicants must meet to apply for physical therapist and, in some states, physical therapist assistant licensure. Graduates of accredited programs should review the materials distributed by the licensing board in the state(s) to which they intend to apply to determine the eligibility requirements in each state.[1]

The Federation of State Boards of Physical Therapy provides a website and extensive resources that explain the licensure process. However, each state administers and controls the licensure process in that state. The address of the Federation of State Boards of Physical Therapy:

Federation of State Boards of Physical Therapy
509 Wythe Street
Alexandria, VA 22314
Telephone: 703/299-3100
Fax: 703/299-3110

To access the State Board of Physical Therapy in your state, check the following website: http://www.fsbpt.org/directory.cfm

The national examination is only one part of the process involved in licensing a therapist to practice. Eligibility for licensure is determined after review of many documents in addition to the National Physical Therapy Examination score. In fact, passing the examination does not guarantee licensure.[2] Licensing requirements may also include an extensive review of educational preparation and transcripts, experience in the field, recommendations of licensed physical therapists, passing a test of state law, screening (fingerprints) for a criminal record, and review of prior convictions. Although it is variable by state, the application process and fees involved for initial licensure often costs the candidate hundreds of dollars.

Once determined eligible by the state licensing authority, the candidate's materials are forwarded to the Federation of State Boards of Physical Therapy (FSBPT). The FSBPT sends the candidate an "authorization to test" letter, which includes instructions for examination scheduling at one of 300 local testing centers in the United States, US territories, and Canada. The candidate must sit for the examination within 60 days of the date on the authorization to test letter.[3] Test center fees are paid at the time that the examination is scheduled.

Table 22-1
STATE-APPROVED CREDENTIALING AGENCIES FOR INTERNATIONALLY EDUCATED THERAPISTS[4]

International Credentialing Associates
1 Progress Plaza, Suite 810
St. Petersburg, FL 33701
Telephone: 727/821-8852
Fax: 727/821-2347

International Education Research Foundation
PO Box 66940
Los Angeles, CA 90066
Telephone: 310/390-6276
Fax: 310/397-7686
http://www.ierf.org

International Consultants of Delaware, Inc.
109 Barksdale Professional Center
Newark, DE 19711
Telephone: 302/737-8715
Fax: 302/737-8756

Foreign Credentialing Commission on Physical Therapy, Inc.
PO Box 25827
Alexandria, VA 22313-9998
Telephone: 703/684-8406
Fax: 703/684-8715
E-mail: fccpt@fsbpt.org

Check with individual state licensing boards for agencies approved by that state.

Reprinted with permission from the American Physical Therapy Association.

Jorge had dreamed of practicing in the United States. Many of his family members had relocated to south Florida. He waited until finishing his university education and training as a physical therapist to join them. He wrote to the state licensing board and began to gather the necessary documentation to meet the requirements.

Internationally Educated Therapists

State laws governing the licensure of foreign educated-therapists also vary by state. All internationally educated therapists will require prescreening of their credentials and English proficiency evaluations (such as TOEFL, TSE, TWE) before being able to apply for licensure to practice.[4] Independent agencies provide credential review. It is important to note that these agencies (Table 22-1) must be approved in the state in which the applicant will apply for physical therapist licensure.

After passing criteria for credential review and English proficiency and meeting all other criteria for state licensure, candidates may sit for the National Physical Therapy Examination. In some states, applicants must also complete a period of supervised clinical internship.

Additionally, work authorization is required for employment in the United States. Physical therapists may apply for a "temporary" nonimmigrant visa, called the H-1B visa, that permits practice as a physical therapist only.[4] There is an annual cap for H-1B visas. For information on visas, please contact the US Department of Justice Immigration and Naturalization Service (website: http://www.ins.usdoj.gov).

Requirements are different for Canadian citizens. Citizens of Canada must request a TN visa at the Canadian-US border. This type of visa requires that applicants offer proof of Canadian citizenship, show a valid US license to practice physical therapy, and possess a letter of employment or contract. The TN visa is valid for 1 year. It must be renewed annually.[4] For more information, contact the US Embassy or Consulate in Canada.

Physical Therapy Practice by Licensure Applicants

Again, state law varies as to what physical therapy license applicants may legally do while waiting to take and hear the results of the examination. Some states permit supervised practice by applicants; others do not. It is important that applicants understand their legal status during the period of application and waiting period before a license is issued (see Chapter 12). The State Board of Physical Therapy in each state can provide this information.

The National Physical Therapy Examination

The National Physical Therapy Examination (NPTE) is a computerized test consisting of 225 multiple-choice questions for physical therapists and 175 questions for physical therapist assistants. Candidates for the physical therapist and physical therapist assistant examinations are allowed 4.5 hours and 3.5 hours, respectively.[5] Candidates are examined individually and must call to schedule an examination date and time.

The examinations are developed by a committee of physical therapy practitioners. Test questions assess the knowledge and abilities required of physical therapists and physical therapist assistants. These questions are developed to reflect a comprehensive analysis of the practice of physical therapists and physical therapist assistants.

Raw exam scores are converted to a scale that ranges from 200 to 800 points. The FSBPT national minimum passing score is 600 points. Since July 1996, all states have adopted the FSBPT passing score.[3]

Exam Content Includes Three Major Areas

1. Assessment and evaluation, including data collection (7%), tests and measurements (11%), and system-specific procedures (6%).
2. Interpretation and planning, including data interpretation (13%), goal-setting, and care planning (9%).
3. Intervention, including preparation (10%), implementation (23%), education/communication/consultation (7%), supporting activities (8%), and system-specific procedures (6%).[6]

A free sample examination is available to download at www.fsbpt.org/files/sylvan.exe

Preparing for the Examination

Gather and Organize Your Resources

Textbooks, class notes, articles, and reading materials all provide a good foundation for examination review. Take care to review your State Practice Act as well. Be sure that your information is current and reflects existing laws in the jurisdiction in which you will practice.

Review Class Notes

Start with your class notes, which are organized by subject area. Look for areas of overlap and begin with a review of terminology. Note indications, contraindications, precautions, and specifications for treatment procedures.

The examination is problem-based, which will require you to review with applications in mind. Ask yourself:

- What is the clinical application of this information?
- If I was given this information about a patient, what difference would it make in my assessment, evaluation, or intervention planning?
- What theories and research-based evidence support this information?

Be sure to consider clinical decision-making regarding all of the following:

- Evaluation and diagnosis of client disorders
- Evidence to document outcomes of intervention, including cost-effectiveness
- Physical therapy interventions, including indications, contraindications, anticipated functional outcome, precautions by diagnosis system
- Ethical and legal considerations
- Psychosocial aspects of illness, injury, and disability

Develop a Realistic Study Schedule

Begin your preparation several months in advance. A study group is a useful way to approach this examination. Determine weekly content to review and plan study for several hours prior to each group session.

Use Active Information Processing Strategies

Your retention is better if you use an active strategy to process information, rather than just re-reading books or notes (see Chapter 9). Take notes from your notes or record key information onto an audiotape. Discuss the information with others periodically to further improve your retention. Review your notes and/or audiotapes at least once weekly.

Take Practice Exams

Practice exams are available through many sources. Be sure that you have covered the content areas included in these examinations.

Review strategies for taking multiple-choice examinations (see Chapter 7). Remember that this is a timed examination. In general, your first answer is the best. Watch for exclusionary words or phrases such as *only, except, never,* or *always.* If English is not your first language, beware of common errors (see Chapter 14).

Courses

There are many review courses available. Although these courses are expensive, they may save the applicant time in identifying key information for review. A course does not take the place of necessary study time, and no course provides a fool-proof mechanism to pass the examination.

Books and Computer Programs

Review books are less expensive and often provide accompanying computer disks to simulate test-taking conditions. A partial listing of these examination preparation resources is provided at the following website: http://www.apta.org/PT_Practice/ptlicensure/license_exam

What Happens if I'm Not Successful?

Although the overall first-time pass rate for candidates educated in US schools is very high (85%), some applicants (15%) are not successful on their first try.[8] In contrast, pass rates for internationally educated therapists have been considerably lower (35%).[8]

State licensing boards determine how often a candidate may take the examination if not successful on the first attempt. Re-examination requires re-application. No candidate may take the examination more than four times in any 12-month period.[3]

If you are not successful, think about the content that presented the most difficulty. Ask your colleagues, supervisors, and faculty for assistance in organizing your studies. Use strategies for active information processing. Enlist the support of others to ensure that you will be successful on a subsequent try.

Summary

Licensure to practice physical therapy requires that candidates meet the criteria required by the state in which they wish to practice. Candidates should check with the state licensing board in their own state to receive applications and regulatory information.

When criteria are met, a computerized national examination with content covering assessment and evaluation, interpretation and planning, and intervention is administered in testing centers by individual appointment. Candidates must be aware of laws governing their practice activities during the licensure application period.

References

1. FSBPT. *Eligibility.* Available at: http://www.fsbpt.org/handbook/eligibility.html. Accessed 8/3/2000.

2. PT Board of California. *Instructions for Completing the Application for Physical Therapist or Physical Therapist Assistant Examination and/or Licensure Webpage.* Available at: http://www.ptb.ca.gov/license/inst.pdf Accessed August 2, 2000.

3. FSBPT. *Frequently Asked Questions Webpage.* Available at: http://www.fsbpt.org/handbook/computerized.html. Accessed August 22, 2000.

4. APTA. *Information for Internationally Educated Therapists.* Available at: http://www.apta.org/About/special_interests/internationalaffairs/info_for_intl_edu_pt. Accessed August 2, 2000.

5. FSBPT. *Examination structure.* Available at: http://www.fsbpt.org/handbook/exam_structure.html. Accessed August 22, 2000.

6. FSBPT. *Rubric PT Test Content Outline.* Available at: http://www.fsbpt.org/PTContent_Outline_99.pdf. Accessed August 26, 2000.

7. APTA. *Licensure Examination Candidate Resources Webpage.* Available at: http://www.apta.org/PT_Practice/ptlicensure/license_exam. Accessed August 2, 2000.

8. FSBPT. *Pass/Fail Rates Webpage.* Available at: http://www.fsbpt.org/exam5.htm. Accessed August 22, 2000.

PUTTING IT INTO PRACTICE

1. Find the website for your state licensing board. Download materials and read them to answer the following questions:
   a. What materials are required as part of the application packet?

   b. What is the fee required with the application?

   c. What limitations are placed on practice of first-time applicants during the application period (look especially for descriptions of terms of temporary licenses, or physical therapist license applicant practice, or prohibition of practice by applicants)?

   d. What are the policies and fees for repeating the examination if not successful the first time?

   e. Are there special requirements for internationally educated therapists?

2. Review your university catalog and list the required courses in your curriculum that meet each of the following content areas:

Content	Course Numbers
Evaluation and diagnosis of client disorders	
Anticipated outcomes of intervention, including cost effectiveness	
Physical therapy interventions, including indications, contraindications, precautions by diagnosis and system, and functional outcome	
Ethical and legal considerations	
Psychosocial aspects of illness, injury, and disability	

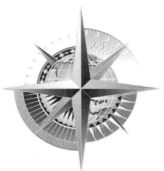

Chapter 23

Entering the Job Market

> *Mark began his job search. He looked over the Sunday paper and saw three ads for part-time physical therapists. They were all in outpatient clinics that seemed to be run by large corporations. He worried, "Which one will be the best for me?" He planned to call each of them on Monday morning. Is this a good strategy?*

Looking for a Job

Employer needs have changed rapidly with health care policy shifts, despite growing societal needs for physical therapy services. In contrast to the situation that existed in the early and mid-1990s, new graduate physical therapists may have to compete with each other for available positions.

Exceptional skills and experiences acquired during the professional education experience may provide an advantage to some graduates. In addition, as new graduate physical therapists take on evolving roles and responsibilities (see Chapter 3), they may also be well suited for positions that use their advanced skills in program development, outcomes evaluation, education, collaboration, or use of technology.

The classified ads are *not* the place to start a job search. Employers who frequently hire physical therapists advertise in professional publications or draw applicant pools from files of therapists who have initiated previous contact with the employer.

Let's start with a different mindset.

New graduates are *beginning their careers in the profession of physical therapy*. Although it is possible to "find a job" in the field of physical therapy, graduates who are more creative and initiate their career path with a strategy in mind are likely to be far more satisfied with the results.

Let's approach this important decision by first asking a few questions.

Create a Picture of Your Ideal Life

Consider the following:

- What is most important to you in your personal life?
- What is most important to you in your career?
- What are your personal goals? Your professional goals?
- How long do you envision yourself staying in one position or one location?

Envision the Ideal Organization

What are the things you consider to be most important in an organization in which you will work? Consider the following:

- What goals or mission of an organization would be most attractive?
- What would this organization contribute to society?

- What size would this organization be?
- What experience will you gain?
- Where is the optimal location of your ideal workplace?
- What are the working conditions?
- With what kinds of people would you most like to work?
- What are the needs of this type of organization in the current climate?

What Do You Have to Offer?

Consider the following:
- What unique skills, abilities, and experiences will you bring to the workplace?
- What problems are you able to solve for the organization, given your unique skills?
- What new programs are you uniquely qualified to develop?
- What changes are you able to offer a potential employer?
- What will colleagues gain by working with you?
- What will clients or patients gain by working with you?

Now that you have an idea of what you want, it will be easier to ask for help and focus your efforts. Before you write a resumé or send a letter, use the following essential strategies of networking and informational interviewing.

Networking

> *Miriam looked at the small stack of business cards she had saved from last year's state APTA conference. She had written to a few of her contacts. How could she work those into a potential job offer?*

Networking is an essential way to develop professional contacts and establish relationships that can be a source of information, collaboration, and future opportunity. There are some key principles that will maximize the effectiveness of your networking efforts.[1,2]

Organize Your Contacts

Be aware of the contacts you already have and organize them in a way to fully take advantage of your resources. Consider your contacts within the field from school, former instructors and students, your former and current colleagues and supervisors, even people you have met at your affiliation sites.

Then, think of the network of your contacts and the entire scope of people who are available to you. Do not overlook social and family contacts, church, community, and others with whom you share special interests. Your potential network is very large.

Use an address book or computer database. Collect business cards and keep them in an organized file. Maintain professional contacts in a way that you can retrieve the addresses and phone numbers easily.

Stay Visible

Establish your visibility among your contacts. This requires an active commitment to establishing and maintaining contact. Keep in touch.

Your network is only available to you if you use it. Decide what you need and where you want to go in the future. Let your contacts know your interests and your goals.

Keep your own business cards with you at all times. Write notes on the back of your business card as a brief reminder of what you talked about or what information you would like the other person to give you. Your card is a very important impression of yourself to leave with someone.

Ask for Help

Ask for help, information, advice, and other contacts. Listen and learn from others. Circulate in many circles. Make an effort to stay in touch frequently. Ask members of your network to go to lunch or dinner. Thank others for their help.

Acknowledge and Promote Others

Acknowledge and promote the accomplishments of others. Share resources and information. Help others in your network succeed in their interests and reach their goals through your contacts. Find out their areas of interest and expertise and periodically review and update your contact lists.

Make Referrals and Help Others

Refer others to people with whom you have contact. Share resources willingly. Send articles of interest to people in your network. Support the skills, expertise, and accomplishments of others. Let others know of your efforts to promote them.

Make your relationships ones of mutual benefit. This is especially helpful if you are networking with competitors.

Informational Interviewing

Students have multiple opportunities to gather information that will support their future job search. Student physical therapists are in a unique position of working with colleagues during clinical internships who have the responsibility to assist their professional development.

Informational interviewing provides answers to questions you may have about opportunities, the job market, key career choices, and strategies for job-seeking. Talk with these clinical contacts to broaden your network, get advice on your resume, and look into opportunities in certain geographical areas.[3] Get the names of their colleagues, school friends, fellow committee members, and previous students to contact. Ask for help in approaching your job search.

Developing Your Resumé

> *Susan worried about being so far away during her clinical affiliations. She wanted to canvas the field in cities in which she wanted to live. She prepared a resumé which indicated her interest in employment in outpatient facilities and then sent her resumé with a cover letter to each facility.*

A *resumé* is a "short account of one's career and qualifications prepared typically by an applicant in a position."[3] A resumé by itself will not land a job, especially in a tightening job market. Some ideas, however, about what a resumé may do for you:

- It may serve as a *calling card*, by giving an employer your contact information.
- It serves a valuable purpose as a *self-inventory*, which will enable you, the job seeker, to assess and present your strengths and experience.
- It may actually provide an *outline* for an interview. You have outlined your accomplishments and capabilities, and your resumé provides a potential employer with a focus for matching your skills with their needs.
- Lastly, it may serve as a *valuable reference* for the employer in considering your candidacy for a position in a pool of applicants.[1]

Your resumé must be first-class, without errors, current, concise, and clear. It should catch the employer's attention and provide a clear match for your skills with an available position. It should demonstrate your competence, experience, and skills in descriptions of actions and achievements and show how you can apply your expertise in a position you are seeking. It should demonstrate your worth to an employer, whether in dollars, contacts, or visibility (Tables 23-1 and 23-2).

The Chronological Resumé

This is a standard resumé format. It is simple to prepare and provides a chronological description of student education and experiences by places, dates, and events. The career objective is employee-focused and global. This resumé may be effective for sending out to prospective employers who have not advertised specific job openings.

Is there anything about the resumé in Table 23-1 that sets apart this applicant? Even though this applicant has done research, presented her findings to colleagues, and even prepared a paper for publication, it does not jump off the page. Those accomplishments are not related to skills that she can offer an employer, nor are they presented as unique or different. Even though she has had unique experiences in research and leadership, this type of resumé fails to illustrate in what way that experience will add to the organization. Her cover letter will be very important to present these points (Table 23-3).

> *Donna read the following job ad:*
>
> *November 26, 2000*
> *(Center City Women's Bulletin)*
> *University-based medical center seeks dynamic physical therapist to join interdisciplinary women's health team. The team will focus on collaborative treatment of high priority women's health issues in NIH-funded project. Research and leadership experience desirable. Contact J. Joyal, University Medical Center, 1001 University Drive, Center City, IL 62667*
>
> *She prepared a position-focused resumé and wrote a cover letter outlining her interests.*

The Position-Focused Resumé

The position-focused resumé encourages the author to address the specifics of the employment listing. This type of resumé outlines the applicant's skills and related accomplishments specific to the requirements and preferences outlined in an employment listing for an available position. See Donna's resumé in Table 23-2.

Table 23-1
CHRONOLOGICAL RESUMÉ

Susan Straightforward

College Address:	Permanent Address:	*Include all contact addresses and include applicable dates for temporary addresses.*
City, State, Zip	Street Address	
Phone	City, State, Zip	
Fax	Home Phone	
E-mail		

Career Objective

An entry-level position in a physical therapy outpatient clinic.

Can be as general or specific as you like.

Education

Mid-State University, Center City, IL
Master of Physical Therapy, 2000

Mid-State University, Center City, IL
Bachelor of Science, Biology, 1996

University name, city, state, degree, major (year, GPA is optional)
In reverse chronological order, most recent first.

Work Experience

Physical Therapy Aide, Middletown Physical Therapy
Middletown, IL January 1997-August 1998
  · Prepared treatment area and assisted with routine
    therapeutic exercise classes
  · Performed inventories, ordered supplies and patient
    education materials
  · Created a database of area resources for patient referrals

Title, employer, city, state, dates. List professional positions prior to physical therapy education or list related positions in the health or human service fields. Give a brief description of your work-related duties. List in reverse chronological order, most recent first.

Clinical Internships

St. John's Hospital, Eastbrook, OK January 31-March 28, 2000
Performed physical therapy evaluation, intervention, and discharge planning for diverse population in acute hospital setting. Provided endurance training for patients post gastric bypass surgery. Presented inservice on lymphedema treatment to 30 staff members.

Facility, city, state, dates. Brief description of clinical responsibilities and accomplishments. List in reverse chronological order, most recent first.

Licensure

Eligible for licensure; will take examination November 2000.

License number, state, and date or indicate your application status.

Presentations

Evidence Supporting Complex Lymphedema Therapy in Treatment of Lymphedema Post Breast Cancer. St. John's Hospital, Eastbrook, OK, March 16, 2000.

List all presentations you have given, including inservice presentations during internships.

Table 23-1, continued

Publications Straightforward S, Dynamic D, Reliable IM. The effect of complex lymphedema therapy: a controlled pilot study. Manuscript in submission for publication. June 1, 2000.	*List publications, including webpages, abstracts, theses, and manuscripts in press.*
Research Activity The effect of complex lymphedema therapy: a controlled pilot study. Collaborative study with Dr. IM Reliable and D Dynamic, performed in partial fulfillment of the requirements for the Master of Physical Therapy degree, received May 2000, Mid-State University.	*List title and collaborators with institutional affiliations.*
Honors and Activities Student Member, American Physical Therapy Association National Student Conclave, October 27-29, 2000, Cherry Hill, NJ Dean's List Fall 1998, Fall 1999, Spring 2000.	*List community activities, clubs, professional organizations, honors and awards. Include dates.*
References References available on request.	*Either list those persons whom you have asked to serve as references or write "References available on request."*

What to Include?

Most students have acquired valuable experiences while in college or graduate school. Voluntary and professional activities, responsibilities, projects, and accomplishments often relate directly to employer needs. Employers want to see that you are a self-starter, have had experience, and can work well with others. Also, if there were large gaps in your activity, you may want to account for those gaps in time with a brief explanation such as, "Part-time university enrollment to fulfill prerequisites for professional education program."

What Not to Include?

Although many resumé writers include a section on personal traits, you do not need to include personal information such as your age, marital status, number of children, citizenship, ethnicity, or your assessment of your personality. In fact, it is illegal for an employer to ask any question that is unrelated to the position for which you are applying. Why create opportunities for biases to enter the picture?

Preparing Your Resumé

Keep your resumé up-to-date as you go through the professional education program. There may be scholarships, part-time work opportunities, graduate or teaching assistantship opportunities that arise. A current and accurate resumé will assist you in your success in these opportunities as well.

After you have prepared a resumé, ask a colleague to look it over. It may also be helpful to ask for feedback from human resource personnel, administrators in a clinical affiliation, or university faculty members. Your university's career placement center undoubtedly offers services that can support your resumé preparation and job search.

Make certain that there are not typographical or grammatical errors in your resumé. Print the document with a high-quality printer and high-quality paper. Take the original to be copied on heavyweight paper at a copy center. It costs only a few cents more per page, and the results are certainly worth it. You want your resumé to work for you. To do that, it must stand out and be read.

Table 23-2

POSITION-FOCUSED RESUMÉ IN RESPONSE TO PUBLISHED EMPLOYMENT LISTING

Donna Dynamic

College Address:	Permanent Address:
Street Address	Street Address
City, State , Zip	City, State, Zip
Phone	Home Phone
Fax	
E-mail	

Include all contact addresses and include applicable dates for temporary addresses.

Objective

Develop and implement physical therapist role on interdisciplinary women's health team.

Focus on specifics of employment listing.

Related Skills and Accomplishments

Women's Health Activities

· Conducted collaborative research, presented and submitted manuscript for publication of study on long-term outcomes of complex lymphedema therapy for women with brachial lymphedema post-breast cancer.

· Participated in organization of Lymphedema Network conference in June 2000.

· Provided peer counseling to over 10 women who experienced rape or domestic abuse. Started a university-based support group for p-346.

Relate to major themes of employment listing. Using action verbs and quantifiable terms, describe your related experiences and skills. What are you trying to show?
"I have experience in the women's health field and have perspectives that go well beyond physical therapy."

Collaborative and Communication Skills

· Practiced as a member of interdisciplinary rehabilitation team at Warm Springs Rehabilitation Center during 9-week internship focusing on neurological rehabilitation.

· Co-authored and edited monthly newsletter for student communications in American Physical Therapy Association.

"Yes, I work well with a team. I get things done."

Research Experience

· Designed and conducted survey of Planned Parenthood volunteers before and after training to determine knowledge base on rape and domestic abuse. Published in corporate newsletter.

· Collected and analyzed data, interpreted results in collaborative research effort on long-term effectiveness of complex lymphedema therapy in women with brachial lymphedema. Co-authored original manuscript and presented research.

I have experience on at least two projects that were successfully completed.

Leadership and Organizational Experience

· Served for 2 years as graduate student American Physical Therapy Association Student Liaison and physical therapy club president, organizing student lecture series and professional events.

· Recruited, trained, and placed over 150 student volunteers in Planned Parenthood agency. Coordinated efforts with staff of 25 professionals in many program areas.

"I take on leadership roles and I'm capable in organizing and directing work-related responsibilities."

Table 23-2, continued

Licensure Licensed physical therapist #000000 IL (Date)	*License number, state, date, or indicate your application status.*
Education Mid-State University, Center City, IL Master of Physical Therapy, 2000 Mid-State University, Center City, IL Bachelor of Science, Psychology, 1994	*University name, city, state, degree, major (year, GPA is optional).* *In reverse chronological order, most recent first.*
Work Experience Peer Counselor (part-time), Women's Resource Center, Mid-State University, February 1998 to June 1999. Provided one-on-one peer counseling relating to rape and domestic abuse. Volunteer Coordinator, Planned Parenthood, West Hills, IL January 1995-August 1997. Recruited, trained, and organized student volunteers for various health-related projects in large nonprofit organization.	*Title, employer, city, state, dates. List professional positions prior to physical therapy education or list related positions in the health or human service fields. Give a brief description of your work-related duties. List in reverse chronological order, most recent first.*
Clinical Internships South Bay Women's Center, Southport, ME January 31, 2000-March 28, 2000. Participated in evaluation and intervention for women with stress incontinence in community-based women's health clinic.	*Facility, city, state, dates, brief description of clinical responsibilities and accomplishments. List in reverse chronological order, most recent first.*
Presentations Complex Lymphedema Therapy in Treatment of Lymphedema Post Breast Cancer, South Cove Women's Center, Westbrook, ME, March 10, 2000.	*List all presentations you have given, including in-service presentations during internships.*
Publications Straightforward S, Dynamic D, Reliable IM. The effect of complex lymphedema therapy—controlled pilot study. Manuscript in submission for publication. June 1, 2000.	*List publications, including webpages, abstracts, theses, and manuscripts in press.*
Honors and Activities Student Liaison, American Physical Therapy Association 1999-2001 President, Campus Physical Therapy Student Organization Dean's List 1998-2001	*List community activities, clubs, professional organizations, honors, and awards. Include dates.*
References References available on request.	*Either list those persons whom you have asked to serve as references for you or write, "References available on request."*

Creating Your Cover Letter

A cover letter is a critical part of your search for employment.

A cover letter must accompany your resumé to show how your individual qualities and experiences set you apart from the rest of the applicants. It should focus on your strongest qualifications, experience, and how you will contribute to the employer's organization. Use the following guidelines:

- Your letter, whether unsolicited or in response to a published employment listing, should be addressed to a specific person in the organization by name and correct title. If necessary, call and ask for spelling and title information. Say, "I would like to send a letter to the director of physical therapy; could you help me with the correct spelling and title for this person?" Use a proper business format in writing the letter, providing your return address, the date, and the address of the recipient. An employment ad might direct you to an individual in the human resources department of a large organization. If so, make initial contact with him or her and write your cover letter to that person.

- The introduction of your letter should indicate your purpose in writing and refer to what attracted you to send the letter and resumé. If appropriate, refer to a published employment listing by date and publication and to the job title listed. If you made a contact at a conference, mention the conference. Even if a specific position is not advertised or available at the current time, indicate what types of positions you are seeking (entry level, staff physical therapist, case manager, full-time, part-time, per diem). Summarize your qualifications and experience in the first paragraph.

- Continue to highlight your experience and education that qualify you for this position in the next few paragraphs. If an employment listing gives several qualifiers, be sure to address each of those. Use action verbs to describe your accomplishments and experience. Use your strongest qualifiers in this section. You can refer the reader to other qualifications in your resumé. Try to stay under four paragraphs (one page) in your letter.

- Conclude the letter with a request to schedule an interview and suggest dates and times that you will be available. This is especially effective if you know that you will be traveling to the employer's location at your own expense and only in town for a few days. Give your telephone number and the dates and times when you can be reached.

Table 23-3 shows the cover letter written by Susan Straightforward in search of possible future openings in practice settings that she desired. She sent her resumé (see Table 23-1) with each personalized cover letter.

Table 23-4 shows the cover letter sent by Donna Dynamic in response to the published employment listing. She also sent the resumé (see Table 23-2), which addresses the specifics of this published employment listing.

Interviewing

Make a Good First Impression

Your first impression is made in a matter of moments. Be careful to make the best impression. Although it might seem obvious, here are a few musts:

- Dress conservatively in clean and pressed professional clothing, shoes, and socks/stockings.
- Avoid excessive or obvious jewelry and accessories, aftershave, or perfumes.
- Take care with your grooming: hair, beard, and nails.
- Take a shower or bathe.
- Brush your teeth and use mouthwash if needed.
- Use deodorant.

Prepare for the Interview

Do your homework and learn as much as possible about the organization and individuals who will be interviewing you. Identify the needs and fears of your potential employer. If you can allay those fears and explain how your presence will meet the needs, you will be more likely to be hired.[1]

Although it may seem that you are the one who needs the job, try to step outside your perspective for a moment. Put yourself in the employer's shoes. The employer may be replacing someone who has left or developing a new position. The employer has an unmet need that created an open position. What, specifically, is the nature of that need? Is it for a certain skill set, temperament, or organizational function? Are there trends in this practice sector that require new knowledge and skills that you have? Think specifically about the projects you have done and papers you have written in your graduate work. How will you fit into the employer's needs?

Table 23-3

SAMPLE COVER LETTER (UNSOLICITED)

Susan Straightforward
556 W. Highland Avenue
Center City, IL 62666
(888)-554-1017

September 1, 2000

Stephen Simpson, Owner
Four Corners Physical Therapy
1500 Reisner Drive
Center City, IL 62667

Dear Mr. Simpson:

Several of my colleagues in graduate school had the opportunity to work with you during their clinical training. Your clinic's reputation for excellent clinical services in orthopedic and sports physical therapy is well known at Mid-State University. I am writing to inquire about potential clinical openings in the next few months. My resumé details my experiences before and during my professional education program. One recent experience confirmed my interests in working in an outpatient sports physical therapy practice setting.

My interest in orthopedics and sports medicine has been long-standing. I recently had the opportunity to work with Jennifer Jacobs at Tri-City Sports Rehabilitation Clinic. I worked with several athletes who were preparing for competition in the Olympic trials. This experience taught me a great deal about goal setting, motivation, and the physical therapist's role in working with elite athletes.

In addition to two internships in outpatient settings, I have gained experience in collaborative research as well as presenting and reporting the outcomes of our research. I am an active student member in the American Physical Therapy Association and am looking forward to representing Mid-State University at this fall's Student Conclave in Cherry Hill, NJ.

Should you anticipate an opening for a physical therapist, please let me know. I am interested in part-time, full-time, or per diem opportunities. You can leave me a message anytime at (888)-554-1017 or reach me by e-mail: sstraightforward@aol.com.

Thank you for your consideration. I hope to hear from you in the near future.

Sincerely,

Susan Straightforward, SPT
Enclosure: resumé

Your current address and telephone at the time of writing the letter.

Date letter is sent.

Name, correct title, and address.

Never write "To Whom It May Concern:"

Include the purpose of writing this letter. Personalize your letter to the person reading it.

Summarize your experience in a sentence and introduce the next paragraph.

What have you found most meaningful and motivating? Who, where, and how did you have this experience? Personalize this section.

What additional experiences support your qualifications? How did you acquire such outstanding skills? Show your enthusiasm in your achievements and accomplishments.

Take action. Remember that the employer has needs which must be met. Be straightforward and indicate your availability to talk. If you don't hear, call periodically and indicate your continued interest.

Table 23-4
SAMPLE COVER LETTER IN RESPONSE TO PUBLISHED EMPLOYMENT LISTING

Donna Dynamic
222 W Hill St.
Center City, IL 62666
(888)-555-6666

December 1, 2000

Janet Joyal, Director
Rehabilitation Services
University Medical Center
1001 University Drive
Center City, IL 62667

Dear Ms. Joyal:

Throughout my professional education experience, I have been impressed with the scope of the clinical services and innovative programs offered at University Medical Center. I am writing to apply for the physical therapist opening in the women's health team, published in the *Center City Women's Health Bulletin* on November 26, 2000. My resumé details my involvement in the women's health field for the past five years in a variety of capacities, including both physical and mental health. I would like to highlight how one of my clinical internships greatly contributed to my experience base and further interested me in the women's health field.

My assignment to the South Bay Women's Center in Southport, ME provided me with a unique opportunity to work with Caroline Coughlin, DPT, and a team of nurse practitioners and physicians. Through this experience, I gained expertise in a growing and important aspect of physical therapy care, the evaluation and treatment of stress incontinence. I worked closely with gynecologists, nurses, and social workers, and thoroughly enjoyed this specialty area. This experience, combined with my previous work, motivated me to seek a career opportunity in women's health.

My research, leadership, and organizational experience also enhances my potential to contribute to new program development in this area. Through my work at Planned Parenthood and at the Women's Resource Center I have developed outstanding organizational and communication skills. My recent research experience includes a collaborative project with Dr. I.M. Reliable on lymphedema management post-breast cancer. I welcomed the opportunity to co-author a research report on this study, and we submitted a manuscript for publication in May 2000.

I look forward to discussing your needs and my qualifications for this position. I am available at (888)-555-6666 every day until 10:00 am, or you can leave a message at this number anytime.

Thank you for your consideration. I hope to hear from you in the near future.

Sincerely,

Donna Dynamic, PT
Enclosure: resumé

Your current address and telephone at the time of writing the letter.

Date letter is sent.

Name, correct title, and address.

Never write "To Whom It May Concern:"

Include the purpose of writing this letter.

Summarize your experience in a sentence and introduce the next paragraph.

What have you found most meaningful and motivating? Who, where, and how did you have this experience? Personalize this section.

What additional experiences support your qualifications? How did you acquire such outstanding skills? Show your enthusiasm in your achievements and accomplishments.

Take action. Remember that the employer has needs which must be met. Be straightforward and indicate your availability to talk. If you don't hear, call Ms. Joyal and inquire about the timetable for the employment search. Indicate your continued interest.

Also, consider the employer's fears. Although you may be the one who is nervous and afraid that you will not be able to pay back your student loans, your potential employer is also afraid. The employer's fears may center around making a poor decision about whether your inexperience will spell trouble for the organization, or about whether you will need excessive help and supervision to come up to speed. The employer might be worried that you will take this job for the time being and move on to something better if it comes along. Your job in this interview is to help your potential employer feel comfortable that you can handle the responsibilities of the position and that you are a great choice.

Now, how do you identify your potential employer's needs and fears? Informational interviewing, of course. Talk with someone in a similar position from a similar organization. Consult your faculty regarding trends in the field. Consult with employees in similar organizations that you may know through your contacts and networks. Find out as much as you can about the position, why it is open, and who had the job last.

Practice responding to potential interview questions directly and concisely. Make good eye contact. Breathe deeply. Imagine yourself succeeding and things going well.

Your interviewer may bring up a salary figure. Do not commit to anything at this point. You have not been offered a position yet! Indicate your interest in knowing the range of salary being considered for this position.

Finish Strongly

Leave a good impression. Thank your interviewer and express continued interest. Find out when a hiring decision will be made. Make yourself useful in providing a list of references without hesitation.

Follow-up Immediately

Go home and immediately write a follow-up letter to your interviewer. Thank your interviewer and restate the areas you would like to emphasize about your background and interests. Be sure to emphasize what you, uniquely, will be able to contribute to the organization. As appropriate, indicate your willingness to relocate, work various hours, or be flexible in waiting for a full-time position to develop.

The Job Offer

When the job offer comes, then you can start negotiating. Look at the terms of employment and the benefits offered. Full health and dental benefits are often valued at 25% to 30% of the total salary package. Negotiate a fair starting salary if you will have to pay benefits yourself. Although a starting salary may be lower than you expected, perhaps there is the potential of career advancement or administrative and program development experience, which will strengthen your future career opportunities. Make a list of the tangible and intangible benefits.

Remember that this is your first position in the profession of physical therapy. Make the most of the opportunities available to you.

Summary

Entry into the job market as a new graduate can be challenging during these uncertain economic times when even experienced physical therapists are having difficulty finding career opportunities. It does not have to be painful or traumatic. Preparing for a career in the profession of physical therapy can be an exciting time of self discovery. Networking and informational interviewing can assist greatly in developing potential employment contacts and opportunities. Thoughtful resumé preparation and construction of appropriate cover letters will enhance personal contacts in opening doors for future opportunities. Prepare for interviews and approach the available opportunities with a positive outlook. Get off to a great start!

References

1. Curtis KA. *Career Survival Skills.* Paper presented at: APTA Annual Conference, Las Vegas, Nev; June 1998.

2. Curtis KA. Wanted: a few good therapists. *Rehab Management.* 1989;2(4):18-22.

3. Bolles RN, Bolles D. *What Color is Your Parachute?* 30th ed. Berkeley, Calif: Ten Speed Press; 2000.

PUTTING IT INTO PRACTICE

1. Interview a partner or colleague and write a brief response to each of the following questions. Give your notes to your partner or colleague.

    Your Ideal Life
    What is most important in your life?
    Consider the following:
    - What is most important to you in your personal life?
    - What is most important to you in your career?
    - What are your personal goals? Your professional goals?
    - How long do you envision yourself staying in one position or one location?

    Envision the Ideal Organization
    What are the things you consider to be most important in an organization in which you will work?
    Consider the following:
    - What goals or mission of an organization would be most attractive?
    - What would this organization contribute to society?
    - What size would this organization be?
    - What experience will you gain?
    - Where is the optimal location of your ideal workplace?
    - What are the working conditions?
    - With what kinds of people would you most like to work?
    - What are the needs of this type of organization in the current climate?

    What Do You Have to Offer?
    Consider the following:
    - What unique skills, abilities, and experiences will you bring to the workplace?
    - What problems are you able to solve for the organization, given your unique skills?
    - What new programs are you uniquely qualified to develop?
    - What changes are you able to offer a potential employer?
    - What will colleagues gain by working with you?
    - What will clients or patients gain by working with you?

2. Identify your network.
    Use the circle below to represent yourself. Write names and draw lines from your circle to individuals you would consider in your network who are readily accessible to you for information, help, and advice. Next, write new names and draw lines to individuals, organizations, and other entities to which your contacts have access. You should have a page filled with ideas and potential contacts. Circle those you feel may be of greatest benefit for information or providing potential contacts in your job search.

                Faculty   **Clinical Instructors**

        Organizations   **Family/Friends**

                                 YOU

3. Informational Interviews.

Who, in your network, could provide you with information about the current needs, employment climate, and trends in the practice sector or geographical location in which you would most like to work? (This is not a person whom you are asking for a position. This is a person whom you are asking for advice in how to approach your job search. You are asking for contacts, access to networks, and information that will help you to succeed.) Make a list below of your best choices:

Call one of those contacts and schedule a convenient time to talk or take this person out for lunch or coffee.

Develop a list of questions below:

4. List your strategies for approaching the job search.

What did you learn from your informational interview?

What new contacts will you make?

What individuals, events, groups, or networks can you approach next?

To whom will you send letters and resumés?

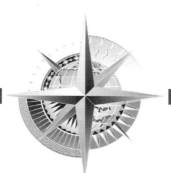

Chapter 24

Challenges for the New Graduate

> Marcie was excited; she was the only one that she knew of her classmates that had landed a job at the county medical center. It was a regional trauma center and had an excellent reputation. She looked forward to starting.
>
> Six weeks later, Marcie had difficulty getting up in the morning. She felt exhausted and depressed. It seemed that so few people really cared about what happened to these patients. She took it so seriously; why was she the only one who cared?
>
> Then there was the physical therapy. She found it hard to believe that she and her colleagues had studied at the same university. Why weren't they doing the things they had learned? It seemed like everyone was just cutting corners and trying to get by with the bare minimum of care. Her supervisor seemed only to care about her productivity, and her patients went home way too soon. She decided to look for a new job in a few months.

Marcie, like many new graduates, is experiencing *reality shock.*[1] What happened here? Did the university medical center take a turn for the worse? Did Marcie have a few bad experiences? It is unlikely that either of these are the cause of Marcie's feelings.

Role Stress

New graduate physical therapists often experience role stress.[1] One source of stress is the conflict-ing values of work and school. This conflict has been called *reality shock*. It is a fairly predictable phenomenon that was first described in the nursing profession in the mid-1970s.[2,3]

What Happens?

Students often study and excel in an idealized environment, where individualized, comprehensive, patient-centered care plans are required, theoretical problem-solving skills are highly valued, and sound professional judgment and professional autonomy are a priority. In contrast, the work environment values safe, efficient care, organization and efficiency, delegation to others, teamwork, cooperation, and accountability.

The phenomenon of reality shock often occurs due to the unexpected differences between the values of the academic world and the working world.[2,3] The behaviors required in the work environment conflict with the idea of individualized, total patient care that students practice in school. The time-consuming, ideal model of patient care presented in school is incompatible with the clinical environment that requires therapists to work within established time and resource constraints. See Table 24-1 for examples of conflicts between school and work values.

In addition to experiencing many difficult conflicts between school and work values, new graduates often leave the university with the impression that there is one correct way to accomplish a task,

Table 24-1

SCHOOL VALUES VS. WORK VALUES

School Values	Work Values
I was required to manage my time, plan my projects, and make my own schedule.	You are responsible to see a patient every 30 minutes.
I was rewarded for being thorough and complete in my work.	You must prioritize because you cannot do everything in the limited time available.
I was encouraged to reflect, read articles, and consider the rationale for my clinical decisions.	You need to follow the protocol as it's written. This is how we do it here.
I was at the top of my class; I have a great memory and strong intuition to know what's right to do.	You need to get feedback from the rest of the team before taking action.
I was encouraged to perform a thorough initial evaluation.	You only have time for screening and triage. We have a long waiting list of patients to be seen.
If I was bored or tired, I could just skip my class or leave early.	You have a responsibility to your patients and colleagues. If you are detached, late, or absent, everyone is short-changed.
I learned all these great manual therapy techniques. Did you ever hear of my professor?	You will need to focus on patient education because you have only one visit.
These exercises would be perfect for this patient's problem.	These exercises require too much assistance and equipment; the patient lives alone.
School was my first priority. I was never late to class.	In addition to arriving on time, you are also responsible for the safety and well-being of all of your patients and for supervising all the support staff who work with your patients.

approach a problem, or address a conflict. In striving to answer test questions correctly, students often believe that their answer is *the* answer, without recognizing that their answer may be *one* answer and that there may be many others as well.

Further, remember that new graduate physical therapists are often comfortable in the world of theory and models, whereas clinicians are more comfortable in reality and recognize what it takes to survive in that world. Consider the situation in the box in the right column.

Both therapists are functioning in their comfort zones. Susan is trying to make sense of this complex and overwhelming problem, using what she is comfortable with—neuroanatomical structures, tracts, and hypothetical lesions. Linda is working in the practical reality of observations and possible inter-

Susan, a new graduate physical therapist, consulted Linda, an experienced therapist who had specialized in neurology, regarding the most appropriate treatment for a young man with a brain injury. They watched the patient's gait together to determine the need for an orthosis. Linda commented on his tone and difficulty flexing the left knee during the push-off phase of gait. She suggested that Susan work with the patient in the kneeling position to try to normalize the patient's tone. Susan was surprised to hear Linda suggest that the patient be discharged without an orthosis. Susan asked where she thought the lesion would be that would cause that specific deficit and felt certain that the patient's safety would be compromised if the orthosis was not ordered.

Table 24-2

COMMON CAUSES OF ROLE STRESS AND BURNOUT

Cause	Feelings that precipitate role stress and burnout
Work overload	I can't possibly get all of this paperwork done.
Understaffing	I'm here alone! How can I see all of these patients this afternoon?
Repetitive tasks	If I get one more of these referrals for ultrasound, I'll scream!
Under-utilization of professional skills	It seems hard to believe it requires a master's degree to turn on a whirlpool!
Role ambiguity	It is so hard to work when I don't know if the patient knows what's going on. I think her doctor should tell her that her femur fracture was from a metastasis, not trauma.
Role conflict	I recommended a certain type of orthosis, and the physician told the patient that it wasn't my decision to make.
Inappropriate helping behavior	I know that I could motivate this patient if he'd just come for his therapy appointments. I think I'll call and remind him about the schedule of the buses that go by his house.
Unrealistic expectations	I could stay on schedule if the nurses would just do their jobs and have all the patients ready by 9:00 am.

ventions. She is thinking about the future and projecting an effect of an intervention and eventual recovery. Susan does not think like Linda at this point in her career (see Chapter 9). The result of this interaction is probably frustration for both therapists.

Doing it All Is Not Easy

Finally, we have to keep in mind that the new physical therapist's role requires skills in several areas that are not highly emphasized in most physical therapy curricula, including time management, caseload management, discharge planning, and interprofessional relationships. The complex demands in the clinical environment may leave many new graduates overwhelmed and exhausted.

Interestingly, many new graduates have been protected from the realities of clinical practice during clinical education as well. Student physical therapists are often responsible for a reduced caseload, infrequently delegate care responsibilities to support personnel, and often see the most interesting "teaching case." It is not surprising that new graduates are

stressed when expectations change with employment!

Burnout

Burnout is a state of emotional and physical exhaustion that results from intense and long-standing professional stress. This is especially prevalent in the helping professions, in which professional demands frequently exceed the resources available to meet them. Burnout may result in a loss of concern for people, a withdrawal from interaction, and alienation from the work environment. Detachment may be either emotional or physical.[4]

Burnout has been documented widely in the profession of physical therapy, often starting during the student years.[5-8] Therapists report feelings of emotional exhaustion, often related to work overload with conflicting time and resource constraints.[7,8] Many issues may result in feelings of burnout. Look at the list in Table 24-2 and see if you can identify any common feelings or situations.

So what can we do?

Resolving Reality Shock Productively

By developing awareness and skills that allow them to adapt to and take an active role in the work environment, new graduates feel better about their work, their colleagues, and the profession of physical therapy.

New graduates who master the skills required for the clinical role are likely to be more satisfied. In contrast, graduates who are unable to resolve the conflicts they face may find themselves dissatisfied and in a constant search for the perfect job. The consequences of unresolved conflict are serious. Check the list in Table 24-3.

Validating Feelings and Conflicts

Role conflict is a normal process that evolves from a predictable set of circumstances. It occurs across professions and even when changing professions. The workplace is likely to require performance that is in *direct conflict* with the recent graduate's experience in professional education.

Graduates must recognize that this stressful period is part of the process of assuming the professional role and joining an organization.[9,10] There are sources of support and strategies that will help graduates to adapt to the realities of clinical practice.

First, recognize that the feelings presented in Tables 24-2 and 24-3 are real. Individual reactions to role conflict may range from disappointment and confusion to outrage. The action that you take as a result of a feeling is what's important. This is where you have a choice.

Second, realize that we often feel frustrated and angry when circumstances that affect us are out of our control. Lashing out is a coping mechanism that absolves us of responsibility for the problems we face. In reality, an individual physical therapist is not responsible for massive cost containment initiatives and restrictive regulations imposed by government agencies. However, individual physical therapists can be responsible for their own thoughts and attitudes, interactions and actions with their patients and colleagues.

Rather than judging your colleagues and coworkers as wrong, lazy, incompetent, thoughtless, or insensitive, recognize that there are thoughts and beliefs that also motivate their behaviors. Focus your energy on changing what is changeable and on the areas in which you have some control and influence.

Making Good Choices

The choices that present themselves in a work day are endless. Let's start with two of the more important choices—time management and caseload management.

You will not feel that you are accomplishing everything that you "should" be doing. Eliminate this from your expectations. Then, concentrate on what is *most important* for your responsibilities to run smoothly and other staff to be able to work effectively with you.

Survival Skills

There are key activities that will lead to a productive and satisfying career in the profession of physical therapy. These survival skills are essential to cope with the many demands of clinical practice.[11] They include:

- Addressing highest priority patient needs
- Referring to post-discharge care providers
- Using effective interpersonal skills with patients
- Choosing effective time- and caseload-management strategies
- Interacting effectively with other health care professionals
- Planning career development

Time Management

Managing your time can be a challenge throughout your professional education and your career. Review some of the key elements of time management in Chapter 11. Table 24-4 lists many useful time management strategies in the clinical setting.

Caseload Management

Sara was worried as she started her new position. Jack, the physical therapist assistant, had worked at the facility for years and was almost 20 years her senior. The rest of the staff in the practice was much more experienced. She wondered how receptive he would be to working with a new graduate.

Caseload management requires identification of patient needs and careful planning to effectively allocate resources and meet high priority patient needs. Delegation is often a difficult skill for the new staff member.

Support personnel may have more clinical experience than new graduates, and this can be intimidat-

Table 24-3

THE COSTS OF ROLE STRESS

Therapist Feelings	Maladaptive Response	Better Response
There must be a better job out there. My friends from school don't have to put up with this.	Early turnover and job hopping from one dissatisfying situation to another.	Share feelings with colleagues and supervisors. Change strategies to deal with challenges. Suggest improvements in working conditions.
I had no idea clinical practice would be this boring.	Leaving the field or pursuing a career change.	Seek new challenges. Join a committee, supervise students, or add a new program development responsibility.
All I've seen for weeks are backs and necks, hips and knees.	Boredom, depersonalization, treating people like backs and necks, hips and knees.	Adopt the point of view that each patient is unique, regardless of the diagnosis. Group patients with similar problems to provide services and education more efficiently.
I am not making the salary I deserve.	Doing the bare minimum to get by.	Request a raise after showing that your work is exemplary and outcomes exceed expectations.
I'm getting nowhere. I've been working on this positioning program for months and it seems like someone on the night shift always forgets.	Giving up; feeling like it's not worth the effort to try; someone always drops the ball.	Find out what happened and work individually with staff members who have responsibilities. Expect accountability and responsibility.
Hospital policy prevents me from spending more than 45 minutes per day with this patient.	Thinking that the patient will have to suffer because of this policy. Why doesn't the administration consider the patient's needs and not just the bottom line? Blindly following the rules.	Recognize that there are exceptions to rules. Present the patient's needs to your supervisor with a plan for meeting them. Consider alternatives such as co-treatment with occupational therapy.
No one cares about the patients as much as I do.	Spending free time after work and on weekends doing paperwork and related job duties. Assuming that others are doing a poor job.	Make appropriate referrals to community agencies. Serve as an advocate for patient needs.

Table 24-4

TIME-MANAGEMENT TECHNIQUES FOR THE NEW GRADUATE[12]

1. Develop a system. List goals and set priorities. If applicable, make subgoals and give each a target date. Keep your list in plain view, over your desk or on a bulletin board or your clipboard. (You may want to do this in conjunction with your supervisor.)

2. Delegate nonessentials for others to do. Be sure to delegate effectively; give authority within the person's capability, set up a feedback system, define limits, and make and stick to a plan for follow-up. Otherwise, delegation will cost you time, and you might as well have done it yourself.

3. Give yourself a time to think and handle problems. This might involve a few minutes before starting your morning and afternoon schedules. Plan on this and make this time a priority, just as important as all your other scheduled responsibilities.

4. Schedule daily paperwork time and a time to return phone calls. Have what you need to do ready to go so that you can use this time most effectively. Do not compromise on this time more than once a week, no matter *how busy* you are.

5. Make a daily "to do" list every day at the same time (on one piece of paper). Post this in a conspicuous place or carry it on a clipboard you have with you all the time.

6. Frequently ask yourself, "What is the best use of my time right now?"

7. For memos, announcements, paperwork:

  A. Handle each piece of paper you receive only once; get rid of it ASAP.
  Either:
  1. Take action (respond, place on to-do list, etc)
  2. Pass it on to others
  3. Read it, absorb it, and destroy it

  B. For patient-related documentation
  1. Document *once* while seeing the patient. Copying over your notes wastes time.

  2. Use *pre-printed forms* or *computerized documentation systems* when possible to help organize your notes and ensure thorough documentation.

  3. *Dictate* if available. Once you get used to doing this it takes less than one-fourth the time of writing the same information!

  4. During daily treatment, include documentation time while the patient is being seen.

8. For phone calls you make or receive:

  A. Use your "on-hold" time to your advantage to do other paperwork or sort mail and papers.

  B. Make several phone calls at once.

  C. If it is not convenient to receive a phone call, request that a message be taken. Ask reception personnel to find out from the caller when the *best time* is for you to return the phone call or give the caller a good time to call you back.

  D. Make a list of questions or points you want to cover during the phone call. Make records of all phone calls in the same location. A daily planner or desk log works well.

9. Do this now.

ing. New graduates may not have had an opportunity to practice delegation as a student physical therapist, because students are often encouraged to take responsibility for the patient's full plan of care or treatment. The following ideas may help in developing effective delegation skills.

Review job responsibilities and educational background of support personnel. It may be helpful to have an orientation meeting with your clinical supervisor, new staff members, and support personnel to make sure that everyone is hearing the same information. Ask support personnel to share details of their training and experience and how it is easiest for them to support care delivery.

Review your caseload frequently with your supervisor and mutually problem-solve for new ideas of caseload management. Table 24-5 addresses delegation techniques.

Peer Support Networks

One of the most effective coping strategies to deal with reality shock is to develop strong support networks of professional colleagues who face similar challenges. It is especially important that new graduates have contact with experienced colleagues who can offer support to help deal with difficult patients, productivity pressures, physician-therapist communication, and other issues about which new graduates express concerns.

Peer support helps to decrease role stress. When workers have positive interpersonal interactions with their coworkers, they tend to feel more satisfied about their work.[3] Create networks of peers who are able to support each other. Organize social events and informal networking, and make an effort to both seek and offer this essential support.

Mentors

Evidence supports the benefits of a relationship with a mentor.[3] A *mentor* is an experienced clinician who is able to validate your experiences and feelings, share strategies, and offer guidance and advice that assist with early career development. This differs from a clinical supervisor in that a supervisor has direct responsibility for your performance.

If there is not a program in place, seek a mentor through either your local chapter of the APTA or clinical networks in your area. Experienced clinicians are more than happy to share their experiences with you.

Choose Your Battles

Although it may seem that most of the requirements, policies, and procedures in the clinical environment are out of your control, think carefully about where and how your time will be best spent. Take action where it counts. Choosing your battles means working smarter and applying effort in areas that are both important and changeable. Remember your role as a change agent in Chapter 3. Take reasoned action proactively and believe in your power. Table 24-6 gives guidelines for choosing issues for maximum effect.

Summary

New graduates face predictable challenges and frustrations as they move from the more controlled environment of professional education into the workplace. The choices that one makes determine one's experience during this stressful time. Practicing effective survival skills, such as time and caseload management, seeking peer and mentor support, and actively choosing when, where, and how to apply effort for change are essential early career strategies. New graduates who develop awareness and skills that allow them to adapt to and take an active role in the work environment are more satisfied with their work, their colleagues, and the profession of physical therapy.

Table 24-5

CASELOAD MANAGEMENT STRATEGIES[12]

1. **Choose a capable person.** Evaluate the assignment and the person. Have reasonable expectations given the role, talents, and experience of the person to whom you will delegate. Communicate your appreciation of his or her skills, which will ensure completion of the assignment.

2. **Explain the objectives of the assignment.** Review the results you wanted, the lines of authority, but with enough flexibility to allow physical therapist assistants or other support personnel to use their own ideas and initiative.

3. **Give the physical therapist assistant or other support personnel the means and authority to do the job.** Explain the limits, where to go for assistance, and what orders or authority may come with the assignment. Notify others who may be affected by this person's area of authority.

4. **Keep in contact.** Establish a feedback and follow-up system. Monitor progress, but beware of holding back authority.

Watch out for:

1. **Your own fear of losing control.** You must let go of the authority to do this job, even if it's not "your" way. You can support, but not do, the job for the other person. Trust is essential.

2. **Your own feelings of indispensability.** You, the physical therapist assistant, or other support personnel may perpetuate this. Encourage independence, even though it may not be as personally satisfying to you; it is necessary to get the job done most efficiently.

3. **Your tendency to hover or meddle.** Once you have delegated the job, avoid appearing unsure that support personnel can handle it.

4. **Over-delegating.** Avoid delegating policy-making, financial authority, and disciplinary authority. You cannot delegate these things and still be in control.

5. **Delegating responsibility.** You remain responsible for each patient's care. You do not delegate responsibility when working with support personnel. Support personnel are still responsible to you, even though they may report the results of the job to your supervisor. **Do not** allow yourself to be bypassed in the processes of communication.

6. **Not delegating enough or delegating too much authority.** The responsibility of performance cannot be greater or less than the delegated authority provides. Be sure that support personnel exercise judgment that is in compliance with laws that govern practice in your jurisdiction. Remember that you are ultimately responsible and that delegated authority is a choice that you make as a physical therapist. If you want to see a patient once weekly, schedule this. If you want to co-treat occasionally, take the initiative to make this happen.

7. **Not seeking specific feedback.** Require regular progress reports and mutually try to solve problems that arise. Conferences that address these issues should be part of the patient's medical record. Be supportive. Help the physical therapist assistant and other support personnel to succeed!

Table 24-6

WORKING SMARTER AS A CHANGE AGENT

Is it important to me, a patient, my colleagues, and the organization in which I work?	Can I/we influence the desired outcome here?	
	YES	**NO**
YES	1. The highest priority for action. Plan carefully and strategize a series of approaches that are likely to result in the desired outcome.	2. Find out who can influence the desired outcome. At what level is a policy or decision being made? Serve as an advocate for patients. Take community-based action. Write letters, make phone calls. Involve your representative in Congress or the Senate.
NO	3. Focus your time and energy on outcomes that make a difference in people's lives.	4. Do not bother. It is not important and it is out of your control.

References

1. Deckard G, Present R. Impact of role stress on physical therapists, emotional and physical well-being. *Phys Ther.* 1989;69:713-718.

2. Kramer M. *Reality Shock.* St. Louis, Mo: The CV Mosby Company; 1974.

3. Schmalenberg C, Kramer, M. *Coping with Reality Shock: The Voices of Experience.* Wakefield, Mass: Nursing Resources, Inc; 1979.

4. Maslach C. *Burnout: The Cost of Caring.* New York, NY: Prentice Hall Press; 1982.

5. Balogun JA, Hoeberlein-Miller TM, Schneider E, Katz JS. Academic performance is not a viable determinant of physical therapy students' burnout. *Percept Mot Skills.* 1996;83(1):21-22.

6. Kolb K. Graduating burnout candidates. *Phys Ther.* 1994;74(3):264-265.

7. Donohoe E, Nawawi A, Wilker L, et al. Factors associated with burnout of physical therapists in Massachusetts rehabilitation hospitals. *Phys Ther.* 1993;73(11):750-761.

8. Wandling BJ, Smith BS. Burnout in orthopaedic physical therapists. *J Orthop Sports Phys Ther.* 1997;26(3):124-130.

9. Smith DM. Organizational socialization of physical therapists. *Phys Ther.* 1989;69(4):282-286.

10. Schwertner RM, Pinkston D, O'Sullivan P, et al. Transition from student to physical therapist. *Phys Ther.* 1987;67(5):695-701.

11. Curtis KA, Martin T. Recruitment and retention in acute care. *Rehab Management.* 1991;69-75.

12. Curtis KA. *Training New Staff for Clinical Survival.* Los Angeles, Calif: Health Directions; 1987.

PUTTING IT INTO PRACTICE

1. Read each of the following and identify the feelings of the graduate. Discuss a strategy or response that addresses the problem presented:

    a. I'm not being given the opportunity to use any of my resources or my education. I don't have my own patients or any responsibility for anything important. I've done a lot more as a student than I'm doing now! There's nothing I've done to make them think that I'm unsafe or incompetent.

    b. I had some training in how to run treatment groups, but doing it is a totally different story. We're so short-staffed that there's no one I can go to for ongoing support and feedback after each group. I'd really like to know what I'm doing wrong and how I can get all of the patients more involved.

    c. I learned how to do this procedure in school. They did it a different way during my clinical affiliations. Now they do it a different way here. To top it all off, the doctor I've been working with does it even another way. I just don't know what's right!

    d. Before I came here, I worked in a much larger facility. I know that part of the experience I had is because of the size of the place, but it really doesn't seem that the standards of care here are anywhere near as high. I'm really worried that something awful is going to happen to one of my patients, especially on the evening and night shift.

    e. It seems that my supervisor never talks to me except to tell me what is going wrong. There's no comment on all the good things I'm doing!

    f. There's an experienced member of our staff who outright lies about the things he's doing. I covered some of his patients this weekend. He says that he's done all these wonderful things and the patients looked at me like I was crazy when I asked them about those same things.

    g. The thing that I find most disturbing is the attitude of the staff toward the patients. I've been working with very severely involved patients and it just doesn't seem like anyone cares whether they do the best job possible. I hope that I never turn into someone like that!

    h. I'm so nervous when I have to ask one of the doctors to change something. I know exactly what I want to say and then it just comes out sounding like I don't know anything.

2. Identify a person who could serve as a mentor. Keep in touch during your first few years of practice.

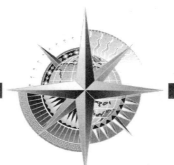

Chapter 25

Planning for Professional Development

> *Carol looked at the brochures for continuing education courses. They all looked so good, and they were all so expensive. She thought, "I've just finished 7 years of college. There is so much that I still need to learn, but how can I pay for all of this?"*

Lifelong Learning

Entry-level education is just the beginning. Learning does not end at the conclusion of formal university education. *Lifelong learning* involves continuing to question, probe, read, assimilate, and apply information that facilitates growth in both personal and professional arenas. It requires reflection, processing of experiences, and integration of new developments into existing knowledge and practices.

Changes in policy require changes in attitudes, practices, and sometimes organizational structures. Research developments, new technology, and collaboration with other professionals expand our horizons and offer us the opportunity to continue to grow and enhance the foundation we have gained during entry-level professional education.

Lifelong learning assures that clinicians and clinical and academic faculty use up-to-date and relevant information on education, technology, administration, and clinical practice parameters.

The Information Age

Information and knowledge are changing at a pace never before experienced. We are bombarded daily by e-mail, the web, voicemail, fax, newspapers and magazines, professional journals, television, unsolicited mail, and telemarketers calling us in our homes and businesses. Information overload has been well-documented. For the first time in history, our capabilities for generating information are far greater than the human capacities to process all the information produced.[1]

Within the physical therapy profession alone, we have seen the emergence of dozens of professional research journals, online publications, listservs, and bulletin boards. How does one know what is most important? How does a practicing clinician access, sift through, prioritize, and decide to use the abundant information that is out there? There are several strategies that can guide professional development.

A Professional Development Plan

Set goals for professional development. What interests do you have? Where do you see your career going in the next few months? The next year? In 5 years? Let's look first at what you find interesting, exciting, and challenging. Consider yourself doing each of the activities in Table 25-1 in the next few years. What intrigues you? In which areas did you score the highest?

The directions in which we choose to go should be consistent with our interests. Interests can change with changes in responsibility and job requirements as well. Therefore, what interests you now may not be what interests you for the future. You may want to return and repeat this inventory periodically to assess changes in your interests.

Check your scores against those of others. The scores in Table 25-2 indicate percentile scores of a group of 150 physical therapists of various experience levels who completed the inventory.

There are many career directions and paths one can take. The questions in Table 25-3 may help you to prioritize your path and direction.

Continuing Education Courses

José lived in Florida, a state which has a continuing education requirement for license renewal. How would he find courses that counted toward his license renewal requirements?

Seminars and Workshops

There are numerous opportunities for physical therapists to participate in short- and long-term seminars, courses, conferences, and online and home study courses. States that require continuing education for license renewal publish a specific listing of the types of organizations, courses, conferences, and professional activities that count toward meeting these requirements. Professional continuing education courses must meet specific criteria and often undergo evaluations to be able to offer continuing education units (CEUs). Check on your state's requirements.

High-quality continuing education courses are well-founded in educational principles and use qualified course faculty, appropriate instructor-to-student ratios, and effective learning activities. Promotional materials often provide sufficient information to evaluate a course. Seek feedback from oth-

ers who have taken the course as well. The guidelines presented in Table 25-4 may assist in deciding which courses to consider taking.

Popular continuing education courses are available in many cities on different dates. The schedule of courses is often known months in advance. Call the continuing education provider to check on upcoming schedules and dates to plan ahead. Courses are publicized by brochures, online listings, and print listings in professional publications.

A listing of continuing education courses is available in *PT Bulletin Online*: http://www.apta.org/bulletin/course_listings.

Online Continuing Education Series

There are various online continuing education courses offered through the APTA and sections. An online continuing education index is available at: http://www.apta.org/ceu/index.html.

Individual sections also offer online and home study courses. Check with their individual websites. All sections can be accessed from the following website: http://www.apta.org/Components/component_home_pages.

Conferences

Attending conferences may be very helpful to foster professional development opportunities. Carefully check the conference program to identify sessions of interest. There may also be pre-conference courses that meet your needs. Review Chapter 21 for information about various types of conferences.

Certificates of Advanced Study

Another option for professional development is to pursue university-based education to obtain a certificate of advanced study in a particular area such as health care management, information systems, or practice management.

Certificates are nondegree programs that offer clusters of related courses, often designed to meet real-life business and organizational needs. These courses may or may not offer university credit hours. Check with your local university extension office to see what is available in your area.

Table 25-1

CAREER INTEREST INVENTORY[2]

1	2	3	4	5	6	7

Not interested   Extremely interested

Using a scale from 1 to 7, rate your interest in each of the following activities:

____ 1. Organize and teach an inservice session for students or staff.

____ 2. Evaluate journal articles and discuss clinical applications with colleagues.

____ 3. Apply new treatment techniques.

____ 4. Project staffing requirements in your area for the next 2 months.

____ 5. Teach an orientation for new employees to prevent back injuries.

____ 6. Present a paper or poster presentation at a professional conference.

____ 7. Modify equipment for a patient's needs.

____ 8. Design new programs to meet department needs.

____ 9. Provide coaching or consultation to colleagues on patient problems.

____ 10. Review all recent studies in the literature on a new type of treatment.

____ 11. Develop standards of clinical competence for physical therapy.

____ 12. Research costs/features and plan a budget to buy needed equipment for your area.

____ 13. Teach part or all of a continuing education course.

____ 14. Save articles of interest from professional journals.

____ 15. Determine the best way to meet an individual patient's needs.

____ 16. Supervise and evaluate performance of other staff members.

____ 17. Provide clinical instruction to PT or PTA students.

____ 18. Collect and analyze data on physical therapy patient outcomes.

____ 19. Interact with a team to determine realistic patient goals.

____ 20. Help other staff members establish performance goals.

____ 21. Develop or revise patient education materials (handouts, pamphlets).

____ 22. Talk with others regarding the feasibility of a clinical research project.

____ 23. Advise other health professionals on the role of physical therapy.

____ 24. Plan methods to increase productivity of a practice site.

____ 25. Organize and publicize continuing education courses or seminars.

____ 26. Survey staff members or patients to obtain information.

____ 27. Document the improvement in a patient's function at discharge.

____ 28. Be involved with interviewing new staff for hiring.

continued

Table 25-1, continued

____ 29. Work on a videotape, CD-ROM, or website to teach new staff or patients.

____ 30. Use high-tech equipment to measure patient function, strength, or flexibility.

____ 31. Develop clinical protocols for evaluation or treatment.

____ 32. Arrange for patient coverage with staff illnesses and vacations.

____ 33. Preview a book or videotape to recommend purchase for the department.

____ 34. Write grants or research proposals to outside agencies for funding.

____ 35. Specialize in an area of clinical practice or disability group.

____ 36. Develop systems for smooth patient transition from inpatient to outpatient physical therapy.

____ 37. Teach a class as part of a physical therapy university course.

____ 38. Design new ways to measure patient outcomes in physical therapy.

____ 39. Be recognized by patients and colleagues as an excellent clinician.

____ 40. Revise and write departmental policies and procedures.

Enter and tally your scores below:

My score	Item	My score	Item	My score	Item	My score	Item
____	1	____	2	____	3	____	4
____	5	____	6	____	7	____	8
____	9	____	10	____	11	____	12
____	13	____	14	____	15	____	16
____	17	____	18	____	19	____	20
____	21	____	22	____	23	____	24
____	25	____	26	____	27	____	28
____	29	____	30	____	31	____	32
____	33	____	34	____	35	____	36
____	37	____	38	____	39	____	40
____	TOTAL	____	TOTAL	____	TOTAL	____	TOTAL
Education		**Research**		**Clinical**		**Administration**	

Clinical Residencies

Janice was unable to find a position in neonatal physical therapy as a new graduate. She talked with a colleague who suggested she pursue a clinical residency in pediatrics for a year.

Post-professional clinical residency programs are emerging as a valuable option for professional development. Clinical residency programs offer an established program of clinical and didactic education. Residency programs enable physical therapists to enhance their preparation in providing clinical services in a specific area of clinical practice. Residents

Table 25-2

CAREER INTEREST INVENTORY SCORING FOR PHYSICAL THERAPISTS[2]

	Percentile Scores			
	0-20	**21-50**	**51-80**	**>80**
Education	10-48	49-54	55-60	61-70
Research	10-33	34-35	46-57	58-70
Clinical	10-54	55-60	61-66	67-70
Administration	10-37	38-48	49-59	60-70
If your score falls within this range...	You are less interested in this area than 80% of all therapists who completed the inventory.	You are less interested in this area than 50% of all therapists who completed the inventory.	You are more interested in this area than 50% of all therapists who completed the inventory.	You are more interested in this area than 80% of all therapists who completed the inventory.

Select your two highest areas of interest by percentile.

Clinical-Education
This is the most common combination. Your interests are combined in working with students. You will also be a natural at developing educational materials for your patients. You work well with groups and will be an excellent clinician.

Administrative-Clinical
With this combination, you are a great resource for any organization. Keep up on changes in health care policy and work proactively as a change agent to help your organization adapt to the changing health care environment. You will enjoy creating new systems that enable you to provide clinical services despite the challenges that face you. You may be happiest in a supervisory position that enables you to continue patient contact, in a consultant role with industry, or as an independent contractor or owning your own private practice.

Education-Research
This combination is particularly well-suited for a career in academia. Be careful to balance these roles. You will probably need to pursue an advanced degree (doctorate) to follow your interests on this career path.

Clinical-Research
Therapists with this combination may be happiest in a clinical setting, working collaboratively with other researchers. There are conflicts inherent in this combination. Clinical care is sanctioned; research is often left to be done on your own time. You need to create some ways of enabling yourself to do research activities in the course of your clinical day. Explore opportunities for advanced degrees that match your interests.

Administrative-Research
Therapists with this combination may be happiest writing and administering grants, directing or evaluating a project. You will probably need to pursue an advanced degree (doctorate) to follow your interests on this career path. You could work happily from either an academic institution or a clinical center.

Administrative-Education
With this combination of interests, you may be well-suited for an administrative position in an academic program, in a clinical center directing a staff development program, or holding a corporate position in the rehabilitation field. Additional education may be indicated.

Table 25-3
SETTING PROFESSIONAL DEVELOPMENT GOALS

Consider your responses to the following questions:

1.   What performance goals would you like to meet in the next year? Draw from your most recent clinical performance evaluation or other sources.

2.   What do you need to be able to do or need to know to reach the above goals?

3.   In what two areas would you like to develop your clinical, administrative, teaching, or research skills in the next year? Be specific.

4.   What is the best way for you to develop these areas? Consider independent study, in-service education at work, mentoring relationships with another person, and outside continuing education courses.

5.   What resources are available in your current workplace that will help you to develop these areas? Consider mentors, practice opportunities, in-service classes, and employee development programs.

6.   What resources are available in the community that will help you to develop these areas? Consider continuing education courses, university programs, self-study courses, and mentors.

7.   What career goals would you like to meet in the next 5 years? What type of position would you like to have in 5 years? What additional skills or training do you need to make this career move? What additional responsibilities can you seek now that would prepare you for these goals?

focus on skills such as examination, evaluation, diagnosis, prognosis, intervention, and management of patients. Residency programs often include experiences in community service, patient education, research, and supervision of other health care providers (professional and paraprofessional).

Credentialed residency programs must be at least 1500 hours and between 9 and 36 months in duration. Following completion of a residency program, a physical therapist may be eligible and more prepared to sit for the American Board of Physical Therapy Specialties (ABPTS) examination in a particular specialty area. A list of credentialed clinical residency programs is available at: http://www.apta.org/Education/clinical/apta_crdtd_clncl_rdncy.

Clinical Specialization

Ahmed had a strong interest in sports physical therapy and had been certified as an athletic trainer prior to pursuing physical therapy education. He wanted most to work with a professional football team. How could he best prepare himself for this career opportunity?

Clinical specialty certification recognizes individuals who have demonstrated advanced clinical knowledge and skills in physical therapy specialty areas. Between 1985 and 2000, the ABPTS certified 2028 physical therapists as clinical specialists. Clinical specialty certification is currently available in seven areas of physical therapy practice:[4,5]
- Cardiopulmonary
- Clinical electrophysiologic
- Geriatric
- Neurologic
- Orthopaedic
- Pediatric
- Sports

Board-certified clinical specialists use the following initials after the "PT" in their titles to designate their area(s) of specialization:
- CCS (Cardiopulmonary Certified Specialist)
- ECS (Clinical Electrophysiologic Certified Specialist)
- GCS (Geriatric Certified Specialist)
- NCS (Neurologic Certified Specialist)
- OCS (Orthopaedic Certified Specialist)
- PCS (Pediatric Certified Specialist)
- SCS (Sports Certified Specialist)

Table 25-4

CRITERIA TO EVALUATE CONTINUING EDUCATION COURSES[3]

	YES	NO
1. Is there a clear rationale for the course? Does this rationale fit with your professional development goals?		
2. Has the target audience been identified? Do you fit within this description?		
3. Has the instructional level been identified? Is this level consistent with your prior knowledge and exposure to this material?		
• Basic (1)—This level assumes that participants have little information within the areas to be covered so that the focus of the activity is a general orientation and increased awareness.		
• Intermediate (2)—This level assumes that the participants have a general familiarity with the topic, so it focuses on increased understanding and application.		
• Advanced (3)—This level assumes thorough familiarity with the topic and focuses on advanced techniques, recent advances, and future directions.		
• Various (0)—This category indicates that a single level cannot be determined. It is intended for programs in which the instructional level may vary.		
4. Have learning outcomes been described? What will you learn? Do these outcomes fit with your professional development goals?		
5. Are objectives achievable, based on the length of the program?		
6. Are the instructional methods appropriate to achieving the learning objectives?		
7. Has the content been outlined and a schedule of presentation provided?		
8. Are CEUs awarded? Is the CEU provider designated with name, address, and telephone number? (CEUs may or may not be required for license renewal, given requirements by state.)		
9. Is certification or credentialing offered? How many courses are required for certification or credentialing? How is performance evaluated? What additional requirements must be met before or after this course?		
10. Is registration restricted (for laboratory and clinical demonstration courses)?		
11. Are faculty qualifications listed? Do faculty qualifications seem appropriate for course content and learning outcomes?		
12. Is the course fee listed, with a clear statement about cancellation policies?		
13. Have other attendees rated the course highly?		

Reprinted with permission from the American Physical Therapy Association.

Advantages of Specialization

Specialty certification provides a mechanism to validate clinical expertise in a practice area. Clinical specialists are often involved in consultation, education, and research in their area of specialization. Although there is not a required salary increase with certification, many clinical specialists assume higher level positions in their organizations that are consistent with their experience and specialty area.

Certification Process

Specialty certification is carried out through electronic testing at various sites nationwide during a specified testing period. Applicants must meet licensure and specified direct patient care experience requirements to be eligible to sit for the examination. The examination is a multiple-choice test of approximately 200 questions. [4,5]

Minimum eligibility requirements are available from the APTA Specialist Certification Department (e-mail: spec-cert@apta.org). A sample of eligibility criteria to sit for the Orthopaedic Clinical Specialist examination is listed in Table 25-5. Check with the current listings for any updates to these criteria.

Advanced Degree Programs

Additional education may be required to meet your long-term career objectives. Explore the career opportunities that may be available by combining a background in physical therapy with public health, business administration, health care or public administration, education, or basic or applied science research.

When and why to go back to school should be a carefully considered decision. Is an additional degree required for your next career move? If your career objectives lead you in these directions, consider these and other degree options:

MPH   Master of Public Health
MBA   Master of Business Administration
PhD   Doctorate of Philosophy—offered in
          many areas
EdD   Doctorate of Education
MPA   Master of Public Administration
DPA   Doctorate of Public Administration

Climbing the Clinical Ladder

Consider for a moment that you could combine lifelong learning, your interests, and your job responsibilities into one fabulous package called your career! The profession of physical therapy offers opportunities to do all this and more.

You *can* craft your career and create opportunities that match your interests and talents. Consider the possible activities and roles to develop your experience base in your first few years in the profession in Table 25-6. Most therapists are based in clinical practice at this time.

Keeping Connected

Patricia had graduated at close to the top of her class. After 6 months of clinical practice, she found herself forgetting the pathophysiology of some common diseases. She didn't recognize the names of the drugs her patient was taking. She found herself so busy that it was impossible for her to keep up with learning about her patient's condition. She had lapsed into the habit of just "going with the flow."

One morning, she failed to take her patient's blood pressure while the patient was sitting at the edge of the bed. She felt she could "talk the patient through" the dizziness she complained of and finish the treatment session in time to meet her colleagues for lunch. Her patient fainted and fell to the floor. Luckily, the patient was not injured. She completed an incident report. In discussion later with her supervisor, she realized how many mistakes she had made.

Continue to Think and Reflect (ie, Don't Lose Your Mind!)

Many practice situations provide new and unexpected challenges. Be careful not to fall into poor habits out of convenience. Your patient's safety comes first. Remember that you are responsible for your patient's well-being whether you or support personnel provide care.

Continue to challenge your critical thinking abilities. Ask yourself key questions that allow you to use all of the information available to you. Never allow yourself to put a patient in danger because you have not had time to find an answer to a question.

Explore the Science as Well as the Art of Clinical Practice

Ask questions of physicians and other health care providers. Be sure that you understand what you are seeing and reading in a patient's medical record. Seek resources and references in the clinical setting. Attend rounds, clinical conferences, and in-service presentations. Ask colleagues if you can observe them to learn more about what they do. Be a team player.

Develop your communication skills. Use effective, clear communication with patients, families, and

Table 25-5
MINIMUM ELIGIBILITY REQUIREMENTS FOR PHYSICAL THERAPY SPECIALIST CERTIFICATION (ORTHOPEDICS)

2001 Exam Administration

1. General

- Applicants must hold a current license to practice physical therapy in the United States or any of its possessions or territories.

- Applicants will be required to pay application review and examination fees.

2. Direct Patient Care Experience

Applicants must meet requirements for Option A or Option B.

- Option A. Applicants must submit evidence of 2000 hours of direct patient care in the specialty area within the last ten (10) years. 25% of these hours must have occurred within the last three years. Direct patient care must include activities in each of the elements of patient/client management applicable to the specialty area and included in the Description of Advanced Clinical Practice (DACP). These elements, as defined in the *Guide to Physical Therapist Practice*, are examination, evaluation, diagnosis, prognosis, and intervention.

- Option B. Applicants must submit evidence of successful completion of an APTA-credentialed post professional clinical residency that has a curriculum plan reflective of the. Experience from residencies in which the curriculum plan reflects only a portion of the DACP (Description of Advanced Clinical Practice) for Orthopedic Physical Therapy will not be considered.

3. Application

Applicants must describe their physical therapy practice experience for each position and facility on the appropriate forms in the application. Applicants must also chart their experience by year to ensure that they meet recency requirements. Applicants must document the number of direct patient care hours in the specialty. The application booklet may be printed at no cost from APTA's Specialist Certification Department Website (http://www.apta.org/Education/specialist/2001_app_booklet.)

Reprinted with permission from the American Physical Therapy Association.

---

staff members. Take the time to introduce yourself and establish collegial relationships with the other health care professionals. The time and effort that you spend in these areas is of critical importance to your professional self-concept and role development.

Maintain an Active APTA Membership

Some new graduates feel that APTA membership is too expensive and drop their membership after graduation. This is one of the biggest mistakes you can make. APTA membership allows you to receive professional publications, stay informed on the latest research and technology, attend professional conferences at a discount, and pursue clinical residencies and specialty certification. APTA membership keeps you informed regarding legislative and political action that supports the profession.

Another reason to maintain your membership: in recent times of diminishing career opportunities, a

Table 25-6
PROFESSIONAL DEVELOPMENT ACTIVITIES FOR THE NEW GRADUATE PHYSICAL THERAPIST

Area	Professional Development Activities
Education	• Provide clinical supervision for a student volunteer, a student physical therapist, or a physical therapist assistant. • Organize and/or present at a continuing education seminar or class. • Seek continuing education and advanced certificates, or prepare for additional degrees that support your long-term career objectives. • Present an in-service for staff or offer to guest lecture in a university class. • Develop content for new patient education materials.
Administration	• Participate in utilization management, peer review, and quality improvement activities. • Develop, market, or evaluate a new program. • Attend a workshop in risk management or information systems. • Hold an office in a professional organization.
Research	• Read and share research articles related to clinical responsibilities. • Attend research presentations at a state or national conference.
Clinical	• Develop and implement guidelines for a new treatment procedure. • Evaluate, revise, and implement an existing protocol. • Gain experience in several clinical areas; collaborate with other professionals. • Direct the activities of support personnel.

greater percentage of APTA members report employment than non-APTA members.[7] Take advantage of the *Career Starter Dues Program* and reduced membership fees for your first few years in practice. Budget and pay dues in installments if needed. Do what you need to do to keep your membership active!

Be a Good Representative of the Profession

Set a good example. Dress, write, and speak professionally. Represent the profession of physical therapy well in the clinical setting, social circles, and in the community. Help others understand what physical therapists do and see, and how effective physical therapy can be. Take the time to get involved in community activities on a pro bono basis.

Keep Your Ties to Your University Network

Be sure to keep in touch with classmates and faculty. They can serve as a valuable network in opening future doors. Those connections can also be a valuable support in your early career experiences. They can provide a bridge from the past to your future. Attend alumni events and help with communications among your classmates.

Summary

Principles of lifelong learning support professional development. Physical therapists should consider their interests in clinical, research, education, and administrative areas in planning their professional development. Seek opportunities that allow you to combine lifelong learning, interests, and job responsibilities. Make the most of your career in the profession of physical therapy!

References

1. Shenk D. *Data Smog*. New York, NY: Harper and Collins; 1997.

2. Curtis KA. *Career Planning in Physical Therapy*. Presented at California Chapter, American Physical Therapy Association Annual Conference, Monterey, Calif, October 8, 1988.

3. APTA. *Guidelines for Evaluating Continuing Education Programs Webpage*. Available at: http://www.apta.org/ Education/continuing_edu/eval_ce_prog.   Accessed September 2, 2000.

4. APTA. *American Board of Physical Therapy Specialties Directory of Certified Clinical Specialists in Physical Therapy 1985-2000 Webpage*. Available at: http:// www.apta.org/Education/specialist/dir_cert_cln_pt-85-97. Accessed September 2, 2000.

5. APTA. *Physical Therapy Specialist Certification-Frequently Asked Questions Webpage*. Available at: http://www.apta.org/Education/clinical/pp_clinical-faq/sportsFAQ. Accessed September 2, 2000.

6. APTA. *Minimum Eligibility Requirements for Physical Therapy Specialist Certification Webpage*. Available at: http://www.apta.org/ Education/specialist/minimum_eligibility/orthopaedics. Accessed September 2, 2000.

7. APTA. *Employment Survey Reveals APTA Members Faring Better Than Their Non-member Colleagues Webpage*. Available at: http://www.apta.org. Accessed August 15, 2000.

PUTTING IT INTO PRACTICE

1. Complete the inventory in Table 25-1. What do the results tell you? Do the results fit with your expectations? What interest areas would you like to emphasize in your professional development?

2. What performance goals would you like to meet in the next year? Draw from your most recent clinical performance evaluation or other sources.

    What do you need to *be able to do* or *need to know* to reach the above goals?

3. In what *two* areas would you like to develop your clinical, research, teaching, or administrative skills in the next year? Be specific.

    What are the best ways for you to develop these areas?
    (Consider independent study, in-services at work, mentoring relationships with another person, and outside continuing education courses.)

    What resources are available in your current workplace that will help you to develop these areas? (Consider mentors, practice opportunities, in-services, classes, and employee development programs.)

    What resources are available in the community that will help you to develop these areas? (Consider continuing education courses, university programs, self-study courses, and mentors.)

4. What career goals would you like to meet in the next 5 years?

5. What type of position would you like to have in 5 years?

    What additional skills or training do you need to make this career move?

    What additional responsibilities can you seek now that would prepare you for these goals?

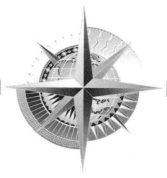

Appendices

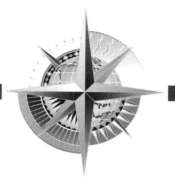

Model Definition of Physical Therapy for State Practice Acts

Physical therapy, which is the care and services provided by or under the direction and supervision of a physical therapist, includes:

1. Examining (history, system review, and tests and measures) individuals with impairment, functional limitation, and disability or other health-related conditions in order to determine a diagnosis, prognosis, and intervention; tests and measures may include the following:

   - aerobic capacity and endurance
   - anthropometric characteristics
   - arousal, attention, and cognition
   - assistive and adaptive devices
   - community and work (job/school/play) integration or reintegration
   - cranial nerve integrity
   - environmental, home, and work (job/school/play) barriers
   - ergonomics and body mechanics
   - gait, locomotion, and balance
   - integumentary integrity
   - joint integrity and mobility
   - motor function
   - muscle performance
   - neuromotor development and sensory integration
   - orthotic, protective, and supportive devices
   - pain
   - posture
   - prosthetic requirements
   - range of motion
   - reflex integrity
   - self-care and home management
   - sensory integrity
   - ventilation, respiration, and circulation

2. Alleviating impairment and functional limitation by designing, implementing, and modifying therapeutic interventions that include, but are not limited to:

   - coordination, communication, and documentation
   - patient/client-related instruction
   - therapeutic exercise (including aerobic conditioning)
   - functional training in self-care and home management (including activities of daily living and instrumental activities of daily living)
   - functional training in community and work (job/school/play) integration or reintegration activities (including instrumental activities of daily living, work hardening, and work conditioning)
   - manual therapy techniques (including mobilization and manipulation)
   - prescription, application, and, as

appropriate, fabrication of assistive, adaptive, orthotic, protective, supportive, and prosthetic devices and equipment

- airway clearance techniques
- wound management
- electrotherapeutic modalities
- physical agents and mechanical modalities

3. Preventing injury, impairment, functional limitation, and disability, including the promotion and maintenance of fitness, health, and quality of life in all age populations

4. Engaging in consultation, education, and research

Reprinted with permission from the American Physical Therapy Association (Program 19) [Amended BOD 02-97-03-06; BOD 03-95-24-64; BOD 06-94-03-04; BOD 03-93-18-46; BOD 03-86-22-85; Initial BOD 11-78-45-132]

An updated version of this document (last amended January 2004) may be found at:
American Physical Therapy Association. *Guide for Professional Conduct.* Available at: http://www.apta.org/governance/HOD/policies/HoDPolicies/Section_4/GUIDEFORPROCONDUCT. Accessed February 6, 2005.

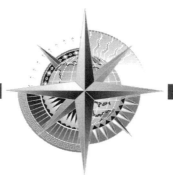

APTA Code of Ethics and Guide for Professional Conduct

Code of Ethics

Preamble

This Code of Ethics sets forth ethical principles for the physical therapy profession. Members of this profession are responsible for maintaining and promoting ethical practice. This Code of Ethics, adopted by the American Physical Therapy Association, shall be binding on physical therapists who are members of the Association.

Principle 1

Physical therapists respect the rights and dignity of all individuals.

Principle 2

Physical therapists comply with the laws and regulations governing the practice of physical therapy.

Principle 3

Physical therapists accept responsibility for the exercise of sound judgment.

Principle 4

Physical therapists maintain and promote high standards for physical therapy practice, education, and research.

Principle 5

Physical therapists seek remuneration for their services that is deserved and reasonable.

Principle 6

Physical therapists provide accurate information to the consumer about the profession and about those services they provide.

Principle 7

Physical therapists accept the responsibility to protect the public and the profession from unethical, incompetent, or illegal acts.

Principle 8

Physical therapists participate in efforts to address the health needs of the public.

Adopted by the House of Delegates, June 1981

Amended June 1987, June 1991

Guide for Professional Conduct

Purpose

This Guide for Professional Conduct (Guide) is intended to serve physical therapists who are members of the American Physical Therapy Association (Association) in interpreting the Code of Ethics (Code) and matters of professional conduct. The Guide provides guidelines by which physical therapists may determine the propriety of their conduct. The Code and the Guide apply to all physical therapists who are Association members. These guidelines are subject to changes as the dynamics of the profession change and as new patterns of health care delivery are developed and accepted by the professional community and the public. This Guide is subject to monitoring and timely revision by the Ethics and Judicial Committee of the Association.

Interpreting Ethical Principles

The interpretations expressed in this Guide are not to be considered all inclusive of situations that could evolve under a specific principle of the Code but reflect the opinions, decisions, and advice of the Judicial Committee. While the statements of ethical principles apply universally, specific circumstances determine their appropriate application. Input related to current interpretations, or situations requiring interpretation, is encouraged from Association members.

Principle 1

Physical therapists respect the rights and dignity of all individuals.

1.1 Attitudes of Physical Therapists

A. Physical therapists shall recognize that each individual is different from all other individuals and shall respect and be responsive to those differences.

B. Physical therapists are to be guided at all times by concern for the physical, psychological, and socioeconomic welfare of those individuals entrusted to their care.

C. Physical therapists shall not engage in conduct that constitutes harassment or abuse of, or discrimination against, colleagues, associates, or others.

1.2 Confidential Information

A. Information relating to the physical therapist-patient relationship is confidential and may not be communicated to a third party not involved in that patient's care without the prior written consent of the patient, subject to applicable law.

B. Information derived from component-sponsored peer review shall be held confidential by the reviewer unless written permission to release the information is obtained from the physical therapist who was reviewed.

C. Information derived from the working relationships of physical therapists shall be held confidential by all parties.

D. Information may be disclosed to appropriate authorities when it is necessary to protect the welfare of an individual or the community. Such disclosure shall be in accordance with applicable law.

1.3 Patient Relations

Physical therapists shall not engage in any sexual relationship or activity, whether consensual or nonconsensual, with any patient while a physical therapist/patient relationship exists.

1.4 Informed Consent

Physical therapists shall obtain patient informed consent before treatment, to include disclosure of: (I) the nature of the proposed intervention; (ii) material risks of harm or complications; (iii) reasonable alternatives to the proposed intervention; and (iv) goals of treatment.

Principle 2

Physical therapists comply with the laws and regulations governing the practice of physical therapy.

2.1 Professional Practice

Physical therapists shall provide consultation, evaluation, treatment, and preventive care, in accordance with the laws and regulations of the jurisdiction(s) in which they practice.

Principle 3

Physical therapists accept responsibility for the exercise of sound judgment.

3.1 Acceptance of Responsibility

A. Upon accepting a patient/client for provision of physical therapy services, physical therapist shall assume the responsibility for examining, evaluating, and diagnosing that individual; prognosis and intervention; re-examination and modification of the plan of care; and maintaining adequate records of the case including progress reports. Physical therapists establish the plan of care and provide and/or supervise the appropriate intervention.

B. If the diagnostic process reveals findings that are outside the scope of the physical therapists knowledge, experience, or expertise, the physical therapist shall so inform the patient/client and refer to an appropriate practitioner.

C. Regardless of practice setting, physical therapists shall maintain the ability to make independent judgments.

D. The physical therapist shall not provide physical therapy services to a patient while under the influence of a substance that impairs his or her ability to do so safely.

E. When the patient is referred from another practitioner, the physical therapist shall communicate the findings of the examination, the diagnosis, the proposed intervention, and reexamination findings (as indicated) to the referring practitioner and any other appropriate individuals involved in the patient's care, while maintaining standards of confidentiality.

3.2 Delegation of Responsibility

A. Physical therapists shall not delegate to a less qualified person any activity which requires the unique skill, knowledge, and judgment of the physical therapist.

B. The primary responsibility for physical therapy care rendered by supportive personnel rests with the supervising physical therapist. Adequate supervision requires, at a minimum, that a supervising physical therapist perform the following activities:

1. Designate or establish channels of written and oral communication.

2. Interpret available information concerning the individual under care.

3. Examine, evaluate, and determine a diagnosis.

4. Develop plan of care, including short- and long-term goals.

5. Select and delegate appropriate tasks of plan of care.

6. Assess competence of supportive personnel

to perform assigned tasks.

7. Direct and supervise supportive personnel in delegated tasks.

8. Identify and document precautions, special problems, contraindications, goals, anticipated progress, and plans for reevaluation.

9. Reevaluate, adjust plan of care when necessary, perform final evaluation, and establish follow-up plan.

3.3 Provision of Services

A. Physical therapists shall recognize the individual's freedom of choice in selection of physical therapy services.

B. Physical therapists' professional practices and their adherence to ethical principles of the Association shall take preference over business practices. Provisions of services for personal financial gain rather than for the need of the individual receiving the services are unethical.

C. When physical therapists judge that an individual will no longer benefit from their services, they shall so inform the individual receiving the services. Physical therapists shall avoid overutilization of their services.

D. In the event of elective termination of a physical therapist/patient relationship by the physical therapist, the therapist should take steps to transfer the care of the patient, as appropriate, to another provider.

E. Physical therapists shall recognize that third-party payer contracts may limit, in one form or another, provision of physical therapy services. Physical therapists shall inform patients of any known limitations. Third-party limitations do not absolve the physical therapist from adherence to ethical principles. Physical therapists shall avoid underutilization of their services.

3.4 Practice Arrangements

A. Participation in a business, partnership, corporation, or other entity does not exempt the physical therapist, whether employer, partner, or stockholder, either individually or collectively, from the obligation of promoting and maintaining the ethical principles of the Association.

B. Physical therapists shall advise their employer(s) of any employer practice which causes a physical therapist to be in conflict with the ethical principles of the Association. Physical therapist employees shall attempt to rectify aspects of their employment which are in conflict with the ethical principles of the Association.

Principle 4

Physical therapists maintain and promote high standards for physical therapy practice, education, and research.

4.1 Continued Education

A. Physical therapists shall participate in educational activities which enhance their basic knowledge and provide new knowledge.

B. Whenever physical therapists provide continuing education, they shall ensure that course content, objectives, and responsibilities of the instructional faculty are accurately reflected in the promotion of the course.

4.2 Review and Self Assessment

A. Physical therapists shall provide for utilization review of their services.

B. Physical therapists shall demonstrate their commitment to quality assurance by peer review and self assessment.

4.3 Research

A. Physical therapists shall support research activities that contribute knowledge for improved patient care.

B. Physical therapists engaged in research shall ensure:

1. the consent of subjects;
2. confidentiality of the data on individual subjects and the personal identities of the subjects;
3. well-being of all subjects in compliance with facility regulations and laws of the jurisdiction in which the research is conducted;
4. the absence of fraud and plagiarism;
5. full disclosure of support received;
6. appropriate acknowledgment of individuals making a contribution to the research;
7. that animal subjects used in research are treated humanely and in compliance with facility regulations and laws of the jurisdiction in which the research experimentation is conducted.

C. Physical therapists shall report to appropriate authorities any acts in the conduct or presentation of research that appear unethical or illegal.

4.4 Education

A. Physical therapists shall support quality education in academic and clinical settings.

B. Physical therapists functioning in the educational role are responsible to the students, the academic institutions and the clinical settings for promoting ethical conduct in educational activities. Whenever possible, the educator shall ensure:

1. the rights of students in the academic and clinical setting;
2. appropriate confidentiality of personal information;
3. professional conduct towards the student during the academic and clinical education processes;
4. assignment to clinical settings prepared to give the student a learning experience.

C. Clinical educators are responsible for reporting to the academic program student conduct which appears to be unethical or illegal.

Principle 5

Physical therapists seek remuneration for their services that is deserved and reasonable.

5.1 Fiscally Sound Remuneration

A. Physical therapists shall never place their own financial interest above the welfare of individuals under their care.

B. Fees for physical therapy services should be reasonable for the service performed, considering the setting in which it is provided, practice costs in the geographic area, judgment of other organizations and other relevant factors.

C. Physical therapists should attempt to ensure that providers, agencies, or other employers adopt physical therapy fee schedules that are reasonable and that encourage access to necessary services.

5.2 Business Practices/Fee Arrangements

A. Physical therapists shall not:

1. directly or indirectly request, receive, or

participate in the dividing, transferring, assigning, rebating of an unearned fee.

2. profit by means of a credit or other valuable consideration, such as an unearned commission, discount, or gratuity in connection with furnishing of physical therapy services.

B. Unless laws impose restrictions to the contrary, physical therapists who provide physical therapy services in a business entity may pool fees and moneys received. Physical therapists may divide or apportion these fees and moneys in accordance with the business agreement.

C. Physical therapists may enter into agreements with organizations to provide physical therapy services if such agreements do not violate the ethical principles of the Association.

5.3 Endorsement of Equipment or Services

A. Physical therapists shall not use influence upon individuals under their care or their families for utilization of equipment or services based upon the direct or indirect financial interest of the physical therapist in such equipment or services. Realizing that these individuals will normally rely on the physical therapists' advice, their best interest must always be maintained as well as their right of free choice relating to the use of any equipment or service. While it cannot be considered unethical for physical therapists to own or have a financial interest in equipment companies, or services, they must act in accordance with law and make full disclosure of their interest whenever such companies or services become the source of equipment or services for individuals under their care.

B. Physical therapists may be remunerated for endorsement or advertisement of equipment or services to the lay public, physical therapists, or other health professionals provided they disclose any financial interest in the production, sale, or distribution of said equipment or services.

C. In endorsing or adverting equipment or services, physical therapists shall use sound professional judgment and shall not give the appearance of Association endorsement.

5.4 Gifts and Other Considerations

A. Physical therapists shall not accept nor offer gifts or other considerations with obligatory conditions attached.

B. Physical therapists shall not accept nor offer gifts or other considerations that affect or give an objective appearance of affecting their professional judgment.

Principle 6

Physical therapists provide accurate information to the consumer about the profession and about those services they provide.

6.1 Information about the Profession

Physical therapists shall endeavor to educate the public to an awareness of the physical therapy profession through such means as publication of articles and participation in seminars, lectures, and civic programs.

6.2 Information about Services

A. Information given to the public shall emphasize that individual problems cannot be treated without individualized evaluation and plans/programs of care.

B. Physical therapists may advertise their services to the public.

C. Physical therapists shall not use, or participate in the use of, any form of communication containing a false, plagiarized, fraudulent, misleading, deceptive, unfair, or sensational statement or claim.

D. A paid advertisement shall be identified as such unless it is apparent from the context that it is a paid advertisement.

Principle 7

Physical therapists accept the responsibility to protect the public and the profession from unethical, incompetent, or illegal acts.

7.1 Consumer Protection

A. Physical therapists shall report any conduct which appears to be unethical, incompetent, or illegal.

B. Physical therapists may not participate in any arrangements in which patients are exploited due to the referring sources enhancing their personal incomes as a result of referring for, prescribing, or recommending physical therapy.

C. Physical therapists shall be obligated to safeguard the public from underutilization or overutilization of physical therapy services.

7.2 Disclosure

The physical therapist shall disclose to the patient if the referring practitioner derives compensation from the provision of physical therapy. The physical therapist shall ensure that the individual has freedom of choice in selecting a provider of physical therapy.

Principle 8

Physical therapists participate in efforts to address the health needs of the public.

8.1 Pro Bono Service

Physical therapists should render pro bono publico (reduced or no fee) services to patients lacking the ability to pay for services, as each physical therapist's practice permits.

Issued by the Ethics and Judicial Committee, October 1981. Amended January 1999. Reprinted with permission from the American Physical Therapy Association.

An updated version of this document (last amended March 2004) may be found at: American Physical Therapy Association. *Guide for Conduct of the Physical Therapist Assistant.* Available at: http://www.apta.org/governance/HOD/policies/HoDPolicies/Section_4/GUIDEFORCONDUCTOF THEPTA . Accessed February 6, 2005.

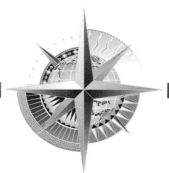

APTA Standards of Ethical Conduct for the Physical Therapist Assistant

Preamble

Physical therapist assistants are responsible for maintaining and promoting high standards of conduct. These Standards of Ethical Conduct for the Physical Therapist Assistant shall be binding on physical therapist assistants who are affiliate members of the Association.

Standard 1

Physical therapist assistants provide services under the supervision of a physical therapist.

Standard 2

Physical therapist assistants respect the rights and dignity of all individuals.

Standard 3

Physical therapist assistants maintain and promote high standards in the provision of services, giving the welfare of patients their highest regard.

Standard 4

Physical therapist assistants provide services within the limits of the law.

Standard 5

Physical therapist assistants make those judgments that are commensurate with their qualifications as physical therapist assistants.

Standard 6

Physical therapist assistants accept the responsibility to protect the public and the profession from unethical, incompetent, or illegal acts.

Adopted by the House of Delegates, June 1982

Amended June 1991

Guide for Conduct of the Affiliate Member

Purpose

This Guide is intended to serve physical therapist assistants who are affiliate members of the American Physical Therapy Association in the interpretation of the Standards of Ethical Conduct for the Physical Therapist Assistant, providing guidelines by which they may determine the propriety of their conduct. These guidelines are subject to change as new patterns of health care delivery are developed and accepted by the professional community and the public. This Guide is subject to monitoring and timely revision by the Ethics and Judicial Committee of the Association.

Interpreting Standards

The interpretations expressed in this Guide are not to be considered all inclusive of situations that could evolve under a specific standard of the Standards of Ethical Conduct for the Physical Therapist Assistant but reflect the opinions, decisions, and advice of the Judicial Committee. While the statements of ethical standards apply universally, specific circumstances determine their appropriate application. Input related to current interpretations, or situations requiring interpretation, is encouraged from APTA members.

Standard 1

Physical therapist assistants provide services under the supervision of a physical therapist.

1.1 Supervisory Relationships

Physical therapist assistants shall work under the supervision and direction of a physical therapist who is properly credentialed in the jurisdiction in which the physical therapist assistant practices.

1.2 Performance of Service

A. Physical therapist assistants may not initiate or alter a treatment program without prior evaluation by and approval of the supervising physical therapist.

B. Physical therapist assistants may modify a specific treatment procedure in accordance with changes in patient status.

C. Physical therapist assistants may not interpret data beyond the scope of their physical therapist assistant education.

D. Physical therapist assistants may respond to inquiries regarding patient status to appropriate parties within the protocol established by a supervising physical therapist.

E. Physical therapist assistants shall refer inquiries regarding patient prognosis to a supervising physical therapist.

Standard 2

Physical therapist assistants respect the rights and dignity of all individuals.

2.1 Attitudes of Physical Therapist Assistants

A. Physical therapist assistants shall recognize that each individual is different from all other individuals and respect and be responsive to those differences.

B. Physical therapist assistants shall be guided at all times by concern for the dignity and welfare of those patients entrusted to their care.

C. Physical therapist assistants shall not engage in conduct that constitutes harassment or abuse of, or discrimination against, colleagues, associates, or others.

2.2 Request for Release of Information

Physical therapist assistants shall refer all requests for release of confidential information to the supervising physical therapist.

2.3 Protection of Privacy

Physical therapist assistants must treat as confidential all information relating to the personal conditions and affairs of the persons whom they serve.

2.4 Patient Relations

Physical therapist assistants shall not engage in any sexual relationship or activity, whether consensual or nonconsensual, with any patient while a physical therapist assistant/patient relationship exists.

Standard 3

Physical therapist assistants maintain and promote high standards in the provision of services giving the welfare of patients their highest regard.

3.1 Information About Services

A. Physical therapist assistants may provide consumers with information regarding provision of services within the protocol established by a supervising physical therapist.

B. Physical therapist assistants may not use, or participate in the use of any form of communication containing a false, fraudulent, misleading, deceptive, unfair, or sensational statement or claim.

3.2 Organizational Employment

Physical therapist assistants shall advise their employer(s) of any employer practice which causes them to be in conflict with the Standards of Ethical Conduct for the Physical Therapist Assistant.

3.3 Endorsement of Equipment

Physical therapist assistants may not endorse equipment or exercise influence on patients or families to purchase or lease equipment except as directed by a physical therapist acting in accord with the stipulation in paragraph 5.3.A. of the Guide for Professional Conduct.

3.4 Financial Considerations

Physical therapist assistants shall never place their own financial interest above the welfare of their patients.

3.5 Exploitation of Patients

Physical therapist assistants shall not participate in any arrangements in which patients are exploited. Such arrangements include situations where referring sources enhance their personal incomes as a result of referring for, delegating, prescribing, or recommending physical therapy services.

Standard 4

Physical therapist assistants provide services within the limits of the law.

4.1 Supervisory Relationships

Physical therapist assistants shall comply with all aspects of law. Regardless of the content of any law, physical therapist assistants shall provide services only under the supervision and direction of a physical therapist who is properly credentialed in the jurisdiction in which the physical therapist assistant practices.

4.2 Representation

Physical therapist assistants shall not hold themselves out as physical therapists.

Standard 5

Physical therapist assistants make those judgments that are commensurate with their qualifications as physical therapist assistants.

5.1 Patient Treatment

Physical therapist assistants shall report all untoward patient responses to a supervising physical therapist.

5.2 Patient Safety

A. Physical therapist assistants may refuse to carry out treatment procedures that they believe to be not in the best interest of the patient.

B. The physical therapist assistant shall not provide physical therapy services to a patient while under the influence of a substance that impairs his or her ability to do so safely.

5.3 Qualifications

Physical therapist assistants may not carry out any procedure that they are not qualified to provide.

5.4 Discontinuance of Treatment Program

Physical therapist assistants shall discontinue immediately any treatment procedures which in their judgment appear to be harmful to the patient.

5.5 Continued Education

Physical therapist assistants shall continue participation in various types of educational activities which enhance their skills and knowledge and provide new skills and knowledge.

Standard 6

Physical therapist assistants accept the responsibility to protect the public and the profession from unethical, incompetent, or illegal acts.

6.1 Consumer Protection

Physical therapist assistants shall report any conduct which appears to be unethical or illegal.

Issued by the Ethics and Judicial Committee, October 1981

Amended January 1996.

Reprinted with permission from the American Physical Therapy Association.

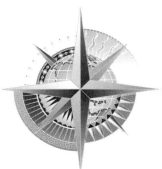

APTA Standards of Practice for Physical Therapy and the Accompanying Criteria

Preamble

The physical therapy profession is committed to providing an optimal level of service delivery and to striving for excellence in practice. The House of Delegates of the American Physical Therapy Association (APTA), as the formal body that represents the profession, attests to this commitment by adopting and promoting the following Standards of Practice for Physical Therapy. These Standards are the profession's statement of conditions and performances that are essential for provision of high-quality physical therapy. The Standards provide a foundation for assessment of physical therapy practice.

The Criteria for the Standards, promulgated by APTA's Board of Directors, are italicized beneath the Standards to which they apply.

I. Legal/Ethical Considerations

A. Legal Considerations

The physical therapist complies with all the legal requirements of jurisdictions regulating the practice of physical therapy.

The physical therapist assistant complies with all the legal requirements of jurisdictions regulating the work of the assistant.

B. Ethical Considerations

The physical therapist practices according to the Code of Ethics of the American Physical Therapy Association.

The physical therapist assistant complies with the Standards of Ethical Conduct for the Physical Therapist Assistant of the American Physical Therapy Association.

II. Administration of the Physical Therapy Service

A. Statement of Mission, Purpose, and Goals

The physical therapy service has a statement of mission, purposes, and goals that reflects the needs and interests of the patients and clients served, the physical therapy personnel affiliated with the service, and the community.

The statement of mission, purposes, and goals:

- Defines the scope and limitations of the physical therapy service.
- Identifies the goals and objectives of the service.
- Is reviewed annually.

B. Organizational Plan

The physical therapy service has a written organizational plan. The organizational plan:

- Describes relationships among components within the physical therapy service and, where the service is part of a larger organization, between the service and the other components of that organization.
- Ensures that the service is directed by a physical therapist.
- Defines supervisory structures within the service.
- Reflects current personnel functions.

C. Policies and Procedures

The physical therapy service has written policies and procedures that reflect the operation of the service and that are consistent with the mission, purposes, and goals of the service.

The written policies and procedures are reviewed regularly and revised as necessary and meet the requirements of state law and external agencies.

Apply to, but are not limited to:

- Clinical education
- Clinical research
- Interdisciplinary collaboration
- Criteria for access to care
- Criteria for initiation and continuation of care
- Criteria for referral to other appropriate health care providers
- Criteria for termination of care
- Equipment maintenance
- Environmental safety
- Fiscal management
- Infection control
- Job/position descriptions
- Competency assessment
- Medical emergencies
- Care of patients and clients, including guidelines
- Rights of patients and clients
- Personnel-related policies
- Improvement of quality of care and performance of services
- Documentation
- Staff orientation

D. Administration

A physical therapist is responsible for the direction of the physical therapy service.

The director of the physical therapy service:

- Ensures compliance with local, state, and federal requirements.
- Ensures compliance with current APTA documents, including Standards of Practice for Physical Therapy and the Criteria, Code of Ethics, Guide for Professional Conduct, Standards of Ethical Conduct for the Physical Therapist Assistant, and Guide for Conduct of the Affiliate Member.
- Ensures that services are consistent with the mission, purposes, and goals of the physical therapy service.
- Ensures that services are provided in accordance with established policies and procedures.
- Reviews and updates policies and procedures.
- Provides for training that ensures continued competence of physical therapy support personnel.
- Provides for continuous in-service training on safety issues and for periodic safety inspection of equipment by qualified individuals.

E. Fiscal Management

The director of the physical therapy service, in consultation with physical therapy staff and appropriate administrative personnel, participates in planning for, and allocation of, resources. Fiscal planning and management of the service is based on sound accounting principles.

The fiscal management plan:

- Includes a budget that provides for optimal use of resources.
- Ensures accurate recording and reporting of financial information.
- Ensures compliance with legal requirements.
- Allows for cost-effective utilization of resources.
- Uses a fee schedule that is consistent with the cost of physical therapy services and that is within customary norms of fairness and reasonableness.

F. Improvement of Quality of Care and Performance

The physical therapy service has a written plan for continuous improvement of quality of care and performance of services.

The improvement plan:
- Provides evidence of ongoing review and evaluation of the physical therapy service.
- Provides a mechanism for documenting improvement in quality of care and performance.
- Is consistent with requirements of external agencies, as applicable.

G. Staffing

The physical therapy personnel affiliated with the physical therapy service have demonstrated competence and are sufficient to achieve the mission, purposes, and goals of the service.

The physical therapy service:
- Meets all legal requirements regarding licensure and certification of appropriate personnel.
- Ensures that the level of expertise within the service is appropriate to the needs of the patients and clients served.
- Provides for appropriate ratios of personnel to patients.
- Provides for appropriate ratios of support personnel to professional personnel.

H. Staff Development

The physical therapy service has a written plan that provides for appropriate and ongoing staff development.

The staff development plan:
- Includes self-assessment, individual goal setting, and organizational needs in directing continuing education and learning activities.
- Includes strategies for lifelong learning and professional and career development.

I. Physical Setting

The physical setting is designed to provide a safe and accessible environment that facilitates fulfillment of the mission, purposes, and goals of the physical therapy service. The equipment is safe and sufficient to achieve the purposes and goals of the service.

The physical setting:

- Meets all applicable legal requirements for health and safety.
- Meets space needs appropriate for the number and type of patients and clients served.

The equipment:
- Meets all applicable legal requirements for health and safety.
- Is inspected routinely.

J. Interdisciplinary Collaboration

The physical therapy service collaborates with all appropriate disciplines.

The collaboration:
- Uses an interdisciplinary team approach to the care of patients and clients.
- Provides interdisciplinary instruction of patients, clients, and families.
- Ensures interdisciplinary professional development and continuing education.

III. Provision of Services

A. Informed Consent

The physical therapist has sole responsibility for providing information to the patient and for obtaining informed consent in accordance with jurisdictional law before initiating intervention.

The information provided to patients:
- Clearly describes the proposed intervention.
- Delineates material (decisional) risks associated with the proposed intervention.
- Identifies expected benefits of the proposed intervention.
- Compares the benefits and risks that are possible both with and without the proposed intervention.
- Explains reasonable alternatives to the proposed intervention.

Informed consent:
- Requires consent of a competent adult.
- Requires consent of a parent/legal guardian as the surrogate decision maker when the adult patient is not competent or when the patient is a minor.

Requires the patient, client, or legal guardian to acknowledge understanding of the intervention and to give consent before intervention is initiated.

B. Initial Examination and Evaluation

The physical therapist performs and documents an initial examination and evaluates the data to identify problems and determine the diagnosis prior to intervention.

The physical therapist examination:

- Is documented, dated, and appropriately authenticated by the physical therapist who performed it.
- Identifies the physical therapy needs of the patient or client.
- Incorporates appropriate tests and measures to facilitate outcome measurement.
- Produces data that are sufficient to allow evaluation, diagnosis, prognosis, and the establishment of a plan of care.
- May result in recommendations for additional services to meet the needs of the patient or client.

C. Plan of Care

The physical therapist establishes and provides a plan of care for the patient based on evaluation of the examination data and patient needs.

The physical therapist involves the patient and appropriate others in the planning, implementation, and assessment of the intervention program.

The physical therapist, in consultation with appropriate disciplines, plans for discharge of the patient, taking into consideration the level of goal attainment, and provides for appropriate follow-up or referral.

The plan of care:

- Is based on the examination, evaluation, diagnosis, and prognosis.
- Identifies anticipated goals and expected outcomes.
- Describes the proposed intervention, including frequency and duration.
- Includes documentation that is dated and appropriately authenticated by the physical therapist who established the plan of care.

D. Intervention/Treatment

The physical therapist provides, or delegates and supervises, the physical therapy intervention in a manner that is consistent with the examination data, the evaluation, and the plan of care.

The physical therapist documents, on an ongoing basis, services provided, responses to services, and changes in the status of the patient relative to the plan of care.

The intervention:

- Is based on the examination, evaluation, diagnosis, prognosis, and plan of care.
- Is provided under the ongoing direct care or supervision of the physical therapist.
- Is provided in such a way that delegated responsibilities are commensurate with the qualifications and the legal limitations of the physical therapy support and professional personnel involved in the intervention.
- Is altered in accordance with changes in response or status.
- Is provided at a level that is consistent with current physical therapy practice.
- Is interdisciplinary when necessary to meet the needs of the patient or client.

Documentation of the intervention:

- Is dated and appropriately authenticated by the physical therapist or, when permissible by law, by the physical therapist assistant, or both.

E. Re-examination and Re-evaluation

The physical therapist continually reexamines the patient, re-evaluates the data, and modifies the plan of care or discontinues the plan of care accordingly.

The physical therapist re-examination:

- Is documented, dated, and appropriately authenticated by the physical therapist who performs it.
- Includes modifications to the plan of care.

F. Discharge/Discontinuation of Intervention

The physical therapist discharges the patient from physical therapy intervention when the goals and projected outcomes have been attained.

Intervention is discontinued when the goals and expected functional outcomes are attained, the patient declines to continue care, the patient is unable to continue receiving care, or the physical therapist determines that intervention is no longer warranted.

Discharge documentation:

- Includes the status of the patient or client at discharge and the goals and functional out comes attained.
- Is dated and appropriately authenticated by the physical therapist who performed the discharge.
- Includes, when a patient or client is dis charged prior to attainment of goals and

functional outcomes, the status of the patient or client and the rationale for discontinuation.

IV. Education

The physical therapist is responsible for individual professional development. The physical therapist assistant is responsible for individual career development.

The physical therapist participates in the education of physical therapist students, physical therapist assistant students, and students in other health professions.

The physical therapist educates and provides consultation to consumers and the general public regarding the purposes and benefits of physical therapy.

The physical therapist educates and provides consultation to consumers and the general public regarding the roles of the physical therapist and the physical therapist assistant.

The physical therapist:
- Educates and provides consultation to consumers and the general public regarding the roles of the physical therapist, the physical therapist assistant, and other support personnel.

V. Research

The physical therapist applies research findings to practice and encourages, participates in, and promotes activities that establish the outcomes of patient/client management provided by the physical therapist.

The physical therapist supports collaborative and interdisciplinary research.

VI. Community Responsibility

The physical therapist demonstrates community responsibility by participating in community and community agency activities, educating the public, formulating public policy, or providing pro bono physical therapy services.

The physical therapist:
- Participates in community and community agency activities.
- Educates the public, including prevention education and health promotion.
- Helps formulate public policy.
- Provides pro bono physical therapy services.

Standards adopted by the House of Delegates, June 1980
Amended June 1985, June 1991, June 1996

Criteria adopted by the Board of Directors, March 1993
Amended November 1994, March 1995

Reprinted with permission from the American Physical Therapy Association.

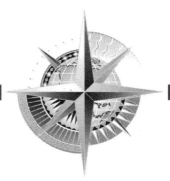

Index

BUILD *Your Library*

This book and many others on numerous different topics are available from SLACK Incorporated. For further information or a copy of our latest catalog, contact us at:

Professional Book Division
SLACK Incorporated
6900 Grove Road
Thorofare, NJ 08086 USA
Telephone: 1-856-848-1000
1-800-257-8290
Fax: 1-856-853-5991
E-mail: orders@slackinc.com
www.slackbooks.com

We accept most major credit cards and checks or money orders in US dollars drawn on a US bank. Most orders are shipped within 72 hours.

Contact us for information on recent releases, forthcoming titles, and bestsellers. If you have a comment about this title or see a need for a new book, direct your correspondence to the Editorial Director at the above address.

Thank you for your interest and we hope you found this work beneficial.